The Philosophical Foundations of Classical Chinese Medicine

The Philosophical Foundations of Classical Chinese Medicine

Philosophy, Methodology, Science

Keekok Lee

LEXINGTON BOOKS
Lanham • Boulder • New York • London

Published by Lexington Books
An imprint of The Rowman & Littlefield Publishing Group, Inc.
4501 Forbes Boulevard, Suite 200, Lanham, Maryland 20706
www.rowman.com

Unit A, Whitacre Mews, 26-34 Stannary Street, London SE11 4AB

British Library Cataloguing in Publication Information Available

Library of Congress Cataloging-in-Publication Data Available
Library of Congress Control Number: 2017937802
ISBN 978-1-4985-3887-9 (cloth : alk. paper)
ISBN 978-1-4985-3888-6 (electronic)

∞™ The paper used in this publication meets the minimum requirements of American National Standard for Information Sciences—Permanence of Paper for Printed Library Materials, ANSI/NISO Z39.48-1992.

Printed in the United States of America

Contents

Acknowledgments

Many acknowledgements are called for, indeed, too many, if every case were to be recalled here. However, there are a few which must be made. The first is to a friend and colleague without whose saintly generosity of spirit in helping me in the matter of computer graphics, this book would not have seen the light of publication, as this poor scholar simply could not rise (or be expected to rise) to become an IT expert; furthermore, the book, even if published (without the computer graphics), would be less than effective, as it would have to make do without the *Xiang* mode of presenting thought. The second is to Zhang Yu and Jiao Bin (Beijing Sanlitun Hospital); without their dedicated help and support, this book could not have been written. Last, but not least, I would like to thank Andriy Vasylchenko (Skovoroda Institute of Philosophy, National Academy of Sciences, Ukraine), for having co-authored with me, the section on **Modern non-classical Logic and *Yinyang/Yao-gua* Implicit *Logic*** in chapter 9, as well as for having made many helpful suggestions to improve clarity throughout the text. I am also grateful to all those, either in conversation or correspondence, who have made insightful comments and suggestions for improvements in the chapter(s) or fragments of chapter(s) shown to them. However, for any flaws and shortcomings which may still exist and, undoubtedly, do exist in this work, I take full responsibility for them.

Preface

汉乐府民歌

长歌行

青青园中葵，朝露待日晞。
阳春布德泽，万物生光辉。
长恐秋节至，焜黄华叶衰。
百川东到海，何时复西归？
少壮不努力，老大徒伤悲。

This is a folk song recorded during the Han Dynasty by the Bureau of Music which had already been set up during the preceding, short-lived Qin dynasty. However, under the eager patronage of Han Wudi of the Western Han period who ruled from 141-87 BCE, the Bureau became very active and vigorous in implementing its remits, one of which was the specific one of collecting and collating folk songs. This means that the song was much older than the Western Han dynasty, and probably had existed for several centuries earlier.

This song talks about the passage of time. Time once gone is gone forever, like the waters of the rivers, which flow into the sea, never to return, like the green leaves of spring turning eventually yellow in the autumn, like the dew drops on the sunflower, which dry and evaporate as the sun grows stronger with the passing of the early morning cool. If in the vim and vigour of your youth, you fail to strive to realize your potential, to realize your various talents, then all that would be left for you in your old age is to sigh sadly with nothing to show for.

The moral is clear, but here one is not interested in this aspect, in this work, but in pointing out that the key tropes invoked in this folk song also happen to refer to the central concepts of Chinese *philosophy*/cosmology and also, therefore, of Classical Chinese *Medicine* (CCM):

1. The daily rhythm of sunrise and (implied) sunset—the sun in the morning is gentle and mild but gets hotter as the day wears on until in the late afternoon it gets weaker, eventually disappearing altogether by the very late afternoon/early evening. This is called the *zhouye jielü* 昼夜节律. This rhythm in Nature is found in ourselves as we, who are living beings, obey, also that *Law of Nature*. (Needless to say, these are not mathematized as the laws of Nature are in modern science—hence, to warn readers that they differ in this profound respect from their Western modern counterparts, this author has italicized the term when used in the Chinese context.)
2. The yearly rhythm of the four seasons: spring and autumn only are mentioned in the folk song. However, in ancient Chinese literature, spring and autumn stand for the passage of the entire year, including summer and winter. This is the *sishi jielü* 四时节律. This rhythm, too, is similarly found in ourselves and we obey that *Law of Nature*, too.
3. CCM contains a key concept called *tianren-xiangying* (天人相应) which includes the two *Laws of Nature* mentioned above.
4. Spring is the time for the first stirring of life on Earth after the die-back of winter; summer is the time for all organisms to grow and develop; autumn is the time for trees to bear fruit and for young animals born in the spring to come to maturity; winter is the time for organisms "to recollect themselves" in rest and tranquillity, even for some to go into hibernation, in preparation for the next cycle in the renewal of life in the following spring. This in CCM is referred to as: *chun sheng xia zhang qiu shou dong cang* 春生夏长秋收冬藏. *Qi* (气) in greater Nature undergoes these four phases in the process of transformation and change; these phases are found in every living organism, including ourselves.
5. The four seasons, involving the phases of change and transformation of *Qi* in the annual cycle, secure the conditions for all life, ensuring the continuity of life forms on Earth. The folk song tells us that this cycle is a gift from Nature or in ancient Chinese terms from Heaven天*tian* and Earth 地 *di*, for which we must be deeply grateful—阳春布德泽, 万

物生光辉. A key text of CCM, the *Huangdi neijing*《黄帝内经》says that *wanwu* 万物 (the myriad things) are the children of Heaven and Earth (Nature), and that Heaven and Earth look after us, as parents look after their own children.

6. The song refers directly to the Sun (*ri*日) and talks indirectly about the sky or the heavens above—the Sun in the heaven/sky above gives forth warmth and light, that is, energy which provides the conditions essential for life.
7. The song also uses the character/word 阳 *yang*, which is another term for the Sun. However, *yang* does not simply stand for Sun but also for *yang qi* 阳气, one of two types of *Qi*. The song also refers to the water (水 *shui*) in rivers (川) and the sea (海) on our planet Earth. In Chinese *philosophy*/cosmology and CCM, water and Earth belong to *yin*, and so are about *yin qi* 阴气. In other words, the song implies the concepts of *yin qi* and *yang qi* as well as *yinyang* 阴阳 which constitute the central concepts of Chinese *philosophy*/cosmology and, therefore, of CCM.
8. The themes referred to at 4, 5, 6, and 7 above may be found in a passage of the *Huangdi neijing*, Chapter 5, which reads: 阴阳者, 天地之道也, 万物之纲纪, 变化, 父母, 生杀之本始, 神明之府也，治病必求于本... (《黄帝内经. 素问. 阴阳应象大论》). This author renders it as follows: *Yinyang* constitutes the *dao* of Heaven and Earth; it embraces *wanwu* within its order and its laws; it is the source of all changes as well as the very foundation of life and growth; it is where the spirit dwells. The physician, in order to heal the sick, must always cut to the root of the illness in terms of *yinyang* and restore its balance in the individual.
9. The reference in the song to the Sun 日, 阳 and its implied reference to Earth may be understood as a reference to Astronomy (Time). A basic aspect of astronomy is the study of the movements of heavenly bodies and Earth's relationships with them. The rising and setting of the Sun on a daily basis is the relationship between Earth and Sun, as only half of Earth's surface is exposed to the Sun at any one time while the other half is in darkness. So, too, does the cycle of the four seasons reflect the relationship between Earth and Sun in the course of the year.
10. The song speaks of the numerous rivers in China, that they, in the main, flow east-west rather than north-south; their headwaters being in the west but flowing into the sea in the east (百川东到海) is a reference to Geography (Space).

11. The song reminds us that time does not wait for anyone, that there is one certainty or constancy in human existence, the law of birth, growth, maturity, decline, and finally death over which we have no choice but to respect （少壮。。。老大。。。). This is a reference to humans who must conduct their lives and their affairs within the constraints imposed by Astronomy (Time) and Geography (Space) on Earth. This implies, in turn, a reference to the three Powers (三才 *sancai*), namely, Heaven above, Earth below and Humans in between.
12. Hence, 9, 10, and 11 above sum up yet another central theme of CCM, namely, that to understand what health is, what illness is, what prevents/cures illnesses, one needs to know Astronomy (Time), Geography (Space) and human affairs. If you knew all three you would not only be wise but you would also live "long and healthily." 上知天文, 下知地理, 中知人事" (*shang zhi tianwen, xia zhi dili, zhong zhi renshi*): to grasp this is basically to grasp what CCM is all about.

This little folk song surprisingly contains key themes in Chinese *philosophy*/cosmology and also some of the essential elements of CCM. This goes to show that these themes and concepts are deeply embedded in Chinese culture and civilization dating from very ancient times and, therefore, that the concepts of CCM must be understood within the framework of Chinese *philosophy*/cosmology.

CHAPTER ONE

Introduction

The 1990s also witnessed the reentry into Chinese medicine of classical philosophy and a self-conscious "return to the sources" that is unashamedly concerned with reworking China's own tradition rather than learning from the West. Scheid, 2002: 194

Background and Nature of Book

This book is a companion volume to *The Philosophical Foundations of Modern Medicine* (Lee, 2012b), which has been written to clarify the philosophical framework within which Biomedicine is conducted and has to be understood. This book attempts an equivalent exploration of Classical Chinese Medicine (CCM).

These two volumes are born out of a common perspective—no scientific activity (including medicine in so far as medicine claims to be scientific) is innocent of philosophy, notwithstanding the claim of positivist philosophy that science is "scientific" only because it has gone beyond the "metaphysical mode" of explanation (Lee, 2012b). One should not be taken in by this piece of blatant positivist propaganda.[1]

While Modern Medicine/Biomedicine emerges from modern Western philosophy since the seventeenth century in Western Europe, CCM has emerged, it will be argued, from philosophical roots which could be said to be at least two and a half thousand—if not more—years old. It may be presumed as a working hypothesis that modern Western philosophy and ancient Chinese *philosophy* are radically different in character; the medicines which ensue from their respective frameworks will also be different.[2] This volume sets out the *philosophical* foundations for CCM; another volume to follow (Lee, in progress/forthcoming) will demonstrate why CCM possesses the specific characteristics it does because of such a *philosophical* framework.[3] This division of labor is called for, as the entire enterprise would lead to such a large volume as to be non-viable. This volume has been written in such a way as to be self-contained, although now and again, wherever appropriate, it would refer to some aspects of CCM, just to remind the reader that their detailed exploration would follow in its sequel. While the latter is predicated upon the former, the former alone could be read as a *philosophical*/cosmological prelude to its sequel from the vantage points to be set out below.

Modern Western philosophy may simplistically be summarized as follows: it is empiricist both in its metaphysics and its epistemology (the metaphysical thesis that only what is ascertainable by means of the five senses and by extension the use of instrumentation is real and exists, the epistemological claim that one can only have knowledge *via* the five senses). Its model of causation is Humean and linear—the phenomenon to be explained, A, is related to one other phenomenon B, its effect, in terms of one cause and one effect, where the causal arrow moves in a straight line only from cause to effect, and cause and effect are associated with each other either as constant conjunction or in terms of probability. It also invokes thing-ontology—it is based on macroscopic/everyday-life objects which have shape, size, and form, are stable, solid, and impenetrable such as mountains, tigers, or tables. Very importantly, modern Western philosophy rests on what Lee (2012b) calls an "ontological *volte-face*"—the universe, and everything in it, including human beings are machines and the science generated from it involves Reductionism, that a whole may "non-mysteriously" be decomposed into its parts while parts can equally "non-mysteriously" be put together (synthesized) to form a whole. The whole is no different than the sum of the parts.

In contrast, the ancient Chinese *philosophy* within which CCM was/is embedded may be said to imply process-ontology—it considers events and processes to be foundational, rather than things. Furthermore, it implies complex causal relationships between events and processes which may be said to be multi-factorial and non-linear. Such a *philosophy* is *Wholist* in orientation—the universe and everything in it, including human beings, constitute *Wholes* which are different from the sum of their parts, and which in turn are related as well as inter-related with other *Wholes*. However, ancient Chinese *philosophy*/cosmology are much more nuanced than such a simplistic account in outline could convey; detailed exploration of aspects of their complexity will be found in specific chapters of this volume.

One must at once enter several caveats. First, this volume does not claim to deal with the whole of ancient Chinese *philosophy*. It has very little to say, *per se*, about the Confucian canon, important though it is normally considered to be. As its remit is very limited, the texts looked at are held to belong to that tradition called Daoism/*Daojia philosophy*/道家, as that tradition is regarded by Chinese scholars down through the ages to be foundational to the《黄帝 内经》/ *Huangdi neijing* (from now on referred to as the *Neijing*), itself regarded as a foundational, if not, *the* foundational text of CCM. This text is considered to be a *Daojia* text. This should not, however, be interpreted to mean that the Confucian tradition has made no contributions to *Daojia philosophy* (or vice versa) as did clearly happen especially during the Han Dynasty (206 BCE—25 CE)—in appropriate places throughout the book, this influence will be pointed out.

Second, the account of the *philosophical*/cosmological underpinning of CCM offered here is intended as no more than an *interpretation*,[4] although its author hopes that such an interpretation would be a plausible and possibly even fruitful contribution to an on-going project undertaken by some Chinese physicians-cum-scholars of late, to go back to cultural/*philosophical* roots; in the words of Scheid, 2002, the project is "the reentry into Chinese medicine of classical philosophy and a self-conscious 'return to the sources.'" What then is this "classical philosophy," this "return to the sources"? This volume can be construed, then, as one such effort to clarify and explore what that *philosophy* and the sources behind it could be and are. The reader must bear in mind that this author is working against a background which is quite different from that which physicians-scholars in China are at the moment engaged with. This author neither lives in China, nor has been educated in China and is not a practitioner of Chinese *Medicine*/中医/*zhongyi* in any known form of that *medicine* set out so clearly by Scheid. The author has only two possibly relevant reasons for this undertaking: first, the interest is a deeply personal one, as the author and family were privileged in having been looked after for up to a quarter of a century by a brilliant physician, trained within a family of several generations of physicians, some of whom even served the imperial household, from time to time, during the Qing Dynasty (1644–1911 CE). Second, as a philosopher with an interest in the philosophy of biology and genetics, a preoccupation with the philosophy of science and technology not to mention environmental philosophy, it is, therefore, not surprising that of late this author has turned to the philosophy of medicine as a domain of exploration.

As a philosopher brought up in the West, within the so-called analytical tradition of Anglo-Saxon philosophy, the author brings to bear whatever skills acquired from this training upon the exploration of Chinese *philosophy*/cosmology which appears to underpin CCM. Whenever relevant, issues in the history of science and the philosophy of science, not to mention contemporary developments at the cutting edge of modern (global) science will be cited to cast light on a matter in hand. At the same time, techniques often relied on by Chinese scholarship which concerns ancient texts, such as tracing a character/word to some of its most ancient scripts in order to get at its meaning are happily relied on. Archaeological discoveries which could shed light on ancient texts will also be brought into play. In a word, the author is happy to live with the charge that the work uses an "eclectic tool-kit" for the task in hand.

It must also be pointed out that this is *not* a sinological work as this author has no professional qualifications in the field, although given the nature of the exercise, it is bound to trespass in some ways into this domain. However, this does not mean that sinologists with an interest in CCM may find it of no relevance to their pre-occupation, in spite of its drawbacks from a strict/purist sinological perspective. The vantage point from which the interpretation of CCM is given here is that of a philosopher trained in the Western analytical school of philosophy whose intention is to make CCM intelligible (in terms of its *philosophy*/cosmology, the methodology of doing *science* which follows from such a foundation) to an English-reading world which is, by and large, unfamiliar with CCM and who may tend to judge CCM to be unscientific, pseudo-scientific, or even downright unintelligible when judged (usually) implicitly by the standards of Biomedicine (or of Newtonian sciences in general). It is an attempt to show in detail how the two medicines are different because they are each embedded within their own respective traditions of philosophy and methodology. Each subscribes to a different paradigm of "scientificity"—judged by that which underpins Biomedicine as a Newtonian science, CCM would necessarily be unscientific. However, all that this demonstrates is that one should not judge a cat show by the standards of a dog show and conclude that a cat is a sub-standard dog, or indeed, not a dog at all. Furthermore, it would show that although the dominant conception of disease in Biomedicine renders it a Newtonian science, not all of Modern Science, since the end of the nineteenth and the twentieth centuries, falls within the Newtonian framework. CCM would be much more readily understandable and understood when looked at from the vantage point of some non-Newtonian sciences such as quantum and relativity physics, not to mention developments within Modern Medicine itself, such as epidemiology (since the nineteenth century) and other areas developed much more recently such as psycho-somatic medicine and Precision/Personalized Medicine. These commonalities are not intended to mask the differences which exist all the same between Biomedicine and CCM—they are meant to argue that each medicine should be respected in its own right, and that it would be a category mistake, simplistically, to judge the one according to the paradigm of scientificity endorsed by the other.

Neither does the volume set out to be an exercise in comparative philosophy *simpliciter*—East/ancient Chinese and West/modern, although it may be read as one. In order to carry out the project, inevitably at times the two have to be juxtaposed and the peculiar features and characteristics of the one are set out against those of the other.

Summary of Structure and Rationale of Chapters in this Volume

Chapter 2

Bibliographical Justification and Clarification of the Main Texts Selected

This is required (a) to make clear that its interpretation of CCM rests on the contention, commonly held among Chinese physicians-cum-scholars that the *Daojia*/道家 tradition had played a key, though not, perhaps, an exclusive role, in its emergence/development. In trying to construct a *philosophical* framework for CCM, it focuses on the *Laozi* 《老子》, the *Zhuangzi* 《庄子》, the *Huainanzi* 《淮南子》; (b) very importantly on the *Yijing* 《易经》 which is part of the *Zhouyi*/ 《周易》 (better known in the West as the *I Ching*) as it is foundational to Chinese culture (and hence crucially relevant to its *philosophy* and its *medicine*); (c) to sort out some key problems regarding some of these ancient texts whose provenance and origins have been subject to debate and controversy through the ages. It has to forego examining the contribution of other traditions, such as the Confucian, the Buddhist, as well as the *Daojiao*/道教 traditions, not to mention the medical traditions of many of the ethnic minority groups over the centuries and millennia—the justification for this principle of economy lies primarily in that this work is not an exercise in the history of CCM *per se* but simply a particular interpretation of the *medicine*, written from certain specific vantage points. Whenever appropriate, it will refer to and acknowledge such relevant contributions.

Chapter 3

Ontology: *Qi* and Its Role in the Lattice of Interweaving Key Concepts

This explores *Qi*/气 as the fundamental ontological category in ancient Chinese *philosophy*. Without a clear grasp of what it entails, one could not hope to understand the notions of *yin qi*/阴气, *yang qi*/阳气, as well as *Yinyang*/阴阳, which everyone agrees are indispensable to all versions of Chinese *Medicine* and therefore of CCM itself. It argues that it is vital to distinguish between the two intimately related modes of manifestation of *Qi*—*Qi*-in-dissipating mode (气散/*qi san*) and *Qi*-in-concentrating mode (气聚/*qi ju*), a nuanced thesis which has very significant implications for the kind of science generated by such an ontological framework.

Chapter 4

Metaphysics: The *Laozi* and the Lattice of Interweaving Key Concepts

This looks at key notions of the *Laozi*: *Ziran*/自然, the Dao/道, *tiandi*/天地 (Heaven which pertains to Astronomy and Time, while Earth pertains to Geography and Space), explores their relationship with *Qi* (the fundamental ontological category) as well as other metaphysical notions such as the distinction between *you*/有 and *wu*/无.

Chapter 5

The *Zhouyi*/the *Yi*: Meanings and Significance

This shows that the *Zhouyi*, being foundational to Chinese culture, is naturally also foundational to its *philosophy* and its *science*. What began as a divinatory text had transformed itself into a set of diagnostic/analytical tools which could be relevant to *philosophical* understanding as well as possess methodological implications for doing *science*. The trigrams and its respective three *yaos*/爻, as well as the hexagrams based on the trigrams (the *Yao-gua*/爻卦 Model), amount to *Wholism*, the philosophical view that the Whole is different from/more than the sum of its parts. It appears to be consonant with what today is called systems thinking.

Chapter 6

The *Yi*: *Yin qi*, *Yang qi*, *Yinyang*, and the *Yao-gua* Model

This develops further the theme of chapter 5, showing in greater detail the relationships between (a) the three meanings of *yi*易 (as found in the *Yijing*), (b) 阴气/*yin qi* and 阳气/*yang qi* (c) between the *Yi* meanings, the two kinds of *qi* (*yin qi* and *yang qi*) on the one hand and the *Yao-gua*/爻卦 Model on the other. It then explores the implications of (a), (b), and (c) for doing *science*.

Chapter 7

Yinyang-Wuxing

This explores the notions of: (a) *Yinyang*/阴阳, (b) *Wuxing*/五行, (c) the joint notion of *Yinyang-Wuxing*, and (d) the implications of this joint metaphysical concept for doing *science*, focusing on the two main modes of interactions in *Wuxing*, the Mutually Engendering/*xiang sheng*/相/生 and the Mutually Constraining/*xiang ke*/相克Cycle and pointing to their relevance in one's understanding of how ecosystems behave and what Ecosystem Thinking amounts to.

Chapter 8
Process Philosophy/Ontology

The preceding chapters which explore the *Yi*, *Qi* in general, *yin qi* and *yang qi* in particular, *Yinyang, Wuxing, Yinyang-Wuxing*, the *Yao-gua* Model will have made it abundantly clear that this kind of *philosophical* orientation cannot be understood within what is called thing-ontology but only within process-ontology. Thing-ontology is the dominant ontology in the Western tradition and has been so for more than two thousand years from ancient Greek philosophy to now. It is the ontology which underpins Newtonian science, focusing on bodies and their motion in absolute space. The first systematic articulation of process-ontology in the West has a history of only several decades. Chinese *philosophy*, in contrast, has always implied process-ontology since the emergence of the *Yijing*, probably more than three thousand years ago. It also looks at two philosophers/scientists in the West, Leibniz and Bohr, who understood implicitly the tradition of process-ontology in ancient Chinese *philosophy* but such understanding was sidelined, misunderstood, and ignored in the West. In the same spirit, it would have occasion to refer to a more recent work by Bohm, 1980, a contribution from a theoretical physicist who, like this author, argues from the standpoint of process philosophy and Wholeness/*Wholeness*.

Chapter 9
Modes of Thinking

This chapter brings the specific characteristics of Chinese thinking in the *Yijing/Daojia* tradition to the fore under the following headings: (a) contextual, (b) dyadic, (c) giving rise to a unique approach which may be called "Contextual-dyadic," and (d) *xiang*/象 mode (endemic in the *Yao-gua* Model), which one may also argue is unique to Chinese *philosophy*. Western philosophy since Descartes has advocated dualistic thinking, unlike Chinese *philosophy* which is dyadic, especially in its Contextual-dyadic manifestation. Given this radical difference, it is not surprising that ancient Chinese *philosophy* neither developed formal logic nor used a two-valued logic (which is classical Western logic)—Chinese *philosophy* implicitly rests on what this author calls *Yinyang/Yao-gua logic* which appears to be an implicit version of many-valued logic (eight values as implied by the eight trigrams). Leibniz and some leading Jesuits who generously claimed that the ancient Chinese were the pioneers of two-valued logic were not entirely correct. While two-valued logic adheres to Aristotle's three laws of thought (the laws of identity, non-contradiction, and excluded middle), *Yinyang/Yao-gua* implicit *logic* does not; from this, one should not and cannot simply conclude that such a logic is "illogical" or that using it commits one to incoherence or unintelligibility as demonstrated by paraconsitent logic. Furthermore, "fuzzy" logic, a form of many-valued logic, appeared in the West in the 1970s; *Yinyang/Yao-gua* implicit *logic* is shown to be an early analog of it.

Chapter 10
***Wholism* in Chinese Terms**
This explores the following: (a) *Qi Wholism: yin qi and yang qi*, *Yinyang*, (b) Macro-micro-cosmic *Wholism* (what sinologists call "Correlative Thinking"), (c) Timespace *Wholism*, and (d) *Ecosystem Wholism*. It also makes clear the difference between what it calls "wholism," "Wholism," and "*Wholism*"—the first is actually the Reductionist thesis in disguise which simply views the whole as an aggregate (the whole is simply the sum of its parts). The second and third are committed to holding that the Whole/*Whole* is different from/ more than the sum of its parts. Wholism is increasingly today being advocated by some scientists although the overwhelming majority of them are still Reductionists (and so are wholists), whereas Chinese *philosophy* has always been *Wholist* ever since the *Yijing*. The Chinese version appears in italics to draw attention to the point that Chinese *philosophy* has its own peculiar characteristics. However, here the focus is on general *philosophical Wholism* which prepares the ground for specific forms of *Wholism* more relevant to a discussion of CCM to be explored in the sequel to this volume.

Chapter 11
Implications of Wholism/*Wholism* for *Science*, Methodology and Ontology
This explores the implications of wholism and Wholism/*Wholism* from the standpoint of the notion of causality. The former is committed to the linear/ Humean model while the latter are committed to non-linearity; in particular, the *philosophy/science* of the ancient Chinese tradition had/has always been conducted within what this author calls a *Wholist*/or "ecosystemic" framework. It looks as if that post-Newtonian sciences especially in the twenty-first century will be conducted as "ecosystem" sciences, in the larger meaning of that term. The ancient Chinese built their "ecosophy" on this wider understanding of "ecosystem" systems, which differs profoundly from the kind of science which modern Western philosophy since the seventeenth century generated, resting on the so-called fact/value distinction. The *Yao-gua* Model as a set of diagnostic/analytical tools is and can be applied in numerous if not all domains of intellectual/practical activities; it also encompasses all aspects of reality. As values are as much a part of reality as so-called facts, why should science/*science* not study such a significant dimension of reality? Science/ *science*, after all, is done by human beings whose conduct in every aspect is

informed by values. From such a perspective, it is the modern Western philosophical tradition which looks odd by so strenuously banishing values from its science, and its science-making.

Conclusion

From the exploration of certain aspects of classical Chinese *philosophy* as delineated here, it appears plausible to infer that, increasingly, it would become easier for those not familiar with it to grasp that it is not so alien after all. A simple reason lies in this: especially in the twenty-first century, science is no longer simply conducted as Newtonian but also as post-Newtonian in numerous domains, which is analogous (though, obviously, not identical to) the *philosophical* framework within which Chinese *science* such as CCM has been conducted. Newtonian sciences are/were conducted within thing-ontology, relying on Humean/linear model of causality; post-Newtonian sciences operate within process-ontology and a non-linear model of causality. Systems thinking in the 1970s was one of the pioneers of generating such a paradigm shift. This book also argues that ecosystems thinking (in the larger sense of that term) is also gaining ground—many different strands and new shoots help to create a new philosophical perspective for doing science, such that the old simplistic divide between what is "scientific," "above suspicion," and what is "unscientific," "pseudo-scientific," "dodgy," or "flaky" would break down, leaving some common space within which it is meaningful to discuss the overlap between the *philosophical* framework for understanding CCM and that for understanding the post-Newtonian sciences which are rapidly gaining ground—after all, there are many different kinds of sciences, depending on their respective philosophical underpinnings. This is the most important thing to grasp should one wish to escape the confines of the limitations imposed by a simplistic approach to the history of philosophy on the one hand as well as the history and philosophy of science on the other—a simplistic approach precisely because it suffers from the self-imposed limitations of time and space.

There is yet another way of understanding the project of this volume; however, to raise it here and now might distract the reader from the prolonged exploration of Chinese *philosophy* and *science* in the ensuing chapters. Hence, it will only be raised in the concluding chapter when the self-imposed task of exploration and clarification is completed and it is clear where the arguments lie.

Before leaving this introduction, there is one more matter which requires some further explanation. This volume is consistently said to give an account of the *philosophical* framework implicitly embedded in Classical Chinese *Medicine* (CCM) and appears to distance itself from a recently emerged version of Chinese *medicine* generally referred to as Traditional Chinese Medicine (TCM), especially in the West but also in China, today. It is not part of the remit of this work nor is this author equipped to do justice to TCM,[5] but, nevertheless, a few words of clarification are called for. The justification for confining this work to CCM relies on three main considerations, the last being the most compelling:

1. The time element: the cut-off point for CCM is very roughly post-Qing, the beginning of the Republican Period, although this guideline can only be used as a crude yardstick, as a matter of convenience only. The Republican Period can itself be divided into two sub-divisions, roughly the first half of the twentieth century and the second half of the last century to the present.
2. Increasingly systematic introduction of Modern Medicine/Biomedicine into China: The first inroad of Modern Medicine into China occurred well before the fall of the Qing Dynasty. It is obvious that this guideline does not coincide too neatly with the time guideline. The original inroad was ignored by the overwhelming majority of Chinese physicians who, on the whole, probably did not even notice its arrival given their own pre-occupations within the context of their own existence; but of the few who were aware of its existence, they were not necessarily hostile and indeed, one, Zhang Xichun/张锡纯 (1860–1933), acknowledged today to be the pioneer in integrating the two medicines (see *Luo, 2014), even made efforts with fruitful results in borrowing from it and incorporating it into the *medicine* of his own culture. However, the first five Republican decades produced a different reaction, one of mutual hostility between the two medicines, indigenous and foreign, as those with political power, in the name of modernization and progress, began a long campaign to suppress—indeed even to eliminate—the former. This strife and hostility was later replaced by peaceful co-existence after the establishment of the People's Republic of China; the government actively pursued/pursues a course of ultimately integrating the two systems. This complicated background involving the relationship between the two medicines—indigenous (therefore seen as "traditional") and modern (imported from the West)—is what makes this author in part concerned to distinguish between CCM and TCM. As the quotation from Scheid, 2002 shows there are physicians in China who are not

altogether happy with the neglect of the cultural and *philosophical* roots of Chinese *Medicine*, a neglect which is bound to occur, given that time is limited and the syllabus is divided between the two medicines in the professional training of the practitioners of Chinese *Medicine* laid on by medical schools in China today. There is a strong undercurrent which urges a return to the cultural and *philosophical* roots upon which Chinese *Medicine* (CM) rests; it is in this spirit that this author uses the term "Classical Chinese Medicine" to distinguish it from that version generally taught in medical schools in China today which in English is called "Traditional Chinese Medicine."

3. The historical dimension: the call for a return to the cultural/*philosophical* roots of CM draws attention to the fact that in its long history down the millennia until the recent emergence of Modern Medicine as a serious rival to it, physicians, especially the scholar-physicians, had been trained (or had trained themselves) not only in the foundational medical texts such as the *Neijing* but also foundational cultural/*philosophical* texts such as the *Yijing/Zhouyi*, the *Laozi*, and the *Zhuangzi* which are all *au fond daojia* texts (chapter 2). The exponents of this call to return to roots are convinced, like the scholar-physicians of yore, that to be an outstanding physician (as opposed to being a merely competent or mediocre one who may excel in having mastered the *medicine* but only as a set of technical skills), one must go beyond the subject as technical expertise to a profound grasp of its *philosophy*, to capture and embody its spirit, its theoretical as well as spiritual dimensions in practice—they are convinced that otherwise CM will sooner or later wither on the vine. Hence their championing of what may be called CCM in English. Two representative works of this strong undercurrent, which have appeared of late, are *Liu, 2003 and *Pan, 2013.
4. The detailed implications for CCM of this set of themes in the chapters outlined above—*Wholism* in its various forms, "ecosystem" *science*, Contextual-dyadic Mode of Thinking, non-linear, multi-factorial mode of causality, *Qi* in its two modes, *Qi*-in-concentrating and *Qi*-in-dissipating modes, thing-ontology/process-ontology, *Yinyang-Wuxing*—will be pursued in greater depth in Lee, (forthcoming).

One final "health warning": this author takes responsibility for foisting the interpretation pursued here upon the writings of scholars, dead or alive, as well as proffering an apology to the latter group in case they find that what they have written or communicated have been misunderstood.

Notes

1. Shapin, 1996: 1 seems, by implication, to challenge this view, as he claims that "There was no such thing as the Scientific Revolution." If correct, then it is neither here nor there that "the Scientific Revolution" requires a new philosophy to support it. After this most provocative beginning, he progressively attenuates it until he ends up with: "I have said that there is nothing like an 'essence' of the Scientific Revolution, and I have sought wherever possible to introduce readers to the heterogeneity, and even the contested status of natural knowledge in the seventeenth century" (161–162). Furthermore, he goes to great lengths to show how a new philosophy was constructed through the efforts of Hobbes, Descartes, among others, who rejected Aristotelianism and that scientists and philosophers alike, the pioneers of the new knowledge about the natural world, departed from the Aristotelian framework. He also writes at great length on the metaphor of nature as machine; unlike this author (Lee, 2012b), he does not see it as an ontological *volte-face*, a crucial component of the new philosophy.

From the standpoint of CCM, this project of excavating and exposing its philosophical foundation accords well with what the very distinguished physician, Zhang Xichun/张锡纯 had written in his essay "On the Relation Between Medicine and Philosophy"—see Fruehauf, 1999.

2. Any reference to "philosophy," "science," "medicine," and other key terms such as "Wholism" will, from now on, be italicized, when they are used in CCM contexts in order to mark the differences between them.

3. This forthcoming volume will contain chapters, among others, on the *Jingluo* Network/the so-called "meridians/channels" (in which *Qi*-in-dissipating-mode operates and whose blockage is the cause of illnesses and pain, according to CCM theory), CCM as Preventive Medicine (the highest expression of *medical* skill), Personhood as a primitive *philosophical* concept (in accordance with Dyadic Thinking which gives meaning to CCM's understanding of illness in terms of a psychosomatic dimension), CCM as Personalised Medicine (which renders Randomised Controlled Trials inappropriate), on *Zheng*/证 and *Fang*/方 (key concepts in CCM diagnostics and therapeutics), the Unity and Coherence of CCM (in terms of its account of the inter-related linkage between *physiology*, illness and therapy), Macro-micro-cosmic *Wholism* (referred to in sinological literature as "Correlative Thinking"), and CCM as *ecosystem science* which all serve to demonstrate the characteristics peculiar and even unique to CCM which are derivative from the *philosophical* and cosmological framework within which CCM is embedded. It will also explore the notion of Integrative Medicine to see if it has meaningful purchase at any level of integration between CCM and Biomedicine.

4. Many other (different) interpretations of ancient Chinese philosophy abound (in English)—one instance of a more recent systematic study is Ziporyn, 2012.

5. See Scheid, 2002 and Sivin, 1987. The status of TCM and its relationship with CCM will be raised in Lee, forthcoming: chapter 11.

CHAPTER TWO

Bibliographical Justification and Clarification of the Main Texts Selected

The exploration of the *philosophical* foundations of CCM, as set out in chapter 1, will consist of two volumes. This volume explores Chinese *philosophy* as found primarily in four Pre-Qin and early Han texts, namely, 《周易》/ the *Zhouyi*, 《老子》/道德经》 the *Laozi*/ the *Daodejing*, 《庄子》/ the *Zhuangzi* and 《淮南子》/ the H*uainanzi*; this exploration will show what way the concepts embodied in them are understood primarily in the *Neijing*, a foundational text in CCM the emergence of which also fell within the same Pre-Qin and early Han period of Chinese history (roughly 1046 BCE– 25 CE).

A major methodological consideration in the historiography of dating an ancient text (such as the first three mentioned above), has to be briefly addressed, as its precise authorship and date of appearance are often unclear. One ought to distinguish between two distinct, though related, aspects of the matter: (a) the actual or part of the content of the text in terms of the notions and concepts discussed, (b) the text in its entirety as a whole mature text. The former (in parts) could predate the latter. One should distinguish between the older/oldest parts of a text (in terms of its content) from the rest of the text as well as the text itself. The issues, surrounding the dating of an ancient text, are not a straightforward matter.

The *Zhouyi*

First, one has to make very clear what names are used in talking about it or parts of it, as usage differs in both Chinese and sinological literature. According to Chinese usage:[1] it contains two parts: (a) the 《易经》/*Yijing*, (b) the 《

易传》/*Yizhuan*. The *Zhouyi*/《周易》 may be translated as the *Zhou Changes*; its older part (a) may be translated as the *Canon of Changes*, while its second/later part (b) may be translated as the *Yi Commentaries* or perhaps more accurately even as the *Yi Treatises*, but it is also called 《十翼》/the *Ten Wings*.[2] Rather confusingly, the name of the text which the Chinese call the *Zhouyi* is rendered normally phonetically in English as the *I Ching* or, more recently, the *Yijing*, and commonly referred to as the *Book of Changes*. This author intends to follow Chinese usage and to adopt the following convention: The *Zhouyi* refers to the extant text which has come down to us and which has two parts. When this composite text is cited in this book, it will simply be referred to as the *Yi*/the *Zhouyi*; when its older part is mentioned, the term the《易经》/ the *Yijing* will be used and when the later part is invoked, it would be referred to as the *Ten Wings*.

The detailed contents are as follows:

The *Yijing* contains (a) the sixty-four hexagrams, (b) their names, (c) the *guaci*/卦辞/*Judgment/Decision of the Hexagrams*, and (d) *yaoci* 爻辞/*Judgment of the Yao*[3] (one for each of the 384 *yaos*).

The *Ten Wings* laid out in sequence are:

1. *Tuan zhuan* 彖传上	*Part I, Treatise on the Judgments of the Hexagrams*
2. *Tuan zhuan* 彖传下	*Part II, Treatise on the Judgments the Hexagrams*
3. *Xiang zhuan* 象传上	*Part I, Treatise on the Xiang*
4. *Xiang zhuan* 象传下	*Part II, Treatise on the Xiang*
5. *Xici zhuan* 系辞上	*Part I, Treatise on the Appended Terms*
6. *Xici zhuan* 系辞下	*Part II, Treatise on the Appended Terms*
7. *Wen yan* 文言 传	*Treatise on the Elaboration of the Words*
8. *Shuo gua zhuan* 说卦传	*Treatise on the Discourses on the Trigrams*
9. *Xu gua zhuan* 序卦传	*Treatise on the Sequence of the Hexagrams*
10. *Za gua zhuan* 杂卦传	*Treatise on the Non-sequence of the Hexagrams*

According to Chinese scholarship, the *Yijing*, since the beginning of the Warring States Period (475–221 BCE), had been received into the Confucian canon. But when did it itself become a mature text? There are three answers in general to this question: (a) beginning of the Western Zhou (1046–771 BCE), (b) end of the Western Zhou, and (c) beginning of the Warring States Period. One Chinese scholar, *Liu, 2008:10 argues for the second view; Smith, 2008 adopts the third.[4]

It is generally agreed that the *Yijing*'s origin is tied up with divination and its techniques (although there is a minority of scholars who disagree with this, and we shall come back to this point later). In the history of

Chinese divination, numerous methods existed, but there were two main ones, which today modern Chinese combines in one word—*zhanbu* 占卜, to refer to the practice of divination in general. Traditionally, *bu* 卜 referred to the practice, especially of the late Shang Dynasty (1600–1046 BCE), although it continued during the early part of the succeeding Zhou Dynasty (1046–771 BCE), of reading the cracks produced in burning specially prepared tortoise shells or ox shoulder blades. Often these lines literally looked like this 卜; that pattern was conveniently taken over as the character/word to stand for this particular method of divination.[5] This practice is sometimes called *guibu*/龟卜which literally means "tortoise shell divination" but which also covers the use of ox shoulder blade. The second major method was *zhan*/占, conducted within the framework of the *gua*/卦 (that is the sixty-four hexagrams of the *Yijing*), using yarrow stalks, *shi*/蓍 to set up the *gua* which was relevant to the situation in hand for which a divinatory outcome was sought. More accurately, this word was used to refer to both the yarrow stalks as well as to the method itself of using such stalks for the purpose of divination; another name for the stalk, also pronounced *shi*, but is written as 筮. The method is called *zhanshi*/占筮).[6] We know for sure just over a century now (since the discovery of the Oracle Bone Script/甲骨文 around the turn of the twentieth-century) that *guibu* existed in late Shang times but that divining by means of *shi* 蓍/筮 had also flourished during late Shang times, if not earlier—see, among other texts, *The Spring and Autumn Annals According to Lü*/《吕氏春秋·勿躬篇》 (239 BCE) and the *Book of Historical Documents*/《尚书·君奭》 (compilation of speeches dating from eleventh century to fourth century BCE). We also know today that the names of all the hexagrams were already known, at the very latest, by the late Shang Dynasty.[7] The trigrams and the hexagrams were built upon such techniques and rituals. Apart from the *Zhouyi*, references to both forms of the *gua* existed elsewhere, such as in 《礼记·礼运篇》/the *Liji*, *The Book of Rites* (attributed to Confucius and written during the Spring and Autumn Period (771–475BCE), about the rites of the early Zhou Dynasty). This text recorded that Confucius visited the state of Song to study the *gua* which had existed since the late Shang Dynasty—a difference between these different versions is that in *The Zhouyi*, the 乾卦/*Qian gua* precedes the 坤卦/*Kun gua*, whereas in the late Shang system of *guas* (the *Gui cang yi*/《归藏易》), the order was the other way round. The *Lian shan yi*/《连山易》 belonging to the Xia Dynasty (2100–1600 BCE) used *gen*/艮 as the lead trigram; however, both had been lost even by the time Confucius himself (551–479 BCE) was born. The oldest parts of the *Yijing* in the *Zhouyi* could be dated to eighth century BCE.

The *Ten Wings* may be regarded as the fruit of the attempt by Confucians to understand and assimilate the *Yijing* into their own system of thought.[8] Its emergence in the form of the *Ten Wings* is separated from that of the *Yijing* by five to six hundred years, making it in the main a work of the late Warring States Period. In the past, Chinese scholarship had not distinguished between them adequately, but for more than half a century, it has agreed that the two parts originated from different periods. Today, in general, scholars agree that the *Zhouyi* with its two parts, as a mature text, appeared to have emerged toward the middle of the Western Han Dynasty, that is, to say it has existed for just over two thousand years only.

What is the exact relationship between the two parts? There is no total consensus, as some scholars hold that their respective contents have nothing in common—the *Yijing* is entirely about divination (up to and including the Spring and Autumn Period, the dominant view regarded it as no more than a divinatory text) whereas the *Ten Wings* is about *philosophy*. Other scholars maintain that their contents overlap and are inextricably entwined because (a) the *Yijing* is itself not simply a divinatory text (contrary to what the early Chinese had believed right up to the Spring and Autumn Period), but also contains *philosophical* and cosmological ideas which the Confucians (though not necessarily Confucius himself) further developed and sophisticated; (b) yet others agreeing with some scholars (such as Xunzi荀子 (c312–230 BCE) who in his book the *Xunzi* held that those dedicated to the text would not use it for divination purposes:善为《易》者不占 (《荀子·大略》) which may be translated as: "Those who truly appreciate the *Yi* would not be using it for the purpose of divination;"[9] they argued that the *Yijing* is really cosmology/*philosophy*, covering branches of the subject such as metaphysics, epistemology, and ethics (in today's terminology). The *Ten Wings* simply carried further this secular orientation away from its original divinatory function to other interpretations and possible functions, relegating the former to the last of four categories (see below) to which a person might understand and use the text. The four categories were: those interested in language would study its terms and phrases; those interested in motion/movement, would look at it from the standpoint of change or changes; those interested in the world of instrumentation would look at *xiang*/象/pictures, while shamans would be interested in using it to divine—see Part I，Treatise on the Appended Words/《系辞上》:《易》有圣人之道四焉:以言者尚其辞, 以动者尚其变, 以制器者尚其象, 以卜筮者尚其占.

The Han philosopher Dong Zhongshu 董仲舒 (ca. 176–ca.104 BCE) was instrumental in getting the *Yi* accepted by the emperor, Han Wudi in 136 BCE, as the leading "Confucian" classic, on the grounds that Confucius himself was said to have been a devoted student of the text; as a result of such an honored status bestowed by the emperor, it came from then on to be called the *Yijing* (*jing* refers to a classic, canonical text). In addition there was the claim (made on his behalf) that he, Confucius, was the author of part, if not of the whole of the *Ten Wings*. (Do note that the Confucian tradition most certainly did not entertain the view that Confucius's own passionate dedication to studying the text had anything remotely to do with divination; the Sage was known to be against the practice of divination on the rational grounds that divination outcomes were not reliable, and as the quotation from Part I, Treatise on the Appended Words cited above shows, to use the text as a plain divination text is, according to the Confucian tradition, the lowest of four possible uses to which the text could be put.)

This raises the matter about the difference between 经/*jing* and 传/*zhuan*. The difference lies in this—the former is canonical, the latter is a treatise written about such a canonical text,[10] elaborating, drawing out, and even extending its ideas, but never in a critical spirit according to tradition. It is rare that a *jing* and its *zhuan* are published together between two covers; the *Zhouyi* is unique in that the *Ten Wings* and the core (canonical text) are put together as a single tome. It was called the *Zhouyi*, although before early Han times, it was simply called the *Yi*, because it was the only surviving *Yi* in Chinese history—the two other works on the subject of *yi*, as already observed, having been lost even before the birth of Confucius. Why it came to be called the *Zhouyi* was, probably, based on more reasons than one. According to tradition, members of the ruling house who founded the Zhou Dynasty had something to do with it. A more theoretical reason involved the meaning of *zhou* /周—apart from being a surname—it is used to delineate a period of time during which certain movements or changes take place in Nature which eventually come round again in a cyclic manner. *Zhousui*/周岁means a year in terms of age, *zhoutian*/周天 in ancient Chinese astronomy refers to the 360 days in which Earth took to complete its cycle of movement. *Zhou er fu shi*/周而复始 refers to what may be called Cyclic Reversion, a notion which as we shall see later is absolutely fundamental to Chinese cosmology and *philosophy*. Furthermore, this text puts the *gua* for *Tian*/Heaven (乾/*Qian*) as the lead *gua*, the beginning of the cycle[11]—this *gua* represents *yang qi* at its highest point, and could imply that the Zhou Dynasty itself was about to attain its highest strength. Hence to call the text the *Zhouyi* would be very appropriate.

Tradition has it that "three sages" had a hand in creating the *Yijing*, but it cannot agree on who they were. One version said it was Fuxi/伏羲, who invented both the trigrams/八卦 and the hexagrams which are referred to respectively also as the *jinggua*/经卦 and the *biegua*/别卦; (b) it was Shennong 神农, the Divine Husbandman, who invented the hexagrams; and (c) yet another version said that it was King Wen/周文王—a founder member of the Zhou Dynasty, who was responsible for the hexagrams as well as the explanatory text which went with each of them called *guaci*/卦辞, not to mention a statement to each of the six components in the configuration of a hexagram, called *yaoci*/爻辞; (d) another view attributed the *yaoci*, to the Duke of Zhou, a son of King Wen, a veritable culture-hero in Chinese history. Modern scholarship, however, considers Fuxi and Shennong, on the whole, to be legendary if not mythological personages, but holds that whether King Wen invented the hexagrams or not, it is plausible to postulate (even in spite of their high degree of mathematical sophistication) they could have emerged at the end of the Shang and the beginning of the Zhou Dynasty. The consensus of contemporary opinion is that the grammar of the *Zhouyi* (in its older part) was already well established by the fourth century BCE. For instance, R. Smith, 2008:30 says:

> . . . by the fourth century BCE at the latest the essential grammar of the *Zhouyi* had been well established. Its languages included wordless symbols (hexagrams, trigrams, and individual lines), as well as written texts (hexagram names, judgments, and line statements). What the next few centuries would bring was a substantial increase in the lexicon of the *Changes*, together with a number of commentaries that amplified the interpretive framework of the *Zhouyi*.[12] These additions, in turn, greatly expanded the interpretative possibilities of the document.

As for Confucius's own hand with the *Ten Wings*, doubt was already cast on it by the distinguished Song scholar-official, Ouyang Xiu欧阳修 (1007–1072 CE). Today, scholars in general are of the opinion that they do not come from a single hand, but from various authors expounding Confucian values, whether these were descendants of Confucius's original disciples or not, and whether what they wrote were handed-down reports of what Confucius's disciples had recorded about the Master's comments or not. The *Ten Wings* is now regarded as a Western Han (206 BCE- 9CE) compilation.[13]

With regard to the issue whether the hexagrams were invented before the trigrams or vice versa, if tradition were adhered to, the trigrams would have preceded the hexagrams as Fuxi was the first of the three legendary sovereigns/三皇 of ancient China, said to have lived during the mid-twenty-ninth century BCE. He was succeeded by Shennong. Among many stories about Fuxi is the reproductive narrative that he and Nüwa/女娲, though siblings, nevertheless copulated and engendered offspring, of which the Chinese (and other human beings) were all their descendants. (chapter 9 explores this myth as instantiating the Contextual-dyadic Mode of Thinking.) Taking the logic of this narrative at its face value, one could argue that he would have preceded Shennong, because, although also legendary, Shennong was credited with the invention of agriculture and established the use of herbal drugs, not to mention the hexagrams. The acknowledgement of procreation as a process would have emerged even as tribal society based on hunting and gathering emerged. Following this logic, the trigrams would have come before the hexagrams.

Regarding the claim that King Wen invented the hexagrams, if this were correct, it would distinctly imply that the trigrams preceded the hexagrams, as King Wen (no mythological character) was a founding father of the Zhou Dynasty and lived long after that period in Chinese history called the Three Sovereigns and Five Kings.

Looking at the relationship between the trigrams and hexagrams outside of the mythological or even historical context, one could argue that it would seem more logical that those ancient Chinese (whoever they might have been) would have attempted a configuration of the trigrams before they stacked them up according to some pretty sophisticated mathematical rules of permutation to create the hexagrams. Also there appears to be some internal evidence to support this derivation which can be found by analyzing a trigram. It consists of three *yaos*/爻: the bottom *yao* stands for Earth, the top *yao* for Heaven, and the middle one for Humans. The triad of Heaven, Earth and Man was called *sancai*/三才, the Three Talents/Powers forming a powerful cluster of concepts in Chinese thought. Each exercised its own domain of influence but that of Humans was inescapably affected by the other two, while it itself did not affect the other two domains (that is, until of late, global climate change being a spectacular first in the history of humankind). Together they form a *Whole*,[14] encompassing the entire universe. However, in each domain, *yin qi*/阴气and *yang qi*/阳气 existed, adding up to a total of six powers, operating in the universe. Each *yao* in the six *yao* hexagram represents one of these six "powers." As a hexagram is the result of stacking one trigram upon another, no other kind of "gram" would be meaningful, such as a "pentagram" or a "septigram." With this as a theoretical base, we can see that there are only sixty-four possible permutations/hexagrams; and given that each hexagram has six *yaos*, the total number of *yaos* is then 384. This in turn means that the *Yijing* had things to say about 384 specific conditions through 64 sets of 6 *yaos* each.[15]

Another relevant piece of evidence may be found in texts which chronicled events covering the period 722–468 BCE, such as the《左传》/

The Chronicle of Zuo (compiled not later than 389 BCE during the Warring States Period), as earlier observed, which frequently mentioned and recorded the use of the trigrams in divinatory practices. Another text, 《国语》/*The Discourses of the States* (chronicling events of the Western Zhou Dynasty until 453 BCE), is said to be somewhat later than *The Chronicle of Zuo* (and if relied on to date the *Yijing* would push the period of compilation to middle of the late Warring States Period[16]) also gave similar examples.[17] Although these two texts and the *Yijing* emerged fairly near in time, nevertheless the former bore witness to the fact that the latter raised a subject matter which had already been in the public domain. Note also that in the *Yijing*, the hexagrams are named according to those of the trigrams.

Although the Mawangdui/马王堆 silk texts (discovered since the early 1970s) do follow a different sequence in presenting the trigrams from that of the *Yijing* and show some other differences from the latter, nevertheless, scholars are agreed that (1) they are not later than the received version and (2) they, too, are compatible with the view that the hexagrams were created by stacking two trigrams, one upon the other.

In view of the evidence cited above, one could make a plausible case for holding that the trigrams had an independent existence from the hexagrams, and that they formed the basis for the creation of the latter.

Daojia Texts

So far, we have been looking at the *Yi* for three reasons:

(a) It is the earliest extant as well as the most influential and seminal text in the development of nearly all domains of Chinese intellectual life and activity.
(b) Down the millennia, many outstanding physicians had insisted on the necessity of studying the *Yi* for a proper understanding of CM. Other physicians, through the centuries, who aspired beyond mediocre competence had/have adhered to such dicta. It is also the case that even if a particular medical book did not explicitly mention the *Yi*, nevertheless, the work could not be fully understood without reference to this "divination" text and its influence upon *medicine*—one instance is the famous Han physician, Zhang Zhongjing/ 张仲景(150–219 CE) and his opus the *Shanghan zha bing lu* /《伤寒杂病论》. Naturally, all physicians must know the foundational text in CCM and this is the *Neijing*, which is said to be a Daoist text. We must, therefore, say something about Daoism before we can go on to explore the relationship between Daoism and Daoist concepts and CCM.
(c) Although the *Laozi*, the *Zhuangzi*, and the *Huainanzi* might not have explicitly mentioned the *Yi*, Chinese scholarship has held, down the ages and holds today, that these *Daojia* texts cannot be understood without an understanding of the *Yi*. The chapters which follow will try to show the basis of such a claim.

This section addresses the following issues:

1. How the term "daoism" is to be understood for the purpose of clarifying the relationship between Daoism and CCM. In this context, one must distinguish between *Daojia* and *Daojiao*.
2. Why for the limited discussion of this book, only three so-called Daoist texts (the *Laozi*, the *Zhuangzi*, and the *Huainanzi*) are chosen for exploring their relationship with the *Yi*.
3. If the distinction mentioned in 1 above is sound, then what do the texts mentioned in 2 above have in common which can be said to support the view that Daoism is *philosophy*, not a mere religion.

One must distinguish between *Daojia*/道家 and *Daojiao*/道教, which Chinese scholarship recognizes, but which is sometimes challenged by sinological literature on the subject of Daoism. "Jiao"/教 means "religion"; hence *Daojiao* clearly refers to the religion called Daoism. On the other hand, *Daojia* is commonly understood to refer to Daoism not as a religion but as cosmology/*philosophy*. The *Neijing* itself is said to be a "Daoist" text, clearly not in the sense that it enjoys canonical status in the domain of Daoist religion, but that as a foundational text in CM/CCM, it embodies certain ideas which can be said to belong to *Daojia*. The term *Daojia* was coined, it is said, by Sima Tan/司马谈 (ca. 165–110 BCE), a historian of the Western Han Dynasty, and used also by his son, Sima Qian/司马迁 (ca. 139–86 BCE), who continued the book already begun by his father, which came to be called the *Shiji*/史记/ the *Historical Records*. In general, the term 家 is translated as "School"—one talks of the *Rujia*儒家 (the Confucian School), the *Yinyangjia* 阴阳家 (the *Yinyang* School), the *Fajia* 法家 (the Legalist School). The *Rujia* focused on moral/social/political ideas; the *Fajia* on using the law as the key concept and tool in governing society; the *Yinyangjia* (unfortunately the original text(s) were lost with only some fragments extant), as far as one could determine, focused on the *Yinyang* pairing. On this analogy, whether one deems such Schools to deal with a subject matter which can be called "philosophy" is immaterial, as the issue is not one about advancing stipulative definitions in order to "win" an argument; definitional moves of such a kind constitute a mere sleight of hand. Furthermore, although their respective teachings differed fundamentally, nevertheless, they were all predicated upon ignoring the existence (or the relevance to their preoccupation) of a transcendent being (god/gods) whose commands must be obeyed. The validity of their teachings was not grounded in the supernatural; indeed, if one prefers not to use the term "philosophy" to characterize these Schools, one could opt for an alternative term, and call their teachings naturalistic or humanistic, in contrast to a world-view which embraces the supernatural orientation. ("Humanism" as well as "Naturalism" are here used to refer to any world-view which is arrived at through the use of human reason alone, without revelation.)

The term "Daoism" in English deserves closer attention as it suggests a set of ideas which anyone who calls him/herself a "Daoist" would share in common, while, perhaps, acknowledging at the same time important differences between various versions of "Daoist" thinking and practices under the broad umbrella "name" of "Daoism." In English, it is meaningful, say, to invoke the term "Protestantism," but that term hides many differences amongst the numerous sects in that large branch of Christianity which defines itself against another big branch of the same religion called Catholicism.[18] In European languages, the suffix "ism" can conveniently be invoked to serve the purpose just outlined. But in the Chinese language and Chinese culture, such an easy maneuvre is not readily available. One can speak of "the Dao" (that is, the "Dao" which the *Laozi* talks about); one can speak of applying "the Dao" to understanding different domains of theory and praxis, such as "the dao of rulership"/君主之道/*jun zhu zhi dao* (which the *Huainanzi* was ultimately interested in), the "dao of the military" (as in Sunzi's *The Art of War*), the "dao of medicine " (医道 *yidao*).[19] In English, one can meaningfully say that the *Neijing* is a "Daoist" text; however, in Chinese, one must say that it is a "Daojia" text, to distinguish it from say *The Correct Classic/Zhengyijing*/《正一经》[20] which is considered to be a "Daojiao" text—one cannot simply blur the differences between these two kinds of text by calling them "Daoist" texts as in English. Sometimes, "Daojiao" texts are also referred to, for short, as "dao shu," but the context always makes it clear that these texts are "Daojiao" and not "Daojia" in character.

Daojia may or may not be a School; call it what you like, but it is not grounded in the supernatural and in a god of some description with temples, monks and rituals; in contrast *Daojiao* must be as it had/has transformed Laozi into a god, whose statue sits upon an altar in a temple, surrounded by burning joss sticks. The traditional account of *Daojiao* traced its formal foundation to the Eastern Han Dynasty, several centuries after the first appearance of the *Laozi*/the *Daodejing* to someone referred to as Zhang Daoling/张道陵 born in 34 CE. His surname was Zhang and his given name was Ling, but as he founded the Daoist religion, he became known later in history as Zhang Dao Ling. In its earliest days, this religion called itself the *Dao* of Five Bushels of Rice/五斗米道[21] or the *Dao* of the Heavenly Master/天师道, while claiming Laozi as its original teacher, and indeed, proclaiming him to be a god. Its basic texts therefore included the *Laozi* among others as these emerged following its foundation; this religion tended to emphasise an other-worldly detachment from reality (脱离现实), achieving immortality via the search for elixirs (*lian dan xiu xian*/炼丹修仙).[22]

It is said that Sima Tan in using the term *Daojia* and in his brief account about it did not mention the name of Laozi; neither did he refer to the text called the *Laozi*; indeed he did not mention the word *dao* at all, apart from it being part of the term *Daojia*.[23] However, it is acknowledged that the two Sima (father and son) would undoubtedly have meant all the same that the *Laozi* belonged to *Daojia*, that it was in two parts, one about *dao* and the other about *de*/德 even if it is true that unlike contemporary scholars, they would have accepted the traditional account about the author who was called Laozi, or Li Dan/李聃. Whatever the agenda of Sima Tan behind his use of the term, it had come to be associated with the rational and the naturalistic which can be found in the Dao of the *Laozi*, distancing itself from the activities of certain practitioners called the *fangshi*方士[24] as well as somewhat from that perspective called *Huanglao*/ 黄老 about which the Mawangdui excavation in 1973 of an early Han tomb revealed some fragments.[25] We have already earlier observed that the rationalist/naturalistic tendency had begun as early as the Spring and Autumn Period; no doubt, Sima Tan was continuing this orientation in Chinese thought, thereby excising what might smack of the supernatural and the superstitious.

It is, therefore, fair to observe that texts such as the *Laozi* and the *Neijing* regarded as belonging to *Daojia* would be very different in character from say *The Correct Classic*. However, acknowledging their differences would not necessarily lead to a denial that *Daojiao* does share some common concepts with them. Our pre-occupation here is simply to say that one could distil from the former set of texts a cluster of cosmological/*philosophical* concepts which have made contribution to the development of the naturalistic mode of thinking down the millennia, a mode, to which the Confucian humanist tradition was hospital when it developed the *Ten Wings* of the *Zhouyi*.

This observation is very much in keeping with the assessment which Isabelle Robinet (the most respected Western scholar of "Taoism") has given of the alleged distinction. Robinet, 2008 writes:

> The main difference between *daojia* and *daojiao* is perhaps that *daojiao* primarily aims at establishing a connection with the sacred, either as a relationship with deities and spirits or as the attainment of personal transcendence. The question of immortality is related to this point. . . .
>
> The *daojia* dimension of Taoism is absent in several Taoist trends and texts, and others appropriated the *Daodejing* without much regard for its many possible meanings. The *Xiang'er* [想尔] commentary exemplified this attitude. Nevertheless, the philosophical spirit and features embraced by the term *daojia*

> are apparent throughout most of the history of Taoism, beginning with the *Taipingjing* [《太平经》] *Scripture of Great Peace*), which may be the earliest extant *daojiao* text. With YinYang and *Wuxing* [五行] cosmology, the *daojia* has given Taoism one of its most basic conceptual frameworks, without which no religion can have a structured and coherent worldview.[26]

For the very limited purpose of this discussion, only three key *Daojia* texts will be briefly examined—the *Laozi* 《老子》/*Daodejing* 《道德经》, the *Zhuangzi*/《庄子》, the *Huainanzi* /《淮南子》. The last is the least problematic from the biographical and bibliographical point of view, as its origin and date can be ascertained more or less precisely. It is a Western Han (206 BCE-9 CE) text, which was sponsored by the king of the state of Huainan, a grandson of the founder of the Han Dynasty, called Liu An 刘安 (179–122 BCE). It is said, some thousands of scholars gathered under his roof and patronage. Naturally, not all of them would have had a hand in writing the pieces finally assembled as the *Huainanzi*; only eight of them have been identified as the most likely contributors to the volume. Although primarily *Daojia* in orientation, it also incorporated material which covered Confucianism, Mohism, Legalism, and the Yinyang School. Its contents included politics/government, economics, military, astronomy, geography, agriculture, biology, music, not to mention even some myths and legends. For this reason, the text has been regarded by some scholars as something of a mixed bag, which in one sense, would not be surprising, as it was intended to be a compendium of knowledge based on texts down the centuries. However, in spite of such a perception, it remains a coherently presented and elegantly written *philosophical* piece of work.[27] Liu An's preoccupation was not solely an intellectual one; on the contrary, he was hoping to influence the central government, the Emperor Wu, his nephew. Unfortunately, in the end, he was charged with plotting against imperial rule, for which he duly committed suicide; his state was dismantled as a result, and Han Wudi (156–87 BCE) went on to establish Confucianism as the official ideology of the Han Dynasty.[28]

The *Zhuangzi* and the *Laozi* are said to be texts which emerged during the Warring States Period. From the biographical standpoint, the former is relatively more straight-forward, as its putative author, Zhuangzi, is acknowledged to be a historical person who lived some time during the fourth century BCE (between 350 and 300 BCE), reputed to be a *Daojia* figure. However, contemporary scholarship would at best credit him with some of the chapters in the text and also claims that five authorial voices could be detected in it.[29]

In contrast, the *Laozi* is even more problematic, as its putative author, Laozi was over the centuries and is today regarded (in some quarters) at best as a legendary if not mythical or fictional character, in spite of Sima Qian's attestation to the contrary in his *Shiji*. However, whoever Laozi was (the very name seems to refer to a kind of general sage, rather than a specific individual, some have argued), and whether he was mixed up with an astrologer called Dan 聃, are issues which appear, in one sense, irrelevant to the existence of the text itself. Up to now, scholarship, on the whole, agrees that it is not the handiwork of one author, whoever he might have been as some of its contents referred to things which happened at the time of Confucius, others to much later matters. (However, this view, at least, among Chinese scholars may be about to change in view of the discussion to follow.) This scholarship is informed by a major discovery in an archaeological excavation which has excited scholars throughout the world. This involves excavation of one of the three early Han tombs at Mawangdui near Changsha in Hunan Province during which two complete editions of the text were uncovered in the form of two versions written on silk, one of which could be dated to not later than 206 BCE, and the other to between 206 and 196 BCE. These enable scholars to date the *Laozi* to the Warring States Period. However, twenty years later in 1993, another excavation took place which involved the *Guodian* Chu bamboo slips/郭店楚简/ the *Guodian chu jian* found in one of the Chu tombs near the village, Guodian, in Hubei Province. This tomb could be dated to the Warring States Period (between mid-fourth century and early third century BCE, or roughly to before 300 BCE). According to one interpretation, this helps to reinforce the evidence found at Mawangdui that the *Laozi* text is a Warring States piece of writing.

That the Chu tomb is dated to the middle of the Warring States Period is not in doubt,[30] but is it so clearly and unproblematically the case that the version of the text was also a Warring States composition? At least, scholarship in China today appears to have come round to the view that it is older than that. For instance, one scholar,[31] who in fact participated in the excavation twenty years ago, now holds that the Guodian version could be put roughly to the same period as Confucius himself. The evidence for such a view includes the following: (a) Difference in content between this version and the extant version(s)—while the latter contain criticisms of Confucians and their thinking, the former does not. If the teachings of the Guodian text were more or less contemporaneous with those of Confucius himself, then this would explain why such a text would not have anything to say about the matter, as the teachings of Confucius did not attain any significance until well after his death. (b) An earlier date for the Guodian version could cast light on some puzzling features about the purported author, his name, as well as when such a person lived. Confucius himself was said to have sought out someone called Li Dan 李 聃 to learn from him, whom we take to be the person whom history has called Laozi—at least according to this account, such a person did exist and was alive when Confucius himself was living; and as Confucius did try to learn from him, one could infer that he had something of importance to teach others, namely, those teachings which posterity called the *Laozi*. Yet tradition has it that a person called Laozi left the service of the Zhou court to pursue his own life of dedicated reclusion, passing through a pass called Hangu/函 谷 during the Warring States Period. The officer in charge of the pass pressed him to write down his thoughts before he passed through the pass to the new life ahead of him. This person was the official Dan (太史儋 *taishi* Dan)—note that this person was also called Dan but the characters for the two similar sounding names are quite different. Now if one were to postulate that *taishi* Dan already was aware of the work of Li Dan (李聃), then he could simply add more to the extant text, incorporating some criticisms of the teachings of Confucius into the text which he then supposedly left behind for the official at the pass. The person whom Confucius sought to learn from and the *taishi* Dan were separated by approximately two hundred years. However, by the time Sima Qian wrote his history, the Guodian text of the *Laozi* had probably already been lost, people had by then got the two Dans confused—as a result, Sima Qian faced with such a tangle of confusion which he was not in a position to disentangle, simply said that the author of the *Laozi* could have lived up to be to two hundred years old or more modestly to about a hundred and fifty years old. Two important Chinese scholars/*philosophers* of the last century Feng Youlan 冯友兰 and Hu Shi 胡适 disagreed on the date of the *Laozi*, with Feng claiming it to be a Warring State work and Hu that it was earlier. It looks as if Chinese scholarship today seems to side with Hu rather than Feng. Maybe, the said Laozi or Li Dan was not after all legendary, that the Guodian text could, single-handedly even be his handiwork. This would, no doubt, not be the last word on the subject of his identity and the question of authorship of the Guodian text as well as the text called the *Laozi* commonly dated to the Warring States Period. We never can rule out whether a new archaeological find may not be on the horizon which can either reinforce this interpretation or undermine it completely—we can but wait and see.

Why have these three texts been selected for special attention? This is because, as mentioned earlier *en passant*, they are perceived by Chinese scholars down the ages to have contributed toward a powerful tradition of Chinese thinking beginning with the *Yijing*, enriching a perspective which is said to be peculiarly Chinese for understanding/apprehending the world both *philosophically* and *scientifically*. They see the *Laozi* to be a continuation/extension of the cosmological/*philosophical* content and methodology embedded in the divination text. This may be spelt out a bit more by noting that the *Laozi* itself had influenced those Confucian scholars who had a hand in writing the *Ten Wings* of the *Yi*; as far as Han scholarship in *Yi* studies was concerned, it had, in a sense, rendered the *Laozi* and the *Yijing* to be compatible and integrated *Daojia* thinking with the latter—they reckoned that the Dao was at one with the principles underlying the *Yijing and the Zhouyi*.[32]

The *Zhuangzi* is considered to be the second foundational text of *Daojia* and at least parts, if not all of it, are said to accord with the *Laozi* in its understanding of the Dao. As Robinet has pointed out, these two texts concur in giving a new meaning to the term "dao" as Ultimate Truth—nothing preceded it and it was the source of everything, and was therefore primal in this sense. It cannot be named as naming it would only result in limiting it. As regards its implied *epistemology*, the Dao advocates that the knower must attempt to get rid from him/herself all obstacles that stand in the way of grasping the Dao, such as one's prejudices, emotions, desires, ambitions, and pre-occupations which could distort one's apprehension of the reality that the Dao embodies. That is why stillness and tranquillity as the appropriate states of mind were so much emphasised.

At the same time, the *Zhuangzi* and the *Huainanzi* spell out a theme endemic in both the *Yijing* and the *Yi* and the *Laozi* but which was not explicitly raised in them, namely, the notion of *Qi*/气 which is best left untranslated for the moment, until we discuss it in chapter 3.

Similarly, it is appropriate here only to raise, but leave for later exploration (chapter 4), another key concept which informs these selected texts, that of *Ziran*/自然 which occurs so prominently and explicitly in the *Laozi*, though only implicitly in the *Yijing*. Again there is no point in translating it right now as a few words cannot do it justice.

The cluster of concepts identified above—the *Yi*/易 (its fundamental meaning in terms of change), the Dao, *Ziran*, *Qi*, *Yinyang* (which the *Laozi* only mentioned once), as well as that of *shi*/时 and *fang*/方 which mercifully could be translated as "time" and "space" without running the danger of being too misleading—are all to be found in these texts, either explicitly or implied. Furthermore, they are central to a proper understanding of what kind of *science* and what kind of *medicine* CCM really is.

Selected Texts and Their Intimate Link with CCM

The preceding two sections have gone through some of the more important reasons for focusing on the texts as foundational to an exploration of Chinese cosmology/*philosophy*. Admittedly, the ultimate justification for concentrating on them is their link with the *Neijing* and other key medical texts as they are, in the main, all *Daojia* texts. However, so far we have omitted to mention the single most relevant reason for opting to focus on three of these four texts, namely, the *Yi*, the *Laozi*, and the *Zhuangzi* as key to understanding the roots and profundity of CM (what today may be called CCM) as understood through the ages.

Let us take a look at the *Yi* and its influence on CCM thinking, other than the *Neijing*, beginning with the Han Dynasty. Zhang Zhongjing's *Shanghan zabing lun* toward the end of the Han Dynasty, considered by scholars to be a key innovative work in the history of CCM, cannot be understood without a reference to the six *yaos* of the *gua* as hexagram, upon which he modeled his diagnosis of illness via the three *yang jing*/阳经 and three *yin jin*/ 阴经 (六经辨证/*liu jing bianzheng*). Coming to the Jin 晋Dynasty (265–420 CE), one could mention Huangfu Mi/皇甫谧 (215–282 CE) who not only was a noted literary talent but also an eminent physician (putting acupuncture on the map) and whose volume《帝王世纪》/ *Diwang shiji* is said to be rooted in the *Yi*. Coming to the Tang Dynasty (618–907 CE), one cannot overlook the comments of 孙思邈 Sun Simiao (581–682? CE), acknowledged to be "the king of pharmacology"/药王. In the first chapter of his first great opus *Essential Prescriptions Worth a Thousand Pieces of Gold for Meeting All Emergencies*/《备急千金要方》/*Beiji qianjin yaofang*, entitled "论大医习业"/"Discourse on the education of a superior physician," he mentioned the *Yi*, among others, as an essential text for intensive study, should one aspire to transcend mediocrity: ". . . 并须精熟, 如此乃得大 医."

During the Song Dynasty (960–1279 CE), the appearance of the familiar *Yinyang* icon of the "black" and "white" fishes (the *Liangyitaijitu*/ 两仪太极图) is sufficient evidence to testify to the persistent influence of the *Yi* in all domains of knowledge including *medicine*.

For the Ming Dynasty (1368–1644 CE), one may invoke two of its famous physicians. The first is 孙一奎/ Sun Yikui (1522–1619) who wrote: " . . . 深于《易》者, 必善于医; 精于医者, 必由通于《易》. 术业有专攻, 而理无二致也," rendered by this author as:

> If one has a deep understanding of the *Yi*, then one necessarily is good at being a physician; but if one were to possess exceptional command of medicine, then that knowledge and expertise must have come from a thorough understanding of the *Yi*. Although one cannot reach commanding heights in all domains, yet within any one domain of which one is in command, theory and practice must rest on the same underlying principle.

This passage is found in a chapter significantly entitled "不知易者不足以言太医论"/*Discourse on how it is impossible to be a superior physician without knowledge of the Yi*, in his work called《医旨绪余》/*Yi zhi xu yu.*

The second is Zhang Jingyue/张景岳(1563–1640). In *Lei jing fu yi*/《类经附翼》is a chapter entitled "Principle concerning medicine and the *Yi*"/ *Yi yi yi*/《 医易义》/, in which he wrote: 天人 一理者, 一此阴阳也; 医易同源者, 同此变化也.岂非医易相通, 理无二致?可以医不知《易》呼? This author renders it as:

> *Tian* (in this context including Earth) and Humans live under a single principle, that is the law of *Yinyang* in Nature. Hence medicine and the concept of *yi* both draw from the same source and as a result, they involve the same patterns of change. Does this not then mean that (the theory and practice) of medicine and *yi* are inextricably linked, that the same principle underlie them both, that one cannot be a physician without knowing the *Yi*?

Also in the Ming Dynasty, Li Shizhen/李时珍 (1518–1593), produced a monumental work on Chinese *materia medica*, called *Ben cao gangmu*/《本草纲目》. This work cannot be understood without bearing in mind the framework within which it was constructed, components of which include the *Yi* and *Yi* related concepts such as Macro-micro-cosmic *Wholism* (*Tianren-heyi*/*Tianren-xiangying* commonly translated as "correlative thinking" in sinological literature), *Yinyang-Wuxing*/阴阳五行.[33]

From the Qing Dynasty, one may cite an eminent physician, Huang Yuanyu/黄元御 (1705–1758). In chapter 1 of one of his numerous books《四圣心源》/*Si sheng xinyuan*, he wrote: 善言天者, 必有验 于人, 然则善言人者, 必有验 于天矣。天人一也, 未识 天道, 焉知人理 which this author renders as:

> On the one hand, those knowledgeable about astronomy (matters pertaining to the heavens) would also have experience of human affairs while, on the other, those knowledgeable about human affairs would also know at first hand astronomy. As the macrocosm (Heaven and Earth) and the microcosm (Humans) form a *Whole*, if one were ignorant about the *dao* of Heaven (and Earth), how could one be knowledgeable about the principles which govern human conduct.

Indeed, the quotation from Huang Yuanyu implies that the three texts, the *Yi*, the *Laozi*, and the *Zhuangzi* were in the mind of the author (and of fellow Chinese through the ages, as he was no pioneer in this matter), seamlessly linked them together, as can be seen in the writings of Sun Simiao of the Tang Dynasty. In the text from which we have earlier quoted, namely, "Discourse on the education of a superior physician," he wrote: 不读《庄》《老》, 不能任真体运, 则吉凶拘忌, 触涂而生, which this author renders as:

> If one does not know (thoroughly) the *Zhuangzi* and the *Laozi*, one would not really grasp the Dao or understand the *Laws of Nature* governing the processes of change and transformation embodied in *Wanwu*/万物. As a result, one would not readily appreciate the constraints imposed by what is permissible (and therefore propitious) and what is not permissible (and therefore unpropitious); such ignorance leads one to run everywhere into obstacles and problems.

In CM through the ages, should a physician aspire to be less than mediocre or merely competent, his education must include the three foundational texts, perceived to be *Daojia* texts, namely, the *Yi*, the *Laozi*, and the *Zhuangzi*. This book simply follows this ancient tradition.[34]

Conclusion

The first section of the chapter has argued for the following claims:

1. One must be very careful in the way in which one refers to the text commonly called the *Zhouyi/I Ching* making it clear which part of this composite text is being talked about and under what name. This author has opted for the Chinese (rather than the sinological) convention of referring to the composite text as the *Yi/Zhouyi*, the older part as the *Yijing*, and the later part, the *Yizhuan*, as the *Ten Wings*.
2. Even if the entirety of the *Yijing* cannot be dated to the beginning of the Zhou Dynasty, it remains correct to observe that Confucius (551–479 BCE) and no doubt other people, too, already were studying it. Hence, it would be reasonable to conclude that its existence would have pre-dated the birth of Confucius, even if cautious scholarship might not wish to endorse that King Wen and his son at the beginning of the Zhou Dynasty had a hand in contributing to it.
3. It is undoubtedly correct to say that the *Yijing* is a divinatory text, that the *Ten Wings* though not intended to aid divination, could be said to be inextricably bound up with it, and that for nearly two millennia, the *Zhouyi* as a whole would have been used in the activity of divination.
4. However, in spite of this undeniable function as a divinatory text, it remains correct to observe and to argue that the process of secularization in Chinese culture had begun as early as the Spring and Autumn Period, when scholars began to see the *Yijing* as something more than a divinatory text. What more it purveyed would be examined in the chapters that follow.

The second and third sections have argued for the following claims:

5. *Daojia* should be distinguished from *Daojiao*; that this distinction is sound in spite of the practice in sinological literature to use the umbrella term "Daoism/Taoism" to cover both the cosmological/*philosophical* and the religious components.
6. The key ideas which inform CCM in its foundational text, the *Neijing*, come primarily from *Daojia* and not *Daojiao*.
7. Four texts have been singled out for discussion—namely, the *Yi*, the *Laozi*, the *Zhuangzi*, and the *Huainanzi*—because it will be argued in the remainder of the volume that they share a cluster of key concepts, some of which are dealt with explicitly and others are implied, but without which the so-called *Daojia* mode of thinking, in general, and the CCM mode of thinking, in particular, cannot be understood.
8. Historically, this linkage has been explicitly made, at the latest, since the beginning of the Han Dynasty. For instance, the *Huainanzi* made it clear that these texts, among several more (some of which though named had now been lost since Han times and others, though relied upon had not been named) had played a role in articulating the themes and their understanding within its own presentation and structure. The *Huainanzi* used what it called the "roots" and "branch" system in classifying its chapters, the first eight coming under the "roots" heading, as they dealt with the Dao, and the remaining falling under the latter category as it dealt with the application of the Dao in particular domains and contexts. However, as far as the authors of the *Huainanzi* were concerned, the *Laozi* was so well-known that they had not bothered to mention it explicitly in chapter 1 which was no more and no less than their setting out an account of the Dao. The *Zhuangzi* was mentioned in chapters 2 and 7 ("roots" heading), whereas the *Yi* was mentioned as falling within the latter category of chapters.[35]

The third section makes the following important point:

9. The single most relevant reason for opting to concentrate on three of those four texts lies in the undeniable fact that the tradition of CM/CCM itself has singled them out for special mention, as texts which could not be ignored should one wish to understand the *medicine* and to rise above mediocrity as a practitioner of that *medicine*.

Notes

1. See *Liu, 2008: 9; *Mou, 1988: 6. Sinological writing appears, on the whole, to follow a different convention—see Smith, 2008: 37, 30; Wang, 2012. Smith says that the received text of the *Yijing*, which gained imperial approval in 134 BCE, consisted of two parts, the much older core part and the later material called the *Ten Wings*; he implies that he is calling the older core part the *Zhouyi*. With this convention, Wang 2012: 63 appears to follow Smith (although neither in the text nor the bibliography of her book, is Smith, 2008 mentioned); she writes:

As is customary, we can call the core part of the text the *Yi* or *Zhouyi* ("the *Yi* of the Zhou Dynasty"), the commentaries on it the *Yizhuan* ("*Yi* Commentaries") and the two together the *Yijing* (the *Classic of Yi* or the *Book of Changes*).

However, Shaughnessy,1999: 292 has written that texts attributed to Zhou Gong and his father King Wen who lived at the beginning of the Zhou Dynasty "include the *Zhouyi* 周易 (Zhou changes; the earliest stratum of the work better known in the West as the *Yi jing*易经, Classic of changes). . . ." It seems that up to a point Shaughnessy agrees with the Chinese convention that the older part is called the《易经》/*Yijing*. However, at the same time, according to the Chinese convention, as the *Zhouyi* 周易 contains the《易经》/*Yijing* as well as《易传》/the *Ten Wings*, King Wen and his son Zhou Gong could not have been responsible for the *Ten Wings*, as these two personages lived well before the *Ten Wings* were written. It makes sense to say that they could have been responsible only for the《易经》/*Yijing*. Furthermore, what the West calls the "the *Yi jing*易经, Classic of Changes" or what is commonly in English called the "*I Ching*" contains both the earliest stratum as well as the *Ten Wings*. Wu, 2003: xxi simply says that the "*Yi Jing* is composed of the *Jing* proper and ten literary works that elaborate and expand on it." For all these reasons, this author prefers to follow quite straightforwardly the Chinese convention.

2. There is this view held by some Chinese that the *Yizhuan* is rather like adding wings to a tiger (如虎添翼). This is probably the source of the term *Ten Wings*.

3. This book prefers not to translate the term *yao*爻 as "line" and to leave it untranslated, as "line" is not unproblematic. All that the reader needs to bear in mind is that a *yao* can be of two kinds, a *yin yao* (- -) or a *yang yao* (—); that a trigram has three of them in any combination of the *yin* and the *yang yao* and that a hexagram has six of them.

4. R. Smith, 2008: 30 says that "by the fourth century BCE at the latest the essential grammar of the *Zhouyi* had been well established." (Bear in mind that by the *Zhouyi*, he is referring to what this book calls the *Yijing*.) By including the operative phrase, "at the latest," Smith's view may be said to be not incompatible with that of Liu, 2008.

5. For a short and accessible read on the subject, see Lee, 2008 on the nature of the Oracle Bone Script; *Wu, D., 2006: 8; *Zhao, 2006: 38–39; *Chen, Z., 2006: 274, 447.

6. In other words, the *Yijing* only used the method of *shi* 蓍/筮, not the method of *bu* 卜. See Wang, 2012: 29 for a rather curious account of the matter which is totally at odds with this one. See also Rutt, 1999.

7. For detailed textual evidence, see *Liu, 2008: 27–29, 432.

8. See Shaughnessy, 1998 for his account of detecting three authorial hands in drawing up the Treatise on the Appended Words and for a quick reference to the debate among scholars as to whether they are Daoist or Confucianist.

9. See chapter 4, note 1, for another example of Xunzi's efforts to establish the secularization process already begun in earlier times.

10. To understand why a canonical text is called *jing*/经, *dian*/典, or *jingdian*/经典, see Lee, 2008: 162–164, 140–141.

11. See *Liu, 2008: 13–14.

12. In this author's terminology, this *Zhouyi* is the *Yijing*.

13. The literature regarding the dating of the two parts is very large; but to name just two instances setting out in detail some of the evidence, in English, see Smith, 2008 and *Mou, 1998.

14. "*Whole*" is italicized in conformity with authorial decision as announced in chapter 1; see chapter 10 for exploration of "whole", "Whole" and "*Whole*".

15. Wu, 2003: 77–78.

16. Pines, 2002: 41.

17. See * Liu, 2008: 28–30, for consideration of examples from these two texts; Rutt, 1999.

18. All forms of Protestantism, in spite of the profound differences between them, reject the Church of Rome and the Pope as God's true representative on earth—for them, divine communication and instruction are *via* the Bible.

19. Chapter 4 makes a distinction between "the Dao" as a metaphysical concept on the one hand and specific, particular *daos*, such as *yidao*/the *dao* of *medicine*, which are empirically grounded, but within the *philosophical framework* of the *Dao*.

20. This is a text which emerged during that period in Chinese history known as the Nanbei Period 南北朝 (420–589 CE) among the followers of the Celestial Masters Dao. Although long lost, it survived in fragments scattered in other texts of the Celestial Masters Dao.

21. Before admission, the would-be adherent must offer that amount of rice to the organization.

22. For an account of the ancestral roots of *Daojiao*, the similarities and differences between *Daojiao* and *Daojia*, see *Daojia and Daojiao*, 2013 (for two different accounts, of which the first is from the Chinese perspective and the second is sinological).

23. See K. Smith, 2003 for Sima Tan's motive in creating the term "Daojia" in order to identify its referent in terms of a set of ideas which were intended to appeal to the Han Emperor Wu, with Sima Tan himself as the paradigmatic "Daojia".

24. It is not easy to give a simple translation of this term, as scholars appear to disagree widely amongst themselves. The *fangshi* were said to be practitioners of certain special arts (flourishing roughly from the third century BCE to the fifth

century CE), which depending on the context, could mean alchemical, astrological, or even magical skills. The term referred to a wide range of people from alchemists to mountebanks. Sometimes, the term is translated as "masters of formulae" or "masters of methods." See Wang, 2012:34–35; Graham, 1986: 13.

25. For a discussion on all these related matters, see K. Smith, 2003. [Note that the *Huanglao* strand also contributed to the scholarship of *Yi* studies, but toward the end of the Eastern Han Dynasty, it was appropriated by *Daojiao*—see *Zhu, 2005: Vol.1, 218.] Another sinologist has observed that four main streams may be distinguished which fed into Daoism in general: philosophy, hygiene, alchemy and Penglai mythology and that the *fangshi* were associated with the last two mentioned. Welch, 1957: 89–90 writes:

> It was probably between 350 and 250 B.C. that the names of Lao Tzu became associated with what we shall call "philosophical Taoism"; their books testified in turn to the existence of a "hygiene school," which cultivated longevity through breathing exercises and gymnastics; early in the same period the theory of the Five Elements was propounded by Tsou Yen, whose followers are thought to have started research on the elixir of life; and lastly, along the northeastern coasts of China, ships began to sail out in search of the Isles of the Blest, hoping to return with the mushroom the "prevented death.

Welch, 1957: 96–97 is also of the opinion that it was the *fangshi* who developed alchemy: "although Tsou Yen gradually acquired alchemistical stature, he himself knew nothing of the art." It was probably developed by those of his followers who became interested in physical experimentation with the Five Elements. However, for an account of the Huang-Lao version, see Eno, 2010.

26. The Chinese characters inserted within square brackets in the quotation are found not necessarily where they are located in the quotation. The text mentioned *Xiang'er* is actually a commentary on the *Laozi*, probably written around 200 CE by the grandson of the founder of *Daojiao*, called Zhang Lu/ 张鲁. Unfortunately, it was lost a few centuries after its first appearance, until in the early twentieth century a fragment of a Six Dynasties copy of the text was found in the Dunhuang Manuscript Cave and now lives in the British Library. Its content is said to be close to that of the *Taipingjing*. In Chinese, the commentary is: 《老子想尔注 》/*Laozi xiang'er zhu*.

27. A translation in English which does justice to these qualities has recently been published, translated and edited by Major et al., 2010.

28. For a detailed analysis of the relationship behind the politics and the cosmological/*philosophical* world-view in the text, see Wang, 2000; for a quick account, see also Wang, 2013.

29. Roth, 2014. Hoffert, 2006 argues that there is more continuity and coherence in the text than is normally credited it by scholars like A.C. Graham when relating it to the theme of the Dao; although only the so-called Inner seven chapters might be said to be the writing of the historical Zhuang Zhou/庄 周 himself, and the rest were the contributions of later Han Daoists whom Graham calls the "Syncretists," pulling ideas from numerous different sources which could be said often to deviate from the

Master's teachings. Hoffert cites a passage from the section called the *Qiwulun*《齐物论》to support his thesis. The passage reads:

> The Great Way is not named; Great Disputations are not spoken; Great Humanity is not humane; Great Modesty is not humble; Great Courage is not aggressive. When the Way is made clear, it is not the Way. When disputations are put into words, they do not suffice. When humanity is a constant principle, it does not succeed. When modesty is transparent, it cannot be trusted. When courage is aggressive, it does not inspire awe. These five are round but tend toward the square. Therefore, understanding that rests in what it does not understand is the highest. Who can understand disputations that are not spoken, the Way that is not a way? If one has the ability to understand this, it is called the Reservoir of Heaven. Pour into it and it won't fill up, dip from it and it won't run dry, yet no one knows the source from which it comes.

This is called the Concealed Light.

See his analysis of the passage above in Hoffert, 2006: 164.

30. Chinese scholars have now come to the conclusion that, in all likelihood, the tomb belonged to the poet/scholar/official Qu Yuan/屈原 (343–278 BCE) of the State of Chu (one of the states during the Warring States Period), and indeed was/is regarded as one of China's greatest poets and patriots—consult **Tansuo faxian* 探索发现, CCTV broadcast on 11 and 12/03/2014 at 12 noon (London time).

31. Guo Qi/ 郭祁—see reference in preceding note.

32. See *Zhu, 2005: Vol.1, 276 for a list of Han scholars who endorsed this view.

33. In the rest of this book, all the concepts mentioned in this section, would be discussed and explored in full.

34. For a detailed account of this tradition, see *Pan, 2013: Vol.1, 9–16.

35. See Major et al., 2013.

CHAPTER THREE

Ontology

Qi and Its Role in the Lattice of Inter-weaving Key Concepts

Chapter 2 links four texts together—the *Yi/Zhouyi*, the *Laozi*, the *Zhuangzi*, and the *Huainanzi*; this, then, permits highlighting a cluster of key concepts which are crucial in providing the general *philosophical* and methodological underpinning for CCM. Some of the concepts so far identified are: *yi*/易, *Ziran*/自然, *Dao*/道, *Qi*/气, *Yinyang*/阴阳, *shi*/时, and *fang* /方.

The single most important methodological consideration guiding the writing of this work, as mentioned in chapter 1, is the thesis that no science (and hence no medicine, in so far as it claims to be scientific) could be articulated, theorized, or practiced without a specific philosophy to underpin it. Quickly to remind readers, the subject of philosophy (following the usual practice in modern Western philosophy) is considered to have four main branches, namely, metaphysics, epistemology, logic, and values. Let us start with metaphysics.

Ontology

This chapter looks at a particular variant of metaphysics called ontology. Very briefly, ontology attempts to answer the question: what are the most basic item(s) of furniture/kinds of being in the universe which can account for the numerous things we observe to exist in the world? With its five senses, humankind has come to know that different kinds of trees and plants as well as animals exist, that heavenly bodies such as Earth, Sun, Moon, and Stars exist, that rainbows, thunder, and lightning exist, and so on. Philosophers attempt to account for all these phenomena, speculating whether a single ontological category is sufficient, namely, the category of Matter. If the answer to that question is "Yes," then one calls such an ontology, Materialism. However, if the answer is "No," then what additional ontological category would be required? In the history of modern Western philosophy, the enquiry took this particular turn: we, human beings, have noticed that we exist somewhat differently from other living beings, such as tigers or apes. While these as well as we, undoubtedly, are material/physical beings, the fundamental difference between us makes it appear necessary to go beyond the ontological category of Matter in order to account for the type of unique consciousness which we possess. This consciousness enables us to discover that Earth goes round the Sun and not the other way round (since the Copernicus Revolution), axiomatize Euclidean geometry, speculate that there may be a transcendent being called God, who created us and the universe, and construct abstractions and speculations of which apes and tigers are incapable. One leading philosopher of the Age of Modernity (René Descartes, 1596–1650) said that apart from Matter, Soul/Mind must exist and that a human being is a combination of two very different kinds of substances Mind/Soul, Body (Matter). This is the famous doctrine of Cartesian dualism. (Chapter 9 explores whether Chinese *philosophy* is also dualist in nature).

Is Chinese *ontology* a form of Materialism, *simpliciter*? Or is it a form of Cartesian dualism? Or is it neither, but instead something much more complex and subtle? We need to begin to address this important issue here, focusing on *Qi*.

What Is *Qi*?

As the key notions mentioned so far form a lattice of inter-weaving concepts, it would not matter too much which of them is selected to kick-start the discussion on the theme of Chinese metaphysics/*ontology*. Upon reflection it is obvious to start with the notion of *Qi*, and in the process of unravelling its philosophical complexity and subtlety, its significance would become clear. Furthermore, the *Daojia* tradition recognized it to play a foundational role in Chinese *philosophy*/cosmology, as it the most basic ontological category in which everything in the universe could be accounted for.

In grappling with a character/word[1] which appears in ancient Chinese texts, it is normal to deconstruct it by looking up older scripts or dictionaries to determine its original meaning.[2] What does the character *qi* look like in the various ancient scripts? See figure below.

A is the Oracle Bone Script/甲骨文; B are three versions in the Bronze Script/金文; and C are the Lesser Seal Script/小篆. The word remains quite unchanged in the scripts which succeeded/succeed, such as the Clerical

Figure 3.1. Character *qi* in various scripts

Script/隶书, the Standard Script/*kaishu*/楷书 looking just like C (in *fanti*/ 繁体, it is氣, *jianti*/简体, it is气).[3] As version A could be easily mistaken for another word 三/*san* meaning "three" (the difference lies in that the three strokes of the former are not of identical length unlike those of the latter), the Bronze Script had introduced some changes. A and B1 are considered to be attempts to depict floating clouds. As such, the original meaning of *Qi* lies in *yunqi*云气, specifically about cloud conditions. B2 and C1 show these conditions even more graphically, that these clouds are fine floating clouds. The Han lexicographer of *Shuowen jiezi*/《说文解字》, Xu Shen/许慎 (c58-c147 CE), who was relying on C1, also explained the word in terms of *yunqi*. Derivative meanings include: the atmosphere in general 空气/*kongqi*; the weather in terms of being cold, hot, rainy, dry, sunny, dull, and so on as in *qihou*/气候, *qixiang*/ 气象 (meteorology); the breath of some living animals when these organisms breathe in and out *qixi*/气息; the mental state of a person as in the expression *chui tong sang qi*/垂头丧气 meaning "dispirited"; *qidu*/气度, *qizhi*/气质, the bearing/character of someone, whether the figure in question is charismatic, authoritative.

Under another entry for the word based on the radical米, B3 which looked no different in reality from the Clerical Script C2, Xu Shen gave another meaning altogether different from that noted earlier. He quoted a passage from a particular text:[4] 齊人來氣諸侯. This can be loosely translated as: "The State of Qi sent to the military of other (feudal) states forage for their animals and food for their soldiers." Xu Shen said that the word itself is composed of two parts: one part comes from the word for "rice" 米, the other comes from 气 which gives it the sound. In other words, it is a *xingsheng zi*/形声字/semantic-phonetic compound. One scholar in particular has commented that Xu Shen appeared to have modified a much older word (to refer to this kind of gift between feudal states), namely, 餼/*xi*—he simply dropped the left-hand component, retaining the right only. In other words餼/氣 referred to food stuff (for humans and animals) given as gifts between states. Whatever the convoluted history about the orthographic development of *qi*, it appeared that sometime after Xu Shen, the practice grew up of writing *qi* no longer as 气 (C1) but as氣 (C2) , until the 1950s when the *jianti* reform took place, reverting to C1.[5]

As early as the Oracle Bone Script, during the late Shang Dynasty, A showed that the word was used to refer to something people could observe in the sky above them. Fine floating clouds appeared to have both shape and size, yet they did not seem to the ancient Chinese to be solid and impenetrable. Although there were, then, no airplanes to fly through clouds, they would have seen on occasions some powerful birds flying into or above them and then through them re-appearing yet again below them. It was obvious that they changed shape and location very quickly. We shall return to these characteristics in a moment.

The meaning of *qi* which Chinese *philosophy* is interested in as an *ontological* category had long left the Shang use of the term *behind*, although so far as one knows, Chinese history had not mentioned any specific date about the transition. Suffice it just simply to remark that by the time the *Yijing* was constructed, the word *qi* could no longer mean what the Shang people had taken it to mean (that is, no more than fine floating clouds in the sky), as the text, even as a straight-forward divinatory one, was based on *yin qi* 阴气 and *yang qi* 阳气 as captured by the image of the *gua* 卦 whether as trigrams or hexagrams. The *yin yao* 阴爻(broken line) and the *yang yao* 阳爻 (unbroken line) bore cosmological meaning if not full *philosophical* import in the early days of the *Yijing*. By the time of the *Laozi*, the *Zhuangzi*, the *Ten Wings*, and the *Huainanzi*, the term had become a fully-fledged *ontological* category. Some scholars maintain that the earliest expression of *Qi* as being metaphysical in character can be found in the *Zhuangzi*,[6] but admittedly in a chapter which is not part of the Inner seven chapters, called《知北游》*Knowledge Roaming North*, but which, nevertheless, accords with the understanding of the Dao, as found in the *Laozi* and other *Daojia* texts.[7] The relevant passage reads: 生也死之徒, 死也生之始, 孰知其纪! 人之生, 气之聚也。聚则为生, 散则为死。若死生为徒, 吾又何患! 故万物一也。。。。故曰: '通天下一气耳, rendered by this author as follows:

> Life is but the companion of death, just as death is the beginning of life, life and death being complementary processes. Who knows the detailed entirety of the process? Life of the human being is but the concentration of *Qi*. *Qi* concentrates, thus life occurs; *Qi* dissipates，death occurs. As life and death are necessary companions, I do not regard death as a disaster. … Thus *Wanwu* (the myriad things) are part of the One, *Qi*. Hence goes the saying: 'Permeating All-under-heaven is *Qi*.

This passage either makes clear or implies several important points:

1. *Qi* is omnipresent in the universe, and is the *ontological* category accounting for *Wanwu*.
2. As such, it cannot therefore be translated by "breath," "air," "gas," nor even straight-forwardly by "energy," which it often is; nor can it be translated by "matter."
3. The notion of *Qi* points to a puzzling feature that it is perhaps both "energy" and "matter" simultaneously.[8]

These points can be related back to the meaning of the word *qi* in the Oracle Bone script, standing for fine, floating clouds. We have imagined what the ancient Chinese would have observed, that clouds had shape and size, yet these characteristics changed quickly from moment to moment (thereby changing location in the process). Yet although they had shape and size (let us call this the A set of properties), clouds were not like other objects which also possessed shape and size, such as mountains, trees, animals—the latter, the ancient observers knew had other properties not possessed by clouds, such as their solidity, impenetrability, and their (relative) stability (let us call this the B set of properties). To say that an object possesses solidity is to say that the stuff it is made of is densely packed, unlike the air in the atmosphere which is not. Dr. Samuel Johnson (1709–84 CE), the famous eighteenth century lexicographer of the English language, famously demonstrated that physical objects such as rocks were real and existed by kicking them in an attempt to refute the skeptic who claimed that they did not exist in the world out there, and were, therefore, not real. Dr Johnson implied that it was their solidity which would make the skeptics regret for having kicked them, as their feet and toes would be agonizingly painful when stubbed. Impenetrability goes with solidity—something impenetrable means that one cannot walk through it, such as a hill, a wooden door. Stability goes with solidity, impenetrability—a hill, a mature tree, a large rock are all stable (or to be more precise, relatively speaking, appear very stable when compared with finely floating clouds). Such objects have weights which can be measured.

When we normally talk about physical objects (mountains, animals), we are talking about those things in the universe which possess both the A and B sets of properties. As such they are said to embody *matter*, and the ontology they presuppose is called *Materialism*. (In modern Western philosophy, the ontological rival to Materialism is *Idealism*—that is to say, that matter is not the ultimate constituent furniture in the universe but are ideas or can be reduced to ideas or mental conceptions entertained by human consciousness such that the ultimate furniture in the universe is no more and no less than ideas.) The ancient Chinese found juxtaposing mountains or tigers with clouds philosophically inspiring and significant, as clouds appeared to them to possess the A but not the B set which could have prompted them to speculate what clouds could instantiate—an interesting category of being appeared to have emerged, which satisfied only the A but not also the B set. In this imagined re-construction of what the ancient Chinese had observed and reflected upon, we have found that they would have wittingly or unwittingly transformed themselves into cosmologists and *philosophers* as they posed to themselves the question: what is the ultimate constituent of the universe? Their attempt to answer such a question would have led them eventually to formulate the following set of related theses:

1. The ultimate *ontological* category might not be Matter *simpliciter*, but something more complex, less simple-minded than Matter in a straight-forward sense, which they called *Qi*. *Qi* is both Matter and its polar opposite, not-Matter. (This is not to say that the ancient Chinese actually entertained a term which can be translated as "ontology;" it is to say that they had the concept, rather than the word for it.)
2. This in turn would have led them to postulate that this *Qi* was capable of two modes of existence or being, as the passage from the *Zhuangzi* cited above, indicated. These two modes of being may be called: (a) *Qi*-in-concentrating-mode (*qi ju*/气聚); (b) *Qi*-in-dissipating-mode (*qi san*/气散).[9]
3. The *Qi*-in-dissipating-mode preceded the *Qi*-in-concentrating mode. In the origin and evolution of the universe, the former existed before the latter. *Yuanqi*/元气/Original *qi*[10] was *Qi*-in-dissipating-mode; it was followed later by the appearance of *Qi*-in-concentrating mode—the one follows upon the other in a seemingly endless cycle of succession.
4. Of the two modes of being, the *Qi*-in-dissipating mode, in contrast to its polar counterpart (*Qi*-in-concentrating-mode) may be said to be the default mode of being, not only because of its existence as *Yuanqi*/Original *qi* but also because, as we shall see, the *qi* "released" through decay or death of the physical object which embodied *Qi*-in-concentrating mode is returned to *Qi*-in-dissipating mode. This would accord well with two (of the three) meanings of the term "易" embedded in the *Yi*, namely, 变易/*bianyi* ("to change"/"change") and 不易/变*buyi* ("not to change"/"no change"). However, this should not be interpreted to mean that the *Qi* in *Qi*-in-dissipating-mode is not itself subject to change (everything in the universe changes including *qi* when expressed as *yin qi* (*qi* of *yin*) or *yang qi* (*qi* of *yang*) which will be explored later), but that in this context of application and under-

standing, as just set out, *Qi*-in-concentrating-mode may be said to be subject to change, whereas *Qi*-in-dissipating-mode is not subject to change, and so is said to remain constant. (Later in the chapter, we shall explore this point further.)

5. *Qi* in its *Qi*-in-concentrating mode as physical things are said to possess "stuff" and "form"—a rendering in English of 有质有形/*you zhi you xing*. That which has both *zhi* and *xing* is Matter. *Xing* can then be said to refer to the A set of properties listed above, that the entity has size, shape and occupies space (location), while *zhi* could be said to refer to the B set of properties, that the entity is solid, impenetrable, stable, has weight, and mass (in today's understanding of physics which will be looked at later in the chapter). That is why too, in ancient Chinese *philosophy* (or at least the *Daojia* tradition of the pre-Qin and early Han times), Matter and material entities belonged to the domain called 形而下/*xingerxia*—this expression appeared for the first time in the *Ten Wings* and may literally be translated as "that which exists at the level of shape and size." In contrast, *Qi* in its *Qi*-in-dissipating-mode was implied to belong to the domain of 形而上/*xingershang* which may literally be translated as "that which exists at the level above/beyond things with shape and size."[11]
6. These two modes of being are inter-related, inter-transformable. As already indicated, "inter-transformable" means that *Qi*-in-dissipating mode can become *Qi*-in-concentrating mode, and after a period of time, *Qi*-in-concentrating mode returns as *Qi*-in-dissipating mode, thereby setting up a cycle of sustainable exchange between the two modes. The causal arrow moves in both directions as follows:

$$\leftrightarrow$$

The passage from the *Zhuangzi* cited above used the life and death of an organism to illustrate the process. The beginning of life is but *Qi*-in-dissipating mode transforming itself into *Qi*-in-concentrating mode while death is but *Qi*-in-concentrating mode transforming itself back into *Qi*-in-dissipating mode—these phases of change mark the birth and death of an organism. But the cycle starts afresh again, with *Qi*-in-dissipating mode transforming itself into *Qi*-in-concentrating mode, in another organism—such a cycle carries on sustainably during the entire evolution of life on Earth (in our Solar system). It is important to note that this unchanging mutual transformation of the two modes of *Qi* occurs not only in the biotic but also abiotic domain—for instance, planets such as Earth did not originally exist as Matter/*Qi*-in-concentrating mode, but as *Qi*-in-dissipating mode.

It should, therefore, be pointed out that the term *Wanwu* can have two meanings—a narrower meaning which refers to organisms but also a broader meaning, referring to entities in both the biotic and the abiotic domains. It is natural to talk about birth and death in the former, less so in the latter. However, the abiotic also has its analogues of birth and death—one can speak of the origin/coming into being of a mountain (orology) and eventually of its decay until the mountain no longer exists and all that is left are some stumps. The Himalayas are so high for the simple reason that in geological terms they are considered to be very young mountains. But eventually they, too, would wear down primarily through weathering, but conceivably even by movements from the center of Earth, changing the crust formation on its surface. Mountains, as high and as big as the Himalayas or the Alps, would eventually be transformed from their *Qi*-in-concentrating mode to become *Qi*-in-dissipating mode. The abiotic as much as the biotic are part of *Wanwu*, of *xingerxia*, and therefore are subject to the same processes of change as the biotic according to the ancient Chinese.

In addition to the above, the *Huainanzi* elaborates further on the notion of *Qi*,[12] presenting an account of the evolution of the cosmos. A relevant passage from the third chapter called "Celestial Patterns"/《淮南子· 天文训》reads:[13]

> 坠未形，冯冯翼翼，洞洞灟灟，故曰太昭。When Heaven and Earth were yet unformed, all was
> ascending and flying, diving and delving. Thus it was called the Grand Inception.
> (Major et al., 2010： 114)
> 道始生虚廓, 虚廓生宇宙, 宇宙生气。The Nebulous Void is the state of the Dao, the Nebulous Void engendered the cosmos, the cosmos in turn engendered *Qi* (or the original *Qi*). (Rendered by this author.)
> 气有涯垠，清阳者薄靡而为天，重浊者凝滞而为地。清妙之合专易，重浊之凝竭难，故天先成而地後定。
> A boundary [divided] the original *qi*.
> That which was pure and bright spread out to form Heaven;
> that which was heavy and turbid congealed to form Earth.
> It is easy for that which is pure and subtle to converge
> but difficult for the heavy and turbid to congeal.
> Therefore
> Heaven was completed first;
> Earth was fixed afterward. (Major et al., 2010: 114)
> 天地之袭精为阴阳—this phrase is left out of the Major translation but is rendered by this author thus: *Yinyang* came about through the essences of Heaven and Earth pairing with each other.

阴阳之专精为四时，四时之散精为万物。积阳之热气生火，火气之精者为日；积阴之寒气为水，水气之精者为月；日月之淫为精者为星辰，天受日月星辰，地受水潦尘埃。

The conjoined essences of yin and yang caused the four seasons.
The scattered essences of the four seasons created the myriad things.
The hot *qi* of accumulated yang produced fire; the essence of fiery *qi* became
the sun.
The cold *qi* of accumulated yin produced water; the essence of watery *qi* became
the moon.
The overflowing *qi* of the essences of the sun and the moon made the stars and planets.
To Heaven belong the sun, moon, stars, and planets;
to Earth belong waters and floods, dust and soil. (Major et al., 2010: 114–115)

The above passage makes clear the following points:

1. The biotic and abiotic, heavenly as well as celestial bodies were all made of *Qi*.
2. Before *Wanwu* (implying the broader meaning) appeared, there was *Qi*.
3. But before *Qi* was produced by *Yuzhou*/宇宙 (the cosmos/universe), the Dao (presented by Major et al.) as the Nebulous Void engendered *Yuzhou*. The line of causal production appears to be like this: the Nebulous Void/the Dao → *Yuzhou* →*Qi* (as *Yuanqi*).
4. The lighter and brighter *Qi* led to the formation of Heaven while the heavier and more turbid *qi* Earth.
5. The lighter and brighter was also called *yang* qi, the heavier and more turbid was called *yin qi*.
6. The mutual reactions and relations between *yin qi* and *yang qi* led to the four seasons which in turn made the emergence and the existence of the myriad things (*Wanwu* implying primarily here the narrower meaning) possible.

We can gloss 3 above as follows: the *Huainanzi* in this passage introduced the notion of the Nebulous Void which the *Zhuangzi* (or the *Laozi*) did not, as well as that of *Yuzhou*, filling in a gap or two left by the passage quoted earlier from the *Zhuangzi*; it also provides the link between the two *Daojia* foundational texts on the one hand and itself as a later *Daojia* text, by explicitly mentioning the Dao in the passage cited above.

First take the following passage from the same chapter (*Knowledge Roaming North*) of the *Zhuangzi* earlier cited: 东郭子问于庄子曰: "所谓道, 恶乎在?" 庄子曰: "无所不在。" 东郭子曰: "期而后可。"庄子曰: "在蝼蚁。"曰: "何其

下邪?" 曰: "在稊稗。" 曰: "何其愈下邪?" 曰: "在瓦甓。"曰: "何其愈甚邪?" 曰: "在屎溺。" This passage is a purported conversation between Zhuangzi and an interrogator called Dong Guozi, and may be rendered (by this author) as follows: "Dong: The so-called Dao, where can it be found? Zhuangzi: It is everywhere. Dong: Would you mind being more specific as that would make things clearer? Zhuangzi: It can be found in ants. Dong: Why is it found in such lowly matter? Zhuangzi: It can be found in this kind of grass (called *bai*) which invades cultivated fields, therefore is regarded as a weed, a pest. Dong: Why, the Dao seems to sink that "low"? Zhuangzi: It exists in earthenware tiles. Dong: Can it be found in anything even "lower" than that? Zhuangzi: Yes, in faeces and urine. To this last retort, Dong fell silent."

If the meaning of the *Zhuangzi*'s response were read in the light of one of the famous passages from the *Laozi*, then the meaning of the *Zhuangzi*'s passage cited above would become clear. That passage from Chapter 42 of the *Laozi* reads: 道生一, 一生二, 二生三, 三生万物《道德经 · 四十二章》. This may be rendered (by this author) as: "The Dao engenders one, one engenders two, two engenders three, three engenders *Wanwu*." Chinese scholars have down the ages interpreted "one" mentioned in the passage either as *Yuanqi*/元气 or equated it with *Taiji*/太极 of the *Yi*, a concept which will be examined chapters 6 and 7. But whether "one" referred to *Yuanqi* or *Taiji* would not interfere with the meaning of "two" as it is understood to refer to the two types of *qi*, *yin qi*, and *yang qi*.

The *Laozi*, unlike the *Zhuangzi* and the *Huainanzi*, explicitly introduced a pair of polarities called *wu* and *you*/无有, commonly translated in sinological discourse as "non-being"[14] and "being." The Dao belongs to the former category while *qi* belongs to the latter—that being comes from "non-being." In other words, the *Laozi*'s account of cosmology could be spelt out as follows (with the arrow → standing for the notion of engendering):

> Dao ("Non-being") → One (Being/*Qi*) → Two (*yin qi* & *yang qi*) →
> Three (co-operation, mutual response and interaction of *Yinyang*) →
> *Wanwu*
> The *Huainanzi*'s account could be spelt out as follows:
> The Nebulous Void/the Dao → the Cosmos → *Qi* →
> *Yinyang* (Heaven and Earth) →
> the Four Seasons (incorporating the Five Transformative Phases/*Wuxing*/ 五行) →
> *Wanwu*

The *Huainanzi*, as the latest historically of these three texts, gives the fullest account (by Han times the concept of *Yinyang* had been conjoined with that of *Wuxing*, a development to be looked at in chapter 7). However, in spite of some differences between them, all the passages cited from the different texts above agreed that *Qi* is the foundation of *Wanwu* both in the wider sense of the biotic and abiotic as well as the narrower sense of the biotic.

The three texts agree that *Qi* can be distinguished in terms of two kinds, *yin* and *yang qi* and that the basis of *Wanwu* is the result of their inter-twining. The *Zhuangzi* goes further than the other two texts by introducing the distinction between two modes of *Qi* operation which are inter-transformable which then leaves us with the puzzling issue of how best to characterize *Qi* as an ontological category. *Qi*-in-concentrating mode would not be mysterious to those familiar with Western ontology, as it clearly denotes Matter, and as such instantiates Materialism. However, *Qi* as *Yuanqi* as well as *Qi*-in-dissipating mode does not fall into this ontological category. The closest notion Western science and philosophy have is that of "energy," a concept, happily and readily understood today because of certain developments in the history of Western science, namely, the science of thermodynamics and Einstein's theory of special and general relativity as well as of quantum physics.[15]

Sadi Carnot (1796–1832), the famous French engineer, was the first to stumble upon what has come to be called the science of thermodynamics.[16] The English had invented the steam engine which went on to fuel the second industrial revolution in general and the railway in particular. Carnot felt that France was being left behind in this race; being patriotic, he decided to study the steam engine in order to increase its efficiency, and thereby to overtake her Anglo-Saxon rival. The English inventors were workmen, some even illiterate such as Robert Stephenson; Carnot thought he could design better steam engines as an engineer with a training in science. He discovered that the efficiency of the engine (admittedly an idealized one) depended only on the difference in temperature between its hottest and its coldest parts which drove the mechanism. Although at first ignored, his finding was later incorporated into thermodynamic theory as developed by the German, Rudolph Clausius in 1850 and the Scots-Irish, William Thomson (later Lord Kelvin) in 1851.

This science is primarily concerned with the conversion of energy between its various forms as well as with the ability of energy to do work for us. Sometimes, it is said to have three laws and sometimes four.[17] But from our limited purpose here, the only relevant one we need to examine in detail is the first law which is called the law of conservation of matter and energy; *this means that matter and energy cannot be destroyed, only transformed, that energy and matter can be converted from one form to another* (for instance, light could be turned into heat and vice versa, solid could become liquid, then gas, and back again), but with the total amount remaining constant. All that we need to concentrate on is that part which this author has underlined.

Our discussion so far of *Qi* shows that it is in agreement with the underlined portion of the First Law of Thermodynamics. *Qi*-in-concentrating mode is Matter and *Qi*-in-dissipating mode would then be energy; the latter is transformable into the former, the former is transformable into the latter. So it is not implausible to claim that *Qi* and its two modes of operation constitute the ancient Chinese version of this law of thermodynamics. But it differs from this law not merely because it is embedded in a different kind of historical, political, and social context but also in a very fundamental aspect. Hence, let us mark this difference by italicizing the Chinese law thus: *the law of thermodynamics* while it appears simply as the First Law of Thermodynamics (in the context of Modern Science since the mid-nineteenth century).

In the context of Western philosophy and modern Western science, Matter is the fundamental ontological category—chapter 8 argues that thing-ontology is the dominant ontological framework in the Western philosophical tradition, whereas process-ontology was endemic in Chinese *philosophy* and the *science* such an *ontological* framework generated from time immemorial. Science in the Western tradition sees energy as something imported from outside the domain of material reality in order to transform it; it is also the case that Matter is transformed by energy to become merely another form of Matter (when wood is burned, it is reduced by the energy of the fire to become ashes, and in turn to become part of soil), while admitting that in the process, energy is released and no longer available for work (the Second Law of Thermodynamics is about the production of this loss of energy for work, existing as "entropy" instead). In contrast, what this author has called the *Chinese law of thermodynamics* was articulated not in the context of technology, of the efficiency of machines which do work on behalf of humankind, but in the context of attempting to understand the processes at work in the natural phenomena which we humans observed and studied. The ancient Chinese, as a result of this kind of orientation, came to appreciate that Matter and so-called energy could not be distinct and separated out from each other, that there was a complex underlying linkage between them. This led them to postulate a dyadic relationship (to be distinguished from a dualist one, a distinction which will be examined and explored in chapter 9) between the two modes of being which *Qi* could take. Such a conception of *Qi* as the basic *ontological* category also implied that *Qi* as *Yuanqi*, of which *Qi*-in-dissipating mode was a part, preceded Matter/*Qi*-in-concentrating mode. Furthermore, the relationship between the two modes of *Qi* is also a dynamic as well as internal one. (These relationships would be spelt out in chapters 6 and 7.)

These points are expressed in Chinese as follows:

(a) 形中有气/*xing zhong you qi*—in form/shape there is *Qi*;
(b) 气中有形/*qi zhong you xing*—in *Qi* there is form/shape;
(c) 气化 形 /*qi hua xing*—*Qi* transforming form;
(d) 形化气/*xing hua qi*—form transforming *Qi*;
(e) 形化形 /*xing hua xing*—form transforming form;
(f) 气化气/*qi hua qi*—*Qi* transforming *Qi*.

An instance of:

(c): *Qi* transforming form: clouds transform as snow
(d): form transforming *Qi*: water from the ocean transforms to become clouds (with help of sunlight)
(e): form transforming form: ice (solid) becoming water (liquid)
(f): *Qi* transforming *Qi*: the *Qi* of water (水气) which constitutes clouds transforms as rainbow

(c) to (f) above are possible expressions of the dynamic relationships between *Qi* in its *Qi*-dissipating mode and *xing* which is *Qi*-in-concentrating mode. These dynamic relationships could occur because of the internal relationship between *Qi* (in its *Qi*-dissipating mode) and *xing* (*Qi*-in-concentrating mode) which is characterized in (a) and (b) above. This is to say that while *xing* embodies *Qi*, *Qi* also embodies *xing*; that *Qi* and *xing* are not mutually exclusive as *ontological* categories. Another way of putting the same point, but this time in Aristotelian terms, is to say that *xing* (Matter) contains *Qi* as well as that it has the potential of transforming itself to become pure *Qi* (*Qi*-in-dissipating mode)—after all, Matter/form is really no more and no less than *Qi*-in-concentrating mode. Similarly *Qi*-in-dissipating mode has the potential to become Matter/form which after all is really *Qi*-in-concentrating mode.

Yet another way of helping those outside the Chinese *philosophical/scientific* mode of thought is to look at Einstein's famous equation, $E = mc^2$ where E=energy, m=mass, c^2=the square of the speed of light. That equation captured Einstein's discovery of the deep connection between energy and mass.[18] However, Einstein's theory had to await confirmation via experiments which was not obtained until 1933 when Irène and Frédéric Joliot-Curie captured in photography the process of energy converting into mass—the photo may be found at the website of the Center for History of physics, American Institute of Physics.[19]

While this was happening in Paris, two scientists in Cambridge University in another experiment demonstrated the reverse process, that of mass converting into pure energy. John Cockcroft and E. T. S. Walton, upon breaking apart an atom, found that its fragments, added together, had slightly less mass than the original atom which had flown apart with great energy. Finally in 2005, the year of the centenary of Einstein's discovery, a team of scientists measured the energy of the gamma-rays emitted by radioactive atoms and found that this energy was equivalent to the change in mass of these atoms before and after the emission of the gamma-rays—the equivalence was to within 4 hundred-thousandths of one percent.[20] This equivalence between mass and energy makes it possible to say that mass is a form of energy; *the law of thermodynamics* could then be said to be in accordance with this conclusion in post-Newtonian physics as enunciated by Einstein in his special theory of relativity in 1905.

Conclusion

In the light of these three important developments in post-Newtonian physics—thermodynamics in the mid-nineteenth century and relativity as well as quantum in the early twentieth century—what the ancient Chinese held about the nature of *Qi* becomes much less mystifying, not at all mystical, and more accessible to the modern mind brought up, by and large, on the Newtonian world-view which nevertheless has got to cope with post-Newtonian physics in particular and post-Newtonian science in general.

This chapter has argued that the ancient Chinese considered *Qi* to be the basic *ontological* category. Barring the option of resisting translating it, how best then should one render *Qi* into English in such a way as to approximate to its reference and use in the original texts? If translate one must, we propose the cumbersome but more accurate term "energy-cum-matter" to do justice to its two modes of being, *Qi*-in-dissipating mode as well as *Qi*-in-concentrating mode. Another way, but even more infelicitous is to coin this barbarism "Em-ism" ("E" for "energy," "m" for "mass" and "ism," the suffix which turns an expression which stands for something concrete, physical, and specific into an abstract concept); this Em-ism does not refer to matter nor to non-matter *simpliciter*, but to a concept which transcends both. Philosophers of science trained in the Western tradition have not, as far as this author can ascertain, thought of formulating a term to capture the ontological distinctiveness of Einstein's physics (linking mass and energy); the ancient Chinese, so to speak, had simply grounded their *physics* on their *ontological* category of *Qi*.[21]

The term "Em-ism" has been coined and put forward not as an instance of what some scholars have called "retrospective privileging;" that is to say, this author is not claiming that the ancient Chinese have scored a brownie point over Einstein regarding the formula "$E = mc^2$," that they had discovered the physics behind that equation some three thousand years before Western scientists. All that this author wishes to do is to draw attention to the following:

1. Cox and Forshaw, 2010: 135 says that in the tradition of Western science "(b)efore Einstein, no one had dreamed that mass could be destroyed and converted into energy because mass and energy seemed to be entirely disconnected entities. After Einstein, everyone had to accept that they are different manifestations of the same type of thing."
2. Before $E = mc^2$, no one had thought mass is a form of latent energy.[22]
3. Put very simplistically, the formula works because the speed of light which is finite is held to be constant (186,000 mi/sec such that someone traveling at the speed of light, would go around the equator approximately 7.5 times in one second), that nothing travels, so to speak, faster than the speed of light.
4. The ancient Chinese had nothing to say about the speed of light in their account of *Qi*; nor did they distinguish carefully between weight and mass; nor did their account permit calculation of a precise nature in the conversion of mass into energy. These are just some outstanding differences between their *Qi ontology* and modern physics.
5. The ancient Chinese, within their own *ontological* account of *Qi*, had themselves made the distinction between *Qi*-in-concentrating mode and *Qi*-in-dissipating mode, and that there was mutual transformation and inter-change between them.
6. As the ancient Chinese did not subscribe to dualistic ontology (see chapter 9 for a discussion of the differences between Western dualism and Chinese dyadism), mass/matter was not separated out from energy (which was the case up to Einstein in the West tradition of philosophy and science); rather *Qi* simply existed and operated as *Qi*-in-concentrating mode as well as *Qi*-in-dissipating mode. These two modes may usefully in the context of appreciating the differences as well as the similarities between different philosophical frameworks generating different forms of science, be regarded, at best, as bearing an analogous resemblance to mass and energy.
7. The ancient Chinese simply adhered to what this author calls *Em-ism*, a term coined as a short and quick snappy label to characterize their *philosophy* and their *science*. Those who do not like it are not obliged to use it as it is not exactly elegant; they could simply spell out the two modes of existence and operation of *Qi*.
8. However, one could perhaps plausibly argue that the ancient Chinese as well as Einstein and scientists after him in the tradition of contemporary

physics are respectively grappling to account for a problem confronting them. That problem, Cox and Forshaw, 2010: 146 put as follows:

> The process of converting mass into energy and energy into mass is . . . absolutely fundamental to the workings of nature; it is an everyday occurrence. For anything to happen at all in the universe, energy and mass must be continually sloshing back and forth. How on earth did anyone manage to explain anything involving energy before we knew this seemingly most basic of facts about the workings of nature?

The ancient Chinese did cope in their own way, not in terms of "mass" and "energy" and the speed of light being constant,[23] but simply in terms of their distinction between *Qi*-in-dissipating mode and *Qi*-in-concentrating mode and the continual "sloshing back and forth" between them.

Carroll, 2016 is a book that is remarkably *Daojia* in spirit; he calls the account of cosmology and physics presented in it "poetic naturalism," an infinitely more elegant and eloquent term than this author's poor offering of "Em-ism."

The interpretation given here is not the only interpretation possible; nor is the meaning of *qi* attempted the only possible one in the totality of Chinese *philosophy* of *Qi*. There are other contexts of its use in theory and practice which the above interpretation does not reflect so well. But in a later chapter, where we shall be exploring the notion of the Dao, we shall raise the matter again.

Notes

1. For an account why a Chinese character may be read as a word or only as a "syllable" in a word, see Lee, 2008.
2. On all the points to follow, see *Wu, Y., 2006: 30; see also *Qi, 2013.
3. For an account of the complicated relation between *jianti* and *fanti*, the so-called "traditional script" today still used in Taiwan, the way in which Chinese characters/words are constructed on a modular basis, as well as of the principles of classification used in understanding how they are constructed and in turn deconstructed, see Lee, 2008: Part II.
4. The text is the 《春秋传》, the *Commentary on the Spring and Autumn Annals*, a text of the Warring States Period, dated not later than 389 BCE, covering that period of Chinese history between 722–408 BCE.
5. For a very different alternative account of this matter, see Wang, 2012: 59. This author would, of course, agree with Wang, 2012 to the very limited extent that

the character can, indeed, be found in the Oracle Bone Script. As for the respective merits of these two accounts, readers should decide for themselves.

6. See Zhang, 1982 in the translation by Ryden, 2002: 49.

7. See Hoffert, 2006.

8. To add to the complexity, there is the trinity of 精 气 神 (*jing*, *qi* and *shen*); the first is (essential) matter which is visible and palpable (in the context of referring to the sperms of the male); the second, in one of its forms at least, as we shall see, is not material (as it is without form or shape and other characteristics possessed by matter) and can in certain contexts be said to refer to energy. The third refers to the spirit, especially when it occurs with *jing* as a two-character word, 精神 and one could use it in much the same way as in the English expression, "her spirit is low."

9. This is the nearest which this author can get to the meaning of the quotation from the *Zhuangzi* earlier cited.

10. There is another meaning which is not relevant to raise here.

11. However, we shall see later that this latter expression is also used to translate the term "metaphysics" into Chinese; its use as such will be then be critically assessed.

12. The Han Dynasty thinkers appeared very keen on the notion of *qi*—the Emperor Xuan 宣汉帝 convened or caused to be convened a seminar on the subject in 51 BCE—see *Zhu, 2005: Vol. 1,130.

13. Very unfortunately, this author felt it is not appropriate to use in its entirety the overall excellent translation provided by Major et al.; in two places, substitute translations have been provided instead.

14. This author prefers the terms (in particular *wu*) to remain untranslated; however, a more accurate translation for *wu* is perhaps something inelegant such as "the domain of great openness" which points to *wu* being that which contains possibilities for being. For now, the term "non-being" will be used within quotation marks.

15. For a very accessible account of the link between thermodynamics, relativity (special and general) as well as quantum physics, both at the experimental and theoretical levels, see Cox and Forshaw, 2010.

16. For a quick account, see *Sadi Carnot*, 2013.

17. For an accessible, brief account see *Three laws of thermodynamics*, 2013; Atkins, 2010.

18. Mass should not be confused with weight. Weight is the measure of the force of gravity acting on a body, and so can vary, as the force of gravity varies from location to location. Mass is the quantity of matter in a body regardless of its volume or of any force or forces acting on the body. In normal circumstances, the mass of a body can be regarded as constant—see *Mass*, 2013.

19. See *Photograph capturing the process of converting mass into energy*, 2013.

20. See *Speed of Light May Not Be Constant*, 2013; Cox and Forshaw, 2010.

21. It would be a bad *philosophical* mistake to consider *Qi* as either plain matter (Materialism) or plain energy. For the former viewpoint, see Byden, 2002: xv.

22. In June 2014, *Nature Photonics* published new research by some physicists at the Imperial College London which shows it is possible to convert light directly into

matter using today's technology (such as high-powered lasers and other equipment); this attempt demonstrates (in principle) what was proven in theory by Gregory Breit and John Wheeler in 1934. See Pike, Mackenroth, Hill and Rose, 2014.

23. Since 2013, some work by researchers show results which appear to challenge Einstein's claim—see *Speed of light may not be constant*, 2013.

CHAPTER FOUR

Metaphysics

The Laozi *and the Lattice of Inter-weaving Key Concepts*

Chapter Three explores the notion of *Qi* as the *ontological* category in ancient Chinese *philosophy* which served to underpin its *science*. This chapter explores other metaphysical concepts, bringing out also the complexities behind the attempt to translate the term "metaphysics" in Western philosophy as the equivalent of the Chinese *xingershang*/ 形而上 ("that which is above form").

Ziran

We begin by looking at another famous passage from the *Laozi* (chapter 25): 人法地，地法天，天法道，道法自然《道德经·二十五章》) which may be translated as: Humankind follows Earth, Earth follows Heaven, Heaven follows Dao, and Dao follows *Ziran*.

It is obvious that the quotation mentions five terms each standing for its own respective concept. For the purpose of the discussion here, let us leave out the term *ren* referring to humankind. For the moment, all that one needs to grasp is that this extended chain of reasoning implies that humans follow first Heaven and Earth, then the Dao and ultimately *Ziran*.

Ziran is the key term in this line of thinking. What exactly is it? It is often translated as "Nature"? Literally, the term does not mean "nature;" it only does so in an implied manner. The two-character word *Ziran* has been literally translated as "self" (the first character) and "what is so" (the second character). Ryden in Zhang, 1982:162 translates it as "what is so of itself," or for short "spontaneous." This author is of the opinion that there is a word which exists in certain European languages derived from the Greek language, which could translate with fair adequacy the Chinese term, and that term is *autopoeisis*. The word itself comes from the Greek *autos* for "self" and *poiein* for "to produce" or "to bring forth" and thus means "self-bringing-forth" or "self-engendering." In the history of Western philosophy, it can be very aptly used in Aristotle's philosophy of biology, to characterize that property peculiar to a living entity, existing as an organizational unity and maintaining its own identity through self-generation, self-renewal, self-regeneration—in Aristotle's view, such beings possessed their own *telos*. In this sense, then, organisms are self-organizing beings. From this, it follows that there is a close enough fit between the two terms *Ziran* and *autopoiesis*.

Having made such an equivalence, one must straightway point out that the reference of the two terms is not identical in the two contexts of use, that of *Ziran* in ancient Chinese *philosophy* and *autopoiesis* when applied to Aristotle's philosophy of biology. Chapter 3 shows that the *ontological* category of *Qi* obtained in both the biotic and abiotic domains, and not merely in the former, as *Wanwu* could have a narrow as well as a broad reference and meaning. In other words, for the ancient Chinese, one could say that *autopoeisis* occurred in both the biotic and abiotic domains; these two domains and the interaction between them would for the ancient Chinese constitute the universe, *Yuzhou*. This meant that the universe exemplified *autopoesis*.

Let us make explicit what is implicit in this account of Chinese cosmology:

1. *Qi* as *Yuanqi*/Original *qi* was engendered by the Nebulous Void (following Major et al.) or the Dao which in turn engendered *Yuzhou* and then *Wanwu*.
2. As humankind is a very specific kind of *Wanwu*, the coming into existence, therefore, of *Wanwu* itself (both biotic and abiotic) had predated the appearance of the human species on Earth. *Yuanqi*, *Yuzhou*, *Wanwu* came into existence totally independent of humankind and would continue to exist independent of humankind. We could conduct a thought experiment and imagine the extinction of the human species to see what consequences would follow—we would find that all the other species (*Wanwu* in the narrow sense) as well as the abiotic domain (the Milky Way, the planets in our solar system, and even outer space—*Wanwu* in the broader sense) would persist and endure.
3. *Yuanqi*, *Yuzhou*, *Wanwu* are *autopoietic* for two reasons, implied ancient Chinese *philosophy*:
   (a) As demonstrated above, they were not the product of human activity;
   (b) Nor were they the product of a transcendent being called God—the texts and others referred to in this book were secular in orienta-

tion. Chapter 5 will show that this process of secularisation had begun as early as, if not earlier than Confucius, that the *Xunzi*, a fourth to third century BCE text, continued in this vein, categorically denying the necessity for invoking the divine/the numinous either for the creation and/or the maintenance of *Yuzhou* and its workings—everything could be explained in non-supernatural, naturalistic terms.[1] Unlike the *Laozi*, the *Xunzi* did not use the term *Ziran*. Although the *Zhuangzi* did not explicitly deal with this issue, yet its contents and its orientation indicated that it would be in the *Laozi* tradition of *Ziran*. The same holds true in the case of the *Huainanzi*. However by the first century CE, after Confucianism had been established by the Han Dynasty as its official ideology for about a hundred and fifty years, *philosophy* had degenerated into superstition, with Confucius and Laozi having been elevated to become gods and be worshipped, with statues of them, in temples (after the establishment of *Daojiao*). To some minds, the rational, naturalistic account of the world and the place of humans in it had to be re-asserted; this challenge was then taken up by a *Daojia* thinker called Wang Chong 王充 (27?—100? CE) in his collected essays entitled *Lunheng* 《论衡》.[2]

4. The term "nature" in the English language is used paradigmatically to refer to what in Chinese is called *Wanwu*, although it can also be used to refer to what in Chinese is called *Yuzhou*. So broadly interpreted, "nature" refers to *Wanwu*-within-*Yuzhou*. Following Lee, 1999: 82–84, this sense of nature may be called Nature_c ("c" hints at the cosmological) and is in keeping with the points made at 2 and 3 above. Following Lee (ibid), the sense of nature as exemplified in *Wanwu* may be called Nature_{nk} ("nk" stands for "natural kinds" both biotic and abiotic—plants and animals, diamonds and aluminium). Chapter 9 will explore these various senses in greater detail.
5. From the above, one see how natural it is to translate *Ziran* as "Nature." For the purpose of ease, simplicity and elegance of translation, the term "Nature" appears fine, yet from the ontological standpoint, it is profoundly unsatisfactory for the following reasons. "Nature," whether spelt with an upper or lower case "n" is a noun. As such, it is used to refer to a physical thing or physical things. Chapter 3 claims that paradigmatically, a physical thing/entity possesses two sets of properties—the A set pertaining to shape, size, and the B set pertaining to solidity, impenetrability, (relative) stability, weight. They are what the ancient Chinese *philosophers* considered to belong to the domain of *xingerxia*, to the domain of what has both substance/stuff (*you zhi*/有质) and form (*you xing*/ 有形), namely, to the domain of matter. In other words, by

translating *Ziran* as "Nature," one would be inserting the former into a framework in which it is not *ontologically* at home. Chapter 3 has also shown that *Wanwu* come from *Qi*; *Qi* is Em-ism, both energy and matter (according to the interpretation which this book espouses), whose dyadic forms of being must then itself be part of *Ziran*. Furthermore, *Ziran* is not so much about thing/things called Nature, but processes the ancient Chinese had detected to be at work which ultimately led to the emergence of *Yuzhou* and *Wanwu*, to their maintenance and sustenance (all of which are neither divinely nor humanly driven). These processes are primarily those of mutual interaction, combining harmoniously two types of *qi*, sometimes called *tian qi* (*qi* of Heaven) and *di qi* (*qi* of Earth) or *yang qi* and *yin qi*. Chapter 8 will demonstrate that Chinese *philosophy* involves what may be called process-ontology whereas Western philosophy advocated and still by and large advocates substance-/thing-ontology. That is why it is important to point out that the translation of *Ziran* into a noun/thing could be misleading. However, it remains correct to observe that Nature paradigmatically manifests *Ziran* processes at work.

6. For these reasons, it is best to translate *Ziran* as *autopoiesis*, "self-engendering processes" or "self-bringing-forth processes." It would also be acceptable to translate it as "spontaneous processes," though, perhaps, less so as "what is spontaneous" or "what is so of itself," for the reasons just made above. Although the term *autopoiesis* may be suitable and desirable, it would only work if readers are prepared to stick firmly to the original and literal meaning of this term, and to rid their minds of secondary cultural/philosophical baggage which the term has unfortunately acquired in certain quarters. For instance, two philosophers of biology, Maturana and Varela, 1980 have used the term "autopoietic" to characterize organisms as "autopoietic machines" which seems to amount to a contradiction in terms. If organisms are indeed self-organizing beings and they embody and manifest the processes of autopoiesis *par excellence*, processes which have nothing to do with human intentionality and activity/interference, then surely, it would appear strange for Maturana and Varela to call organisms "autopoietic machines." Machines, *ex hypothesi*, are artifacts deliberately made by humans, thereby embodying human intentionality and human ingenuity. What could be their motive for doing so? In the opinion of Lee, 1999: 140–148, it is to turn organisms which are paradigmatically naturally-occurring beings or "self-engendering living dynamic systems" via biotechnological techniques into human-made artefacts, to transform organisms which are autopoietic beings into technological entities controlled, manipulated by humankind to fulfill

human desires and purposes—in other words, it is to substitute extrinsic teleology (a trajectory and an orientation which is imposed from outside the organism by humans) for intrinsic teleology (a trajectory and an orientation which is endemic to or inherent in the organism *qua* organism).[3] Lee, 2012b, has also argued that what made the Scientific Revolution beginning in the seventeenth century in Western Europe possible was a philosophical revolution which, if not preceding was simultaneous with its emergence, and which underpinned it; this philosophical revolution is the ontological *volte face* of regarding organisms as machines. The single all-important methodological axiom which informs the thinking and writing of this project and its 2012b companion volume on Biomedicine is that science is never innocent of philosophy—a new philosophy had to be put in place to underpin the new science/medicine.

Heaven and Earth

The quotation from the *Laozi* (chapter 25) cited at the beginning illustrates a persistent theme which runs through Chinese culture and its classical texts, namely, the three concepts and the relationship between them: 天/*tian*/ Heaven, 地/*Di*/Earth, and 人/*Ren*/Humankind, called, as already mentioned 三才/*sancai*, the Three Talents or the Three Powers. In the *Xunzi*, we find that Xunzi 荀子 (ca 312–230 BCE) had written these phrases: 上失天时, 下失地利, 中失人和 *shang shi tianshi, xia shi deli, zhong shi renhe* (《荀子·富国》). This set of phrases was meant to point to the most important piece of wisdom in life and can be rendered generally in terms of two versions. The quotation above casts it in a negative form: all affairs would turn out disastrous should one ignore or violate the patterns or regularities of Heaven (Time), the advantageous locations afforded by geography on Earth below (Space) and/or deviate from harmonious conduct between fellow humans (the domain of human affairs). Cast in a positive form, it could read: all affairs would turn out fine provided one does not ignore or violate the patterns or regularities of Heaven above, the advantageous geographical locations/positions on Earth below and/or deviate from harmonious conduct between fellow humans. A more common or popular version runs as follows: 上知天文,下知地理, 中知人事 *shang zhi tianwen, xia zhi dili, zhong zhi renshi*. This can be rendered as: Know astronomy (Time), know geography (Space) and know human affairs (human domain). The passages may loosely be summed up (by this author) as follows:

> All human knowledge is encompassed within astronomy and geography. To know what there is to be known about what happens in Heaven above and what happens on Earth below is to know everything, and in particular, the relationship

> between astronomical phenomena, on the one hand, and terrestrial phenomena, on the other. Also equally important, if one also knows the nature of humans and their place within this web of relationships between Heaven and Earth, then one would not simply be a walking encyclopedia but wise.

This, in a nutshell, is Chinese cosmology and Chinese *philosophy*.

Let us then first look at Heaven. What do the ancient Chinese know about astronomy? According to tradition, China's first astronomer was called 阏伯E Bo, who lived about four thousand years ago. Many legends surround his life; one said he was born from an egg of a bird, the bird swooping down to the river in which his mother was bathing, impregnating her with its egg. He helped the great Yu (in the Xia Dynasty) to control the floods of the Yellow River. He established his observatory in Henan Province, and was responsible for the lunar calendar to help determine the times for planting and harvesting as well as the twenty-four divisions of the year, called 二十四节气/*ershisi jie· qi*.[4] Upon his death, people honored him as a god. Today his temple (E Bo Tai/ 阏伯台or Huo Shen Miao/ 火神庙) in Henan Province is dated from the Yuan Dynasty (1279–1368 CE). Legend had it that he was buried in the site of the temple. Archaeologists recently have excavated it but they found no burial; however, they did find a lot of pot shards belonging to the Spring and Autumn Period (of the Zhou Dynasty), which shows that the cult of honouring him had already begun then, if not earlier. He was guided by his study of the passage in the sky of the star, Antares (which the ancient Chinese called 大火 星*dahuoxing*) in the Scorpio Constellation (心宿 /*xīn xiŭ*), to help him draw up the lunar calendar and determine its main features.[5]

Archaeological research in China in the last six decades or so has made great strides forward in ancient Chinese astronomy. In 1958, a Neolithic burial site belonging to the late Neolithic Longshan Culture (龙/龍山文化, ca. 2300–1900 BCE) was first excavated at Taosi in Shanxi Province (山西陶寺). After several decades of study, Chinese archaeologists announced in 2005 that they have identified a structure on the site which points to it being a solar observatory; of late, one of China's leading astronomers has even claimed that it could be the earliest observatory in Chinese history. In 1987, another Neolithic burial with astronomical information dated even earlier, was excavated in 1987 at Xishuipo, Puyang, in Henan Province/河南濮阳西水坡, belonging to the Yangshao Culture/仰韶文化 (ca. 5000–2800 BCE). One of the graves has preserved intact details in the burial arrangement which have cosmological and astronomical significance. The body, probably that of a tribal chief or even shaman/astronomer, was laid out in such a way that the southern face above the head was round while the northern face at the foot of the body was square. This is entirely in conformity with Chinese cosmology which held that Heaven was round and Earth square, (although this expression, as we shall see, later in chapter 7, is not to be taken literally). Flanking the body to the East is the outline in white mussel shells of the dragon, and to the West that of the tiger. These referred to constellations in the Chinese sky. The *Beidouxing*/ Northern Ladle ("Plough")/Great Bear/Big Dipper was represented, pointing toward the head of the dragon. After carbon 14 as well as tree ring dating, the consensus is that the tomb arrangement appears to be a representation of the Chinese sky at the time of the burial, nearly 6,500 years ago. (But if this claim is upheld, then it would even predate the usual date given for the beginning of the Yangshao Culture.) All this suggests that the Yangshao people were knowledgeable about astronomy, at least, to the extent that they were attempting to orientate the tomb in accordance with the movement of the Great Bear.[6]

The Chinese were noted for having kept excellently accurate records of astronomical phenomena such as solar eclipses, comets, supernovae, over four thousand years, some dating from as early as the Shang Dynasty.[7] But they are not generally credited with having made "theoretical" contributions to the subject of astronomy itself. The Copernican Revolution is often cited as the beginning of modern astronomy as a proper science. It is true that the ancient Chinese did not articulate heliocentrism, but there are passages which exist in some texts which imply that they have an implicit grasp, almost, of that thesis. Take the passage in the《尚书》/*Shang Shu*, *Classic/Book of Documents*, considered probably to be China's earliest traditional literature, with material dating from the Western Zhou Dynasty,[8] which reads: 地有四游，冬至地上行北而西三万里，夏至地下行南而东三万里，春秋二分是其中矣。地恒动而人不知，譬如闭舟而行不觉舟之运也。《尚书纬.考灵曜》This author's rendering reads:

> Earth makes four journeys. By the winter solstice, it would have moved in a north-westerly direction for thirty thousand *li*; by the summer solstice, it would have moved in a south-easterly direction for thirty thousand *li*. For the two equinoxes, spring and autumn, it would have moved half the distance between the two solstices. The Earth moved, yet we on it did not feel it to move—it was like being shut in the middle of a boat, in an enclosed viewless space when we, too, would not feel the boat move.

It clearly stated that Earth moved, and implied a fairly good grasp of the relation between Earth and Sun, although it did not say that it moved around the Sun, while the Sun stood still.

A passage which displays some theoretical insights regarding planetary motion can be found in the *Neijing* (a foundational text in Chinese *medicine*, as we know). The first reads: 九星悬郎，七曜周旋。《素问：天元纪大论. This author's rendering reads: "The nine stars illuminate the skies and the seven heavenly bodies revolve in space (that is, interstellar space)." The second is about Earth's position in astronomical space: 帝曰：地之为下否乎？岐伯曰：地为人之下，太虚之中者也。帝曰：冯凭乎？岐伯曰：大气举之也。《素问：五运行大论》This author's rendering reads: "Yellow Emperor: Earth is below (Heaven), is it not? Qibo: Humans are upon Earth, and Earth is in (interstellar) space. Yellow Emperor: Is Earth supported by something? Qibo: It is supported by (Nature's) *qi* (in space in the sky)."

For the ancient Chinese, the passage of time was marked primarily by the motion of the Sun as observed from its daily rising and its setting (*zhouye jielü*/昼夜节律), as well as by the passage of the four seasons (*sishi jielü*/四时节律). Let us first talk a little about how time was measured in ancient China which was predicated upon the (apparent) motion of the Sun. However, as usual, it would be fitting to follow a general point in Chinese scholarship, namely, to look at the terms used to express concepts from the history of their philological beginnings in order to extract meanings and implications from them. To recap briefly, to date, in the history of Chinese writing,[9] the earliest systematic, mature form is what is called the Oracle Bone Script dating from the late Shang dynasty, for which there is plentiful archaeological evidence. There are numerous scripts later than that which we shall also have occasion to look at. Another source consulted ancient dictionaries, especially that by the Han philologist Xu Shen which was completed in 100 CE—this work is still considered today to be authoritative in spite of the fact that it is known to contain errors. In the light of these general remarks, let us turn to see how in the various scripts,[10] the character for time (*shi*) was written—see figure 4.1 below.

A is the Oracle Bone Script; its bottom component is the character for "sun" (see Figure 4.5); the top component is the word for 之 which means "moving about." The word then really referred to the sun's passage across the sky. This portrayed the daily rhythm of day and night (*zhouye jielü*). In B (Lesser Seal Script) and C (Clerical Script), there had been a change in the construction of the word, showing an enrichment of meaning. In B, the graph for "sun" had moved to the left (now functioning as the radical for the word); the right component itself had two parts to it—the top being the word for 之, and the bottom showed the word for "hand." However, in this version, the new meaning is not too clear although in C, matters have clarified. The richer meaning embedded in the construction in this version may

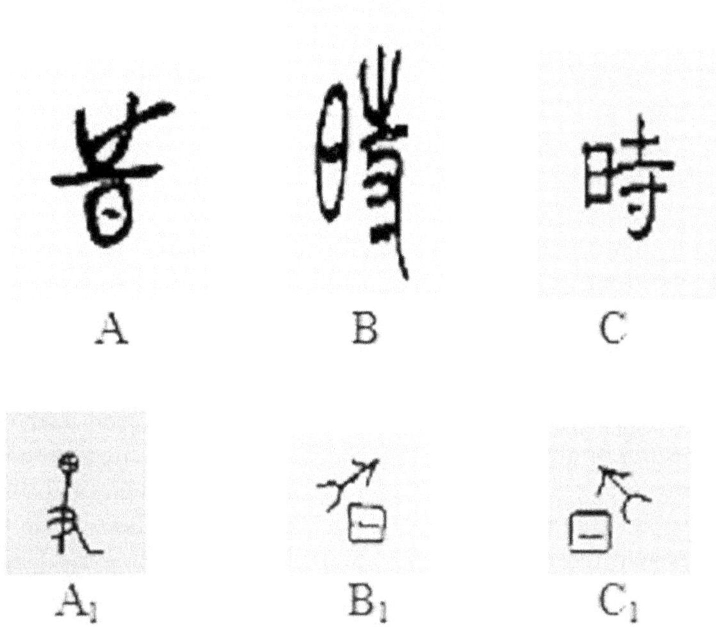

Figure 4.1. Character "shi" in various scripts

be interpreted in two ways.[11] The first simply said that the radical for "sun" 日 on the left obviously showed that the word was connected with the Sun and its activity; the second component on the right 寺 *sì* contributed the sound. The word refers basically then to ceremonies to mark the seasons—at each season, the king/emperor had to perform certain rituals to welcome the Spring, to thank Heaven for the harvest in the Autumn and so on.

However, there is another interpretation, a more interesting and complicated analysis. One finds that the right component had two parts—the top component on the right was for Earth or the ground 土 *tu*; the bottom component on the right for a unit of measurement, the Chinese inch which was 寸/*cun*. What they are telling us is that time was measured (on Earth) in terms of the motion of the Sun (or in today's correct astronomical language, the apparent motion of the Sun) in the course of the day as well as in the course of a year across the heavens. In other words, this new construction introduced two innovations: the word for Earth or ground as well as that for a unit of measurement. These in turn brought out two further points: first that the notion of time, since the Oracle Bone Script version, had come to be understood not simply as an astronomical matter (about the movement of the Sun) but also an astronomical matter which involved Earth. That is to say, it is both an astronomical (Time) as well as a terrestrial matter (Space), as the Sun's (apparent) movements were related to Earth and could be ascertained on Earth, that what was important to grasp was the relationship between Heaven and Earth.[12] Second, the new construction embodied a technique for measuring the (apparent) motion of the Sun. The *Zhou bi suan jing/The Arithmetical Classic of the Zhou Gnomon and the Circular Paths of the Heavens* mentioned, among other things, such a technique.

What then was this technique and what sort of instrument did the ancient Chinese use to measure the passage of time? The instrument was the gnomon,[13] called 碑*bei* or 表*biao*. In its simplest form, it was nothing but a long pole whose length varied from ten Chinese feet in the early period, to eight over a very long period of more than a thousand years, before reverting to ten in the Qing Dynasty with the arrival of Jesuit astronomers at the Qing court. This was firmly planted in the ground. In setting up the gnomon, care must be taken to ensure that the pole was absolutely straight and that the ground was absolutely level. To get the latter right, even before Han times, the astronomers looked at the level of water in a bowl. Before the Tang Dynasty, they used to tie eight cords from the top of the pole forming four angles and stretching to four points on the ground, so that they faced one another exactly. In the course of the day, from sunrise to sunset, as the sun shone on the pole, the ancient Chinese astronomers would notice that the pole cast a shadow on the ground. In figure 4.1, A_1 is the Oracle Bone Script, which shows a hand holding what looks like a long pole. The other two, B_1 and C_1, show the sun and a person's shadow at different angles in the course of the day. The shadow got shorter and shorter as the sun rose higher and higher in the heavens until at noon or round about noon, the shadow was at its shortest; but after the sun had reached the zenith at noon, the shadow would correspondingly get longer and longer as the afternoon wore on. At sunrise and at sunset, one would mark the shadows cast by the pole. If one were to join up the two markings, one would get the east-west direction. Scholars have pointed out that the *Book of Odes/Poerty*《诗经》*Shijing*, of the early Western Zhou Dynasty, already mentioned how to determine the east-west direction. If one were to draw the shortest line from the base of the pole to the east-west line, this would point to the north (in the northern hemisphere).

By measuring the length of the sun's shadow each day, in the course of the year, the ancient Chinese astronomers would also have noticed that the shadows measured differently, and were thus able to determine the solstices which by Shang times were called *zhì*/至. This shows that as early as the Shang Dynasty, the ancient Chinese knew about the summer and winter solstices (夏至/*xiazhi* and冬至/*dongzhi*). The ancient Chinese also worked out the spring equinox, 春分/*chnnfen* (around 1100 BCE) and the autumn equinox, 秋分*qiufen* (*fen* means, in this context, that day and night are equally divided). For instance, in *The Spring and Autumn Annals and the Tradition of the Zuo Commentary*《春秋左传》(*Chunqiu zuo zhuan*, a chronicle of events in the state of Lu, during the Spring and Autumn Period), there is a passage, which referred not only to the solstices, but also to the equinoxes: 凡分至启闭必书云物《左传僖公五年》.[14]

To observe the shadow of the pole and to measure it, the Chinese used a measuring tablet called the 土圭*tugui*. This device was as ancient as the gnomon as it was also mentioned in the *Zhou li*《周礼》*The Rites of Zhou*, probably dated to the third century BCE, and the *Kaogongji* 《考工记》*The Manual of Crafts*, which was the first important official book detailing the arts and crafts industries, such as leatherwork, metalwork, dyes, carpentry, pottery, and scraping in ancient China, dated to the latter part of the Spring and Autumn Period. In reality, the ancient astronomers only measured the shadow for the summer solstice as it would be somewhat inconvenient to measure the much longer shadow in the winter. They simply calculated the date of the winter solstice rather than use observational data to determine it. The Chinese believed that the shadow of a gnomon of eight Chinese feet at the summer solstice would diminish by a (Chinese) inch for every thousand Chinese miles as one moved southward, and that it increased by an inch for every thousand miles as one moved toward the north.[15]

There is an expression which implicitly refers to the two solstices: 立竿见影 *lì gan jian ying*. At the summer solstice, the sun is at its zenith over (what today we call) the Tropic of Cancer, and that is why the northern hemisphere enjoys its longest hours of sunlight. The reverse obtains at the winter solstice when the sun is at its zenith over the Tropic of Capricorn, and that is why the northern hemisphere is exposed to the shortest hours of sunlight or daylight. At the summer solstice, at noon, the pole cast no shadows at the Tropic of Cancer, but at the winter solstice, the pole would cast the longest shadow in the northern hemisphere. This method of measuring the apparent motion of the Sun served as a metaphor which amounted to saying that a certain action taken or policy implemented was immediately effective.

We next need to say something briefly about some words which are so ancient that it looks as if they had existed even before the emergence of the Oracle Bone Script, although it is true that they only existed as severely limited fragments today. For instance, one such word is 日 *ri*, which means "sun." This word is highly significant in any attempt to understand Chinese cosmology and *philosophy* because it would not be too far from the truth to say that the Chinese mode of thought was/is deeply informed by the Sun and its effects on our planet, Earth. The earliest forms of the word are found in a Neolithic culture—one of many in pre-historical China—called the Dawenkou Culture/大汶口文化 (4500–2500 BCE), named after the place in which many artifacts have been found, in today's Shandong Province. In the 1960s, a farmer, turning over the soil in the Juxian County[16] found some pottery with some "drawings" on them. A well-known palaeographer then thought that these were not mere drawings but were inscriptions. However, this view was not taken up seriously until the discovery in the 1980s of some thirty tombs belonging to the late Dawenkou Culture, and some wine vessels were excavated with twenty similar stylised "pictures" or "drawings." By 2000, scholars were able to announce that they had identified fourteen of them as proper writing and deciphered them as seven characters for *fan*/凡/"ordinary," *nan*/ 南/"south," *xiang*/ 享/"enjoy." Three other characters deciphered are related to "sun":

A is the simplest, with a round sun floating on what might be a cloud. B shows the sun having risen over the top of a mountain—there is indeed a mountain due east of Juxian County and the graph could be the word for 旦/*dan*/"dawn"—this would reflect what the Neolithic people saw, the sun rising above the mountain in question, when they looked East. C seems to show the sun's rays spreading out in all directions.

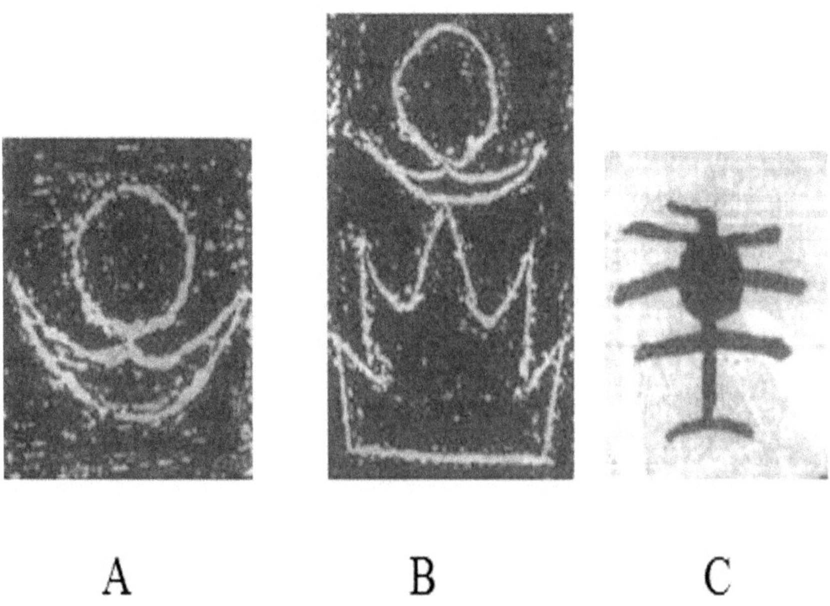

Figure 4.2. Pictograms related to "sun" in Dawenkou Culture

Archaeologists and palaeographers have also found that these characters share similarities and meanings with the forms in the Oracle Bone Script and other scripts and that the latter had evolved from the former;[17] so we need to look at those (the character *ri*), too.

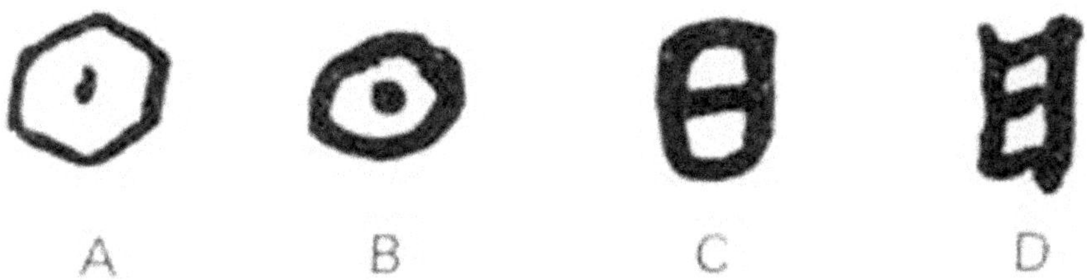

Figure 4.3. Character "ri" in various scripts

A is Oracle Bone Script. Why does it differ from the earlier Dawenkou representation of the Sun by being either hexagonal or pentagonal, and not round? This is not because the ancient Chinese had suddenly misperceived the Sun to be six- or five-sided. Rather it is because the script had to be carved on hard material, either ox shoulder blade or tortoise shell; as such, the scribe found doing a circle almost impossible to achieve. In the Bronze Script (used in bronze vessels)—see B—where the scribe wrote on a soft mould of earth/clay (like the Dawenkou potters) before the vessel could be cast in bronze, the character was round/roundish. C is Lesser Seal Script which followed another set of rules for writing characters, rendering them more stretched length-wise as well as more square-ish at the same time. This process of altering the shape of the written character was carried out even further by later scripts until we get to D, looking distinctly rectangular, a shape the word has retained up to today. Another point worth making is that a dot appeared in the middle in A and B (which later appeared as a line in C and D)—this concerned the way in which the ancient Chinese came to observe the sun. Apart from looking at it in the sky (before the sun got too bright for gazing at directly by noon), another common way of observing it was via its reflection in water which showed it to be round with a dark spot in the middle of the circle. B is a perfect pictograph of it.[18]

Another heavenly body which pre-occupied the ancient Chinese greatly is the Moon. In the various scripts, the character (*yue*) is shown in figure 4.4.

A is in the Oracle Bone Script, which represented the moon as a crescent, not a full moon. This was for two reasons: (a) the crescent moon occurred twice in a month whereas the full moon only once; (b) more importantly, if the full moon were to be used to represent the moon, then

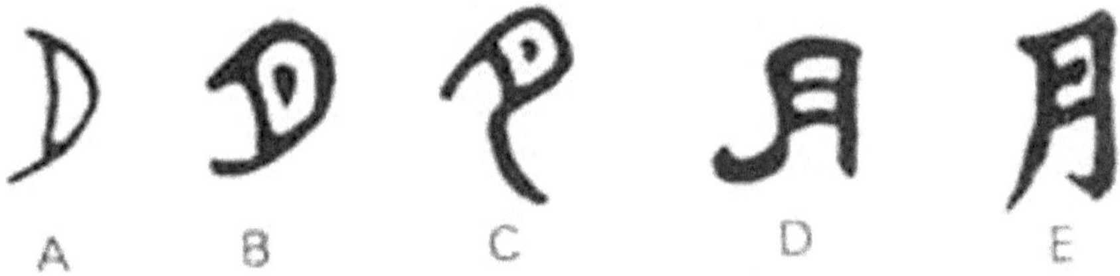

Figure 4.4. Character "yue" in various scripts

it was very easy to get it confused with the script for "sun." B is the Bronze script; by then people had added a dot to the middle of the crescent moon to represent what they could see on the surface of the Moon when conditions were ripe. C is the Lesser Seal Script, D the Clerical Script, while E is the Standard Script which simply shows the developmental stages in accordance with the general rules in the evolution of the Chinese scripts.[19] A and B reflected how carefully and accurately the Chinese people in earlier times observed the Moon.

We have already earlier referred to the astronomical achievements of the Yangshao Culture regarding what in the West is called the Great Bear, but which in *Daojia* literature is called *tiangang*/天罡.

In today's astronomical maps, this configuration (strictly speaking an asterism) is called *Ursa Major*/the Great Bear.

The seven stars are listed in the map above; their Chinese names are: *Tianshu*/天枢, *Tianxuan*/天旋, *Tianji*/天玑, *Tianquan*/天权, *Yuheng*/玉衡, *Kaiyang*/开阳, *Yaokuang*/摇光.[20] Like many other civilisations, the ancient Chinese used the Polestar (*bei ji xing*) as their point of reference; if one were to draw an imaginary line in the map above from Merak to Dubhe

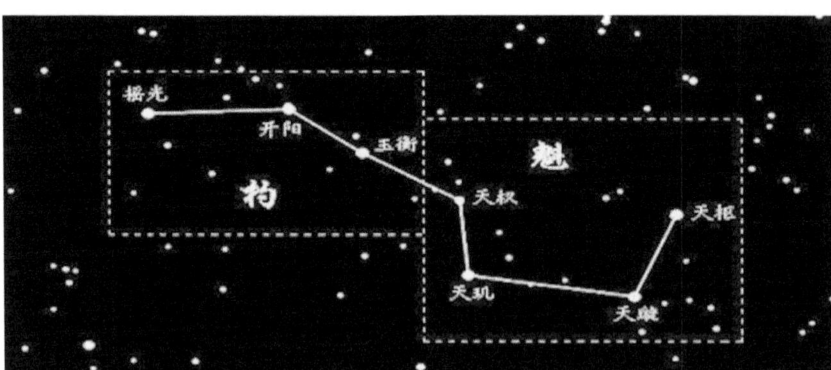

Figure 4.5. Daoist tiangang formation

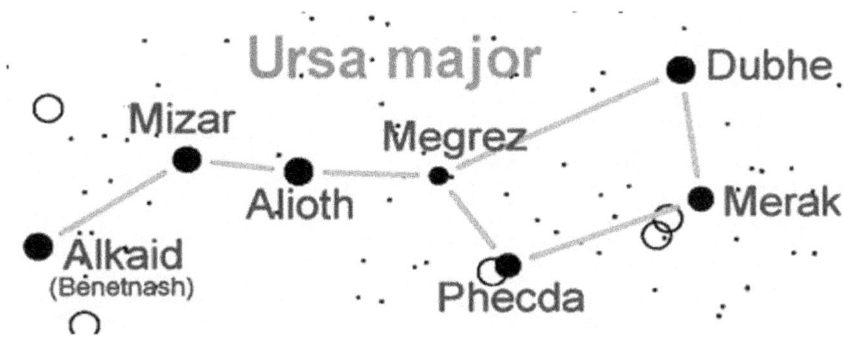

Figure 4.6. Ursa Major/Great Bear

and then out of "the cup," and continuing five times the distance between Merak and Dubhe, one should arrive at the Polestar/Polaris. The ancient Chinese observed that relative to the Polestar, the *beidouxing* moved in a certain way around it during the course of the year. In a text which can be dated probably to the Warring States Period called the *Heguanzi*/《鶡冠子》/*Pheasant Cape Master*,[21] a passage reads: 斗柄东指，天下皆春，斗柄南指，天下皆夏，斗柄西指，天下皆秋，斗柄北指，天下皆冬. "If it (that is, the handle of the Seven Dippers) points east; in the world it will be spring, if it points north, in the world it will be summer; if it points to west, in the world it will be fall; if it points to north, in the world it will be winter (Wang, 2012: 26)."

This passage may conveniently be used to introduce the important theme in Chinese thought that astronomical and terrestrial phenomena were inextricably linked, that Heaven and Earth cannot be understood except in this light—one, therefore, has to know not only astronomy but also geography. Heaven was about astronomy (Time) and Earth about geography (Space), Time and Space being interlinked. However, what was of crucial significance was the relationship between them, namely, that the seasons on Earth (which were of such importance to the survival of Life on Earth) were related to events which happened in Heaven. (Chapter 10 discusses Timespace *Wholism*.)

Geographical locations on Earth are broadly determined by the four compass points, what in the West are conventionally sequenced as North/South/East/West, but which the Chinese sequence as East/South/West/North. What do the words for the four directions look like in the various scripts in the history of Chinese writing?[22]

East/*dong*/东 is, of course, where the Sun rises; it is a place one associates with daylight and sunlight; sunlight makes things grow.[23] The word looks

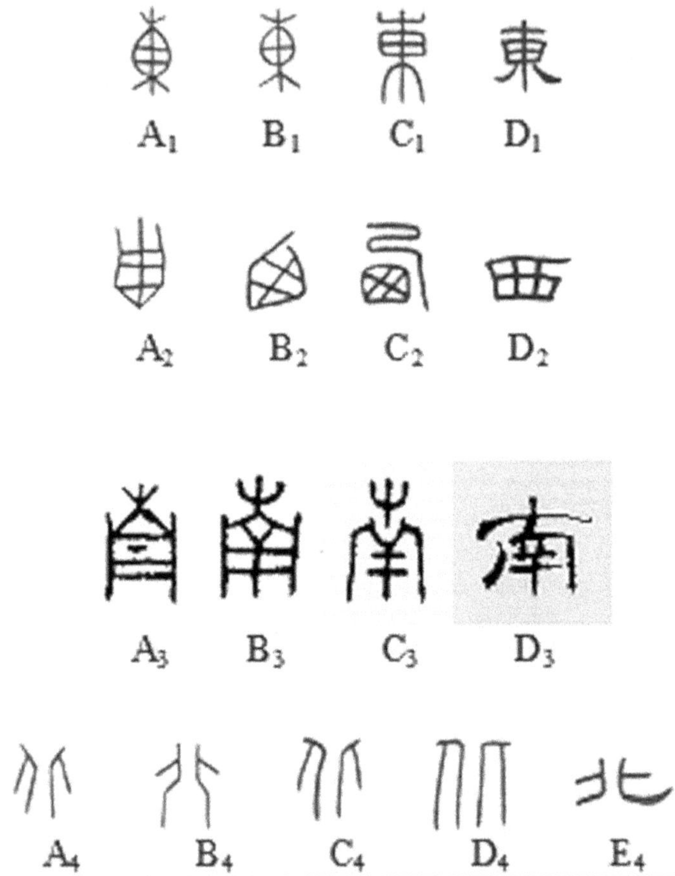

Figure 4.7. Characters denoting the four main compass points in various scripts

like this: A_1, the Oracle Bone Script and B_1, the Bronze Script, were fairly similar; they seemed to show an enlarged bulbous stem with leaves at the top and roots down below. By C_1, the Lesser Seal Script and D_1, the Clerical Script, it is easy to see that the word had two components: one for "sun" 日*ri* and the other for "wood" (derivatively "tree")/木/*mu*, the one being superimposed on the other. The word created was then called a meaning compound/会意字/ *huiyi zi*. It suggests the sun coming through the trees in a forest and is compatible with the notion that plants grow where and when the Sun rises.

West/*xi*/西 is where the Sun sets; and when the Sun sets, the birds return to their nests, their resting place for the night. In A_2 and B_2 (Oracle Bone and Bronze Scripts), the word looks like a bird's nest. To appreciate the image in A_2, you have to turn the page counterclockwise so that it is horizontal. C_2, the Lesser Seal Script, had an additional bit to the nest to show more explicitly that it was a bird's nest, the extra bit "hovering" over the nest represented the bird. By D_2, the Clerical Script, the word had become abstract and stylised, looking like today's writing of it.

The character for *nan*/South/南 in various scripts are shown in A_3 (Oracle Bone), B_3 (Bronze), C_3 (Lesser Seal), and D_3 (Clerical).These had given rise to different interpretations, but the one which is pertinent to our concern here had two components. The first component was the word for "door" and inside that was the word 幸/*xing*, meaning "good fortune." In the history of Chinese architecture from time immemorial, the door faced South, in order to get the sun. To live facing South—enjoying the warmth of the sun, where things grow—is to enjoy good fortunes, which explains the construction of the character for "south."

The character for "north"—北/*bei*—follows the logic of the explanation for "south." The sunny position is the south-facing one with the north side being sunless, cold, and dark. Hence, when one sits, one faces south, with one's back to the north. The character for "north" embodies this fact, as can be seen in its various forms below (E_4 is simply the Standard Script which is still used today, since the early Han Dynasty, while A_4, B_4, C_4, and D_4 are the Oracle Bone, Bronze, Lesser Seal, and Clerical Scripts. The original meaning of 北*bei* was "to run counter" (showing two people going in opposite directions) and was related to the word 背/*bei*, meaning "back," whose top component, as you can see, is北/*bei*. In the context of the general environment as well as of architecture, north was the direction, as already commented on, to which people turned their back, as that was the side from which the bitterly cold winds come sweeping from the Mongolian steppes.

Two words which have even greater cosmological significance than those we have so far looked at are 天 *tian* (Heaven) and 地*di* (Earth).

Tian[24] looks like this (see first line of figure 4.8): A1/A2 are two different forms of the Oracle Bone Script, while B is the Lesser Seal and C, the Clerical Script. In A1, a square sits on top of the character for "large," 大/*da*. The square represented the head of a person. Hence, the original basic meaning of 天 *tian* was "the top of the head." In B, there is a change—the head is replaced by a line over the character 大. As a result, Xu Shen (who worked with the Lesser Seal Script of his time) wrote that *tian* not only stood as the polar contrast of Earth but also derivatively as that for which nothing could be higher, the highest. In Chinese cosmological understanding, *tian* is supreme, and humans, no matter how grand or important they

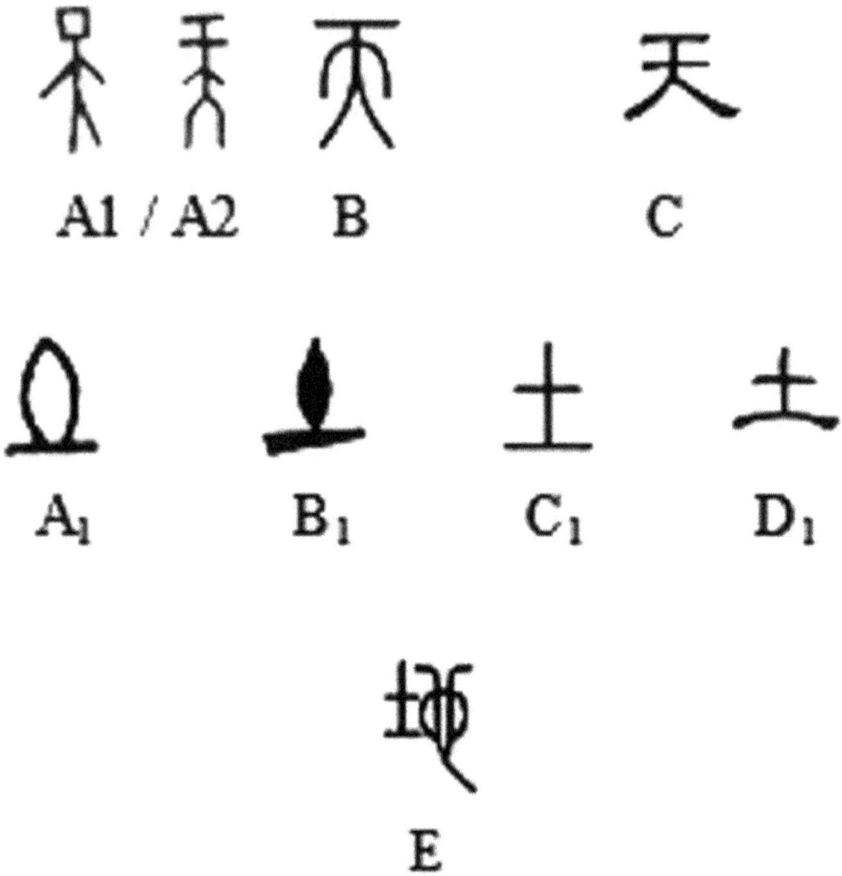

Figure 4.8. Characters "tian," "tu" and "di" in various scripts

fancy themselves to be, are subject to the constraints of *tian*. *Tian* watches over us, and humans turn to it for protection. When they suffer injustices for which they get no redress from emperors/officials/enemies/uncivilized neighbors, they hope that *tian* might dispense justice on their behalf. Not even the most mighty emperor would dare to put himself above *tian*; he humbly called himself "Son of Heaven" 天子/*tianzi* and he ruled only by the grace of the Mandate of Heaven 天命/*tianming*, a political concept of legitimation invented by the Zhou Dynasty. Chinese culture, ever since the demise of the Shang Dynasty, has turned its back, by and large, on the notion of a transcendent being, called God; instead it has opted for *tian* to ground not merely its cosmology but also its morality. *Tian*, together with *di*/Earth, constitute the concept of *Ziran* (or in an implied manner Nature), a concept which has profoundly informed and shaped Chinese *philosophy*, Chinese *science*, indeed, every aspect of Chinese life over the millennia.

A cognate term of *di* is 土/*tu* (see second line of figure 4.8) which means soil/earth; in modern Chinese, the two words are put together to form one word *tudi* to refer not only to cultivated land but also to territory. In figure 4.8 A_1-D_1 show the various scripts for *tu*. Basically, A_1 and B_1 (Oracle Bone and Bronze Scripts) seem to show a mound of earth—the bottom horizontal line represents the ground on which the mound stands. In C_1, the Lesser Seal Script, the mound has disappeared. In its place is another horizontal line which represents the topsoil while the bottom horizontal line, the soil below ground; the vertical line represents a plant sticking out of the soil. Not all scholars agree with this interpretation, but it seems a plausible one.[25] Naturally, good wholesome soil is absolutely essential for cultivation. We must, therefore, respect the soil. D_1 is the Clerical Script.

Let us now look at the main character for Earth, 地/*di*[26] in the Lesser Seal Script (E in figure 4.8). The word has two components: the *tu* radical is on the left and the second on the right refers to the female genitals and its parts. This then shows very clearly that the ancient Chinese considered the soil/earth as the source of all life. We know that plants are basic to terrestrial food chains: plants, herbivores, then carnivores. There can be no carnivores if there were no herbivores and there cannot be herbivores without plants. In that crucial sense, *di* makes Life possible; it is therefore, Life's womb, just as in the case of mammals, without females there can be no reproduction and no birth. Earth is then Mother Earth (many other cultures share this view from time immemorial). So it is all very fitting that Mother Earth should be respected. We, humans, are Earth- and earth-rooted beings; as such, we cannot, for a moment, whether we are carnivores, vegans or omnivores keep ourselves alive without Earth. We live on Earth. Apart from food, we also make use of its other resources, wood, fuel, water. Where do we get them? From the ground. Wood comes from trees, and trees grow in the soil. Fire comes from burning wood while peat, coal, ultimately, come from trees and plants which once grew in the soil. We are beings beholden to Earth in all ways. Significantly, too, we cannot live without water; but the relationship between water on the one hand and vegetation and soil is a complex and intimate one—without water/水/*shui*, nothing would grow, nothing would thrive, but without soil for plants to grow on, water would also diminish or even disappear altogether. In sum, to understand 水土/*shuitu*, is to understand Life. It is also to understand the place of humans in that ecological web of life.

We know, too, that even if Earth is fertile, its fertility would remain a potentiality unless the Sun gives Earth heat as well as light. The ancient Chinese might not have a science called photosynthesis but all the same, they showed an excellent grasp of what that science today tells us. That is why in Chinese cosmology, *Tian* and *Di* are such supremely important concepts. It is no exaggeration to say that all aspects of Chinese culture (including Chinese *philosophy* and Chinese *science*) rest on our understanding of the ways of *Tian* and *Di*, the complex relationships between them, and our own place in it. That is why it seems fitting to call Chinese cosmology and Chinese *philosophy* an "ecosophy" and the science implied by such a framework "ecosystem science"—but more of that, as the book unfolds, especially in chapters 10 and 11.

Why is it so important to know about *Ziran* processes at work and the regularities which we humans could detect and discover in the natural phenomena around us and to act in accordance with them? One answer usually given is that Chinese culture and civilization were based on agriculture; the harvest depended on knowing as much as one could about weather conditions and anticipating the changes to them as the year or the seasons unfolded. This explanation is undoubtedly correct, but only up to a point. From archaeological evidence, as already pointed out, the Neolithic peoples occupying part of what today we call China were not primarily/wholly agriculture-based, but depended on hunting, gathering, yet they knew their astronomy. One could also explain their interest in astronomy as basically tied up with their interest in astrology—this, too, would be correct. Another attempt to explain such a pre-occupation is to say that the successful conduct of military affairs presupposed availability of such knowledge. That, too, would be correct, by Shang times, if not during the Neolithic period of Chinese history. However, no matter how intimate the link between astrology and astronomy, between astrology/astronomy and the military, between astrology/astronomy and hunting/gathering or sedentary agriculture, one should still be able to distinguish the motive for wanting to have such knowledge from the knowledge itself; furthermore, it remains plausible for one to argue that the astronomical observations and understanding of these ancient peoples could be evaluated in their own rights as their attempt to do *science*.

Let us engage in another thought experiment: suppose we simply stumbled upon the Neolithic burials but had no knowledge whatsoever about any cultural beliefs about such peoples, the existence of shamans in their lives, that the shamans were held by them to mediate between humans and the gods above and so on. It is not impossible nor implausible to imagine a dedicated team of astronomers today who is also informed by the history of astronomy in their own and other cultures to work out eventually what the astronomical framework within which those Neolithic peoples had set out the burial of their dead. In other words, it is possible to "excavate" the astronomy behind the astrology. As a matter of fact, as the process of secularization kicked in in ancient China, thinkers of one description or other (whether they called themselves *Daojia* or *Rujia*) began to detach to a greater or lesser extent the astronomy from the astrology. This, however, should not be interpreted as the denial, nevertheless, of a persistent link between astronomy and astrology. When the *Laozi* declared that humankind must follow Heaven's *dao*, Earth's *dao*, the Dao and *Ziran*, what it appeared to tell us to comply with, and not violate, was not some shamanic astrological findings and instructions, but simply the patterns and the regularities which could be detected and discovered in *Ziran* processes. Hence above all, the wisdom of following the Dao/*Ziran* was not simply relevant to limited, specific pre-occupations and interests such as ensuring the success of hunting, fighting battles, harvesting, divining, astrological/shamanic mediating/communicating with the god or gods above, but that following the Dao/*Ziran* was the only method available to a people/civilization which had departed from the ready path of Revelation. To this topic, this book will return in due course.

Some further concluding remarks about the limited discussion above of the concepts of *Tian* and *Di* must be made in order to prevent misunderstanding about this particular interpretation of them:

1. As we have already commented upon, it focuses on them from the angle entirely of astronomy and geography and the relationship between the two. As such, it is not meant to deny that in ancient Chinese thought, as just now emphasized but bears repeating, astrology and astronomy were intimately linked. This aspect of the subject is acknowledged in chapter 5 in which the *Yijing* is presented as *au fond* a divinatory text. Nevertheless, the point to grasp is that it is not merely and only such a text, as the divination itself rested on an understanding of the processes at work in the cosmos, in what in the *Laozi* is called *Ziran* which stood for the patterns and the regularities in which the heavenly bodies moved or appeared to move, the effects of such movements on Earth, their implication for Life on Earth and so on. Today's astronomy might not be over impressed by astronomy done with the naked eye but all the same, this lack of high tech did not prevent even the Neolithic peoples from making accurate observations and inferences from them. Similarly, we moderns might not be overimpressed by the low tech methods used by early ancestors to make observations and inferences based on them about the north, the south, the east, and the west in terms of the passage of night and day, of the four seasons in a year. However primitive the technology involved, it remains true

that the ancient Chinese observers did do their astronomy and their geography (that is their *science*) to further their divination activity but that this *science* had gone hand in hand with their *philosophy* of *Ziran*, as articulated by the author(s), for example, of the *Laozi*, but which were already present in an implicit form in the *Yijing*, the divinatory text itself.

2. Furthermore, as we shall go on to show in the chapters to follow, how the *philosophy* which can be excavated from the divination text itself has methodological implications for doing Chinese *science* (and therefore also Chinese *Medicine*)—indeed, it has yielded a very powerful set of analytical tools not only for doing *science* in the Baconian understanding of the term "science" but also in the broader understanding of the term as "wissenschaft." As such it has yielded *sciences* in numerous and very different domains, such as rulership, military affairs, conflict resolution, and management, just to mention a few.
3. We also must bear in mind that the *Ten Wings* of the *Yi* have made additional meanings to the terms *Tian* and *Di*, naming them respectively *Qian*/乾 and *Kun*/坤, each with its own distinctive properties, understanding of which entered into numerous domains including *medicine*, rulership, military affairs, gender relationships, as well as divination.
4. In general, one would like the reader to bear in mind that this discussion here is but a very partial and limited understanding of the concepts of *Tian* and Di in the entirety of Chinese thought on the subject of their relationship as well as between them and humankind. However, a possible and plausible justification of this partial account rests on drawing attention to the fact that the *Yijing* is not a simple divinatory text per se, but that the divination could be said to rest on something which had to do with an understanding of astronomy (*Tian*) and geography (*Di*) as well as a grasp of *Ziran* processes (not withstanding that the concept *Ziran* is not found in the *Yijing* itself nor for that matter in the *Yi*) embedded in the unfolding of the phenomena which the ancient Chinese people observed around them.

Dao

We have so far given an interpretation of *Ziran*, *Tian*, and *Di*. From the *Laozi* quotation cited at the beginning of the chapter, the Dao is said to follow *Ziran*. Why is there a need to interpolate another term between *Tian* and *Di* on the one hand and *Ziran* on the other? If it is intended to do real work, what could it mean and imply?

Once again, we begin by looking into its deconstruction, calling up the word in the various ancient scripts—see figure 4.9. Scholars have noticed that so far their study of the Oracle Bone Script has not enabled them to decipher the word for *dao*—it is, therefore, "not proven" whether the word existed in the Oracle Bone Script.[27]

The earliest versions so far located were in the Bronze Script, one of which is shown as A; B is the Lesser Seal Script, and C, the Clerical Script. Note that the Bronze Script version is distinctly different from B and C but which, from our point of view, is more interesting. This is because it exhibits two components which show more clearly the meaning of *dao*, usually translated as "way." One component has something to do with the word *xing* written today as 行. So we need to elucidate this component/word first. A_1 is the Oracle Bone Script; B_1, the Bronze Script; C_1, the Lesser Seal Script; and D_1, the Clerical Script. (Note how today's script for the word [行] is not really different from D_1.) A_1 and B_1 show very clearly that what is represented is a major crossroad, with through roads from East to West

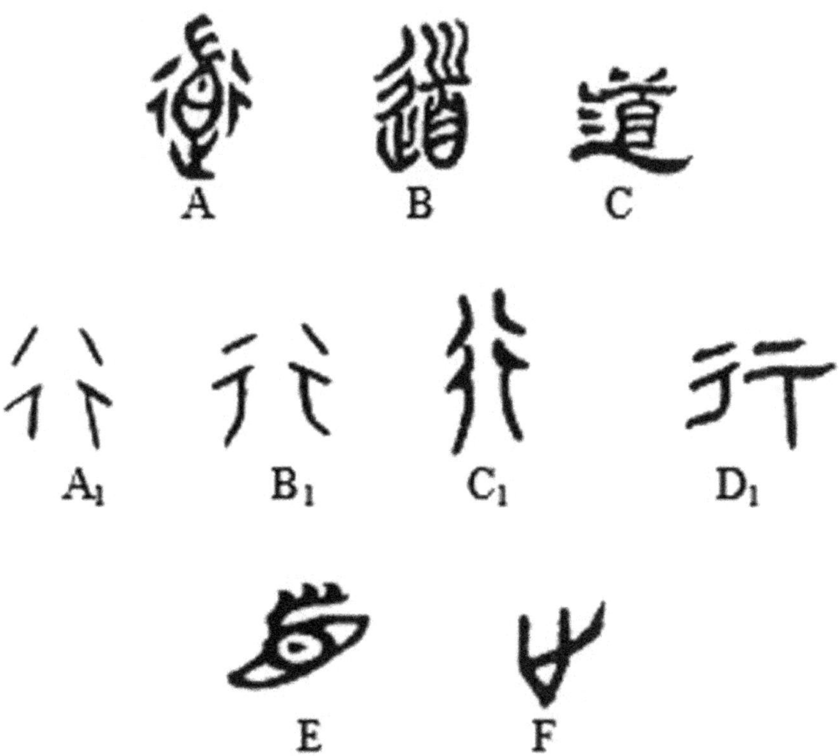

Figure 4.9. Character "dao" and its components in various scripts

and from South to North; hence its original meaning is "road" (as a noun). When humans walk, they walk along a road; hence, a derivative meaning is "to walk" (as a verb), which is the meaning given by Xu Shen in his dictionary, though acknowledged by him to be a derivative meaning of the word. Do bear in mind that Xu Shen was working with the Lesser Seal Script, C_1 above, and he did not know that the Oracle Bone Script had existed much earlier. But since the discovery of that more ancient script at the turn of the twentieth century, scholars could see more clearly the original meaning of the word.[28]

The word for *dao* involves two words in its construction, that for *xing* (commented on above) and that for *shou* 首meaning "head," both coming from the Bronze Script.[29] We can see this is so by examining closely A and B above for *dao*. We see a head as shown under E in figure 4.9[30] inserted between the two arms of *xing*. Invoking the head is simply a well-known exercise in synecdoche, a figure of speech, in which a part is used to stand for the whole; the head stands for the whole human being along the road. (In turn, *shou* is also used to refer to a leader.)

Another interpretation to which Version A of *dao*, in particular, may be prone is as follows: *dao* actually represents the process of birth in mammals: it shows the emergence of the head of the baby through the birth canal. This in turn is used to stand for the capability of Heaven and Earth to support and sustain the continuity of life on Earth. Such a way of looking at *dao* would then be in keeping with the *Laozi*'s concept of the Dao, which is said to engender all life forms, to be the basis of Life. A passage in chapter 6 of the *Laozi* appears to hint at this interpretation: 谷神不死, 是谓玄牝。玄牝之门, 是谓天地根。绵绵若存, 用 之 不勤。One translation reads:

> The valley spirit never dies;
> It is the woman, primal mother.
> Her gateway is the root of heaven and earth.
> It is like a well barely seen.
> Use it; it will never fail. (Feng and English, 1989)

The reference to the valley and its spirit, to root, as well as to the womb as the portal of the female, regarded as mysterious, profound, dark, or secret are analogies of Heaven and Earth as the source of *Wanwu*.

The Bronze Script for *dao* introduces a component right at the bottom of the word which is the word for "foot," 止 *zhi* shown under F in figure 4.9. This appears to justify also looking at *dao* in terms of the motion of walking along the road, and hence of following it. By version B (Lesser Seal Script), this understanding had been transformed somewhat, as B combines the component on the right 首with its left component looking like this, *chuo* 辵 which means "walking, then halting." By version C (Clerical Script), the left hand component has evolved to look like this: 辶.These developments, too, would be in keeping with the *Laozi* and the general Chinese *philosophical* outlook which advocate that humankind must walk along the true path, although each school of *philosophy* advocates its own conception of what the correct"dao" is.

The above shows that *dao*, apart from straightforwardly being a road, path, or way, also signifies that humans in life must traverse such a road/roads, whether interpreted literally, figuratively, or *philosophically*. This very brief summary of the rather complicated philological understanding of *dao* would, as we shall see later, stand us in good stead in grasping the importance of two other terms related to *dao* in CCM, its *philosophy*, its *science* and its methodology—通/*tong*, meaning "to move through with no obstacle standing in the way" and 透/*tou*, meaning "clear and transparent." Note that these three words 道，通，透 share the same radical辶; this radical indicates movement/motion, implying a dynamic (not static) state—this shows that Chinese cosmology/*philosophy* is primarily interested in the dynamic, not so much the static mode of operation or existence, a fundamental theme which would be explored in great detail in the course of this book (chapters 5, 6, 7 in particular).

It may be appropriate at this point to distinguish between two uses of the word "dao," namely, a specific or particular *dao*, on the one hand, and the general/*philosophical dao* on the other. We propose to call the latter "the Dao" and the former "dao" preceded by the specific domain to which that use is applied. We can elicit such a distinction from the quotation cited at the beginning of this chapter which says that *Tian* and *Di* follow the Dao. This implies that the Dao in this context is the general/*philosophical* version whereas the *dao* of Heaven (天道 *tiandao*) and the *dao* of Earth (地道*didao*) are used more specifically and each respectively is restricted to that domain alone, whereas the Dao would include here both the *dao* of Heaven, the *dao* of Earth, the *dao* of Humankind (人道/*rendao*). All these specific *daos* would entail following/complying with the Dao and would together form part of the Dao, though not the whole of it.

This reading would be compatible with the other important quotation from chapter 42 of the *Laozi*: The Dao engenders one, one engenders two, two engenders three, three engenders *Wanwu*. In chapter 3, we have shown that "one" could be said to refer to *Yuanqi*/元气 which in turn engendered *yin qi* and *yang qi* ("two"), whose co-operation, mutual response and interaction as *Yinyang* ("three") ultimately engendered *Wanwu*. There, we have also pointed out that the Nebulous Void (on one interpretation) could be said to be synonymous with the Dao, that the Dao is *wu*, that *wu* engenders *you*, that *Wanwu* in turn are engendered by *you*—the *Laozi*, chapter 40 reads: 天下万物生于有, 有生于无。

Chapter 3 presents an account of *Qi* as the fundamental *ontological* category of Chinese *philosophy* and *science*, which is neither simple matter nor energy but best referred to as Em-ism. In the light of the proposed distinction above between the Dao on the one hand and a specific, particular *dao* on the other, we can characterize the account of *Qi* as *ontological* category as an instance of the latter and call it *qidao*, the *dao* of *qi*. This specific, particular *qidao* belongs to the domain of *you*, but was engendered by *wu*. But the Dao, as such, cannot be identified with it or indeed with any number of other specific, particular *daos*, which all belong to the domain of *you* which one could say is the domain which *science* (whether as what we today call physics or medicine/*medicine*), in general, studies, whereas the Dao as presented by the *Laozi* is above *science*, to be metaphysics in the recent but non-abusive sense of that term and not in the original sense of "meta" as simply "after." For historical and other reasons, "metaphysics" is not an appropriate translation of the Chinese term *xingershang* which strictly speaking refers only to what is above form while its counterpart *xingerxia* 形而下 refers to what has form (shape and other properties). The philosophical baggage of the Western use of the term—the distinction between physics/science and metaphysics (what is above/beyond physics/science)—does not neatly coincide with the distinction between *xingerxia* and *xingershang*. Take *Qi* which manifests itself in two modes of being, *Qi*-in-concentrating-mode and *Qi*-in-dissipating-mode; the former mode is matter but the latter mode is not matter, but may at best be translated as energy, if one must, in talking about *Qi*-in-dissipating-mode in certain contexts. Yet both are forms of being. To put it into Chinese terms, one could say that *metaphysics*, being beyond and above physics, would belong to the domain of *wu* and not *you*. In other words, the Dao is a *metaphysical* notion, not a notion which is simply *xingershang*. The Dao as *metaphysics* resides on a different existential plane than that simply of *xingershang*. To mark this difference in existential planes, this author proposes to modify the term *xingershang*, rendering it as 形而上之上 *xingershangzhishang*—that which is beyond what itself is above form, as a possible term to refer to the notion of *metaphysics* in Chinese.

We next return to chapter 25 of the *Laozi* to look at what precedes the quotation cited right at the beginning of this chapter. It reads: 有物混成, 先天地生。寂兮 寥兮, 独立不改, 周行而不殆, 可以为天下母。吾不知其名, 字之曰道. Rendered broadly by this author, it reads: "Something undefined yet complete first engendered Heaven then Earth. How still and empty it is, standing on its own, unchanging, yet moving ceaselessly, inexhaustibly. It could be regarded as the Mother of All-under-Heaven. I do not know its name but I use the term 'the Dao' to refer to it."

This is the metaphysical Dao which is all-embracing, limitless unlike specific, particular *daos*. The specific *daos* are aspects of the Dao, are different expressions of the Dao; that is why, it is held that their difference lies in the different names or labels that they wear (此两者, 同出异名). However, names are human linguistic and conceptual constructs to differentiate what in reality is undifferentiated (《庄子》· 齐物论: 道之所以亏也—see the *Zhuangzi: Qiwulun*).

The Dao is *wu* (which in the opinion of this author is best said to refer to the domain of great openness), yet it can give rise to *you*/有 (being)—when one traces everything back along the "unbroken thread" mentioned in the passage to follow, one would find that *you* comes from *wu*. This interpretation appears to accord with chapter 14 which reads: 视之不 见, 名曰夷; 听之不闻, 名曰希; 搏之 不 得, 名曰微 。此三者不可致诘, 故混而为一。其上不皦, 其下不昧。绳绳不可名, 复归于无 物。是谓无状之状, 无物直象, 是谓惚恍。迎之不见其首, 随之不见其后。执古之道，以御今之有。能知古始, 是谓道纪。Feng & English, 1989 translate as:

> Look, it cannot be seen—it is beyond form.
> Listen, it cannot be heard—it is beyond sound.
> Grasp, it cannot be held—it is intangible.
> These three are indefinable;
> Therefore they are joined in one.
> From above it is not bright;
> From below it is not dark.
> An unbroken thread beyond description.
> It returns to nothingness.
> The form of the formless.
> The image of the imageless,
> It is called indefinable and beyond imagination.
> Stand before it and there is no beginning.
> Follow it and there is no end.
> Stay with the ancient Dao.
> Move with the present.
> Knowing the ancient beginning is the essence of Dao.

This interpretation also appears to accord with the very famous opening chapter of the *Laozi* : 道可道, 非常 道。 名可名, 非常 名。 无名天地之始; 有名万物之母。 故 常无欲, 以观其妙: 常有欲, 以观其徼。 此两者, 同出

异名，同谓 之玄。玄之又玄，众妙之门。This author's rough rendering is as follows:

> The specific *dao* which can be laid out/written about in detail is not the Dao, which is limitless, enduring and unchanging. A name which can be named is a specific name and is not the Name which cannot be named which is beyond the limits of specific names. The Name, which cannot be named, has engendered Heaven and Earth. What can be named such as Heaven and Earth is the Mother of *Wanwu*. The Marvel that is the Dao only reveals itself to those who have rid themselves of all distorting desires and specific names; those who are unable entirely to escape the reach of desires and specific names may at best only catch a glimpse of the Marvel of the Dao. The two are stages of the same process of grasping the Marvel/the Mystery that is the Dao, but we give them different names to mark the differences between them. When we get beyond the specific named *dao* or *daos* to the gate of the nameless Dao itself, all that is subtle and wonderful would be revealed to us.[31]

The *metaphysical* Dao cannot be exhaustively reduced or tied down to any one interpretation of what it is. This is so, not only because the Dao embraces each and every specific understanding but because each specific understanding and conception of it necessarily imposes certain constraints and restrictions upon our perception of the world, thereby ruling out other possibilities of which the Dao is capable. In that sense, not only are our desires standing in the way of grasping the Dao, it is also the case that every attempt we make by tying it down to a specific understanding of it in a specific context by way of language may prevent us from appreciating the Dao in another context, even in contexts not yet dreamt of. In chapter 1, we cited the *Zhuangzi* as holding a similar view, "squaring" concepts which are "round" produces distortion. The specific *daos* may be regarded as "square" and the Dao as "round;" as Hoffert, 2006 points out, such a procedure diminishes the Greatness of the Dao, and is a grave misunderstanding of its true nature. Language necessarily lays down conceptual boundaries, thereby excluding any other conception. Philosophers, the world over, intra and inter traditions, ought constantly to remind themselves that all conceptions of philosophy lay down constraints and boundaries, their own specific, particularistic *dao* of philosophising. Elevating one specific *dao* of philosophing runs the risk of distorting the metaphysical Dao of the *Laozi*.

That is why the *Laozi* holds that the Dao is beyond words, or at least, is not tied down to particular words. In chapter 34, we find: 万物恃之而生而不辞，功成不名有。"The Dao engenders and nourishes *Wanwu* but does so silently, without declaiming its success." Chapter 35 reads: 道之出口，淡乎

其 无味，视之不足见，听之不足闻，用之不足既。"Talking about/describing the Dao renders it insipid and tasteless. One may look for the Dao but not see it, one may listen but not hear it. Yet one may use it and not exhaust it." Chapter 41 says: 道 隐无名. "The Dao is hidden and nameless." (These renderings are by this author.)

Where then is the Dao hidden (if it makes sense to ask such a question)? The *Laozi* appears to suggest that it could be hidden in the Great Unhewn or the Great Uncarved[32] (wood, but literally a wood from a particular type of tree called "po," but the word also means simplicity 朴 *pu*). In several places, it invokes that image to stand for the Dao—for instance, see chapter 28: 复归于朴—Return to Great Unhewn or the Great Uncarved; in chapter 32, the Great Unhewn or the Great Uncarved is implied rather than explicitly mentioned: 道常无名。曰朴 虽小，天下莫能臣也 which reads (as rendered by this author) as: "the (*metaphysical*) Dao defies being named. Small it might be (in one sense), (yet) it cannot be grasped by (the mightiest He in the realm), the Minister of State." The *Laozi* could have just as readily used the image of jade ore to stand for the Great Uncarved but it chose not to do so. (After all, the author(s) of the *Laozi* were keen to emphasise that wisdom in life consisted of resisting the desire for ever-increasing appropriation of material goods both in quantity and quality.) In Chinese culture, jade holds pride of place; the jade carver confronted with a lump of the ore would entertain the potentialities inherent in it. One must bear in mind that images, no matter how appropriate in one limited aspect to illustrate a point, could be misleading in other aspects. So in this context of characterizing the *metaphysical* Dao, one must not think of the Great Uncarved or the Great Unhewn as a limited lump of jade ore, marble, or a piece of wood, no matter how large (which sustains only one carving or at best several carvings only), as the Dao is inexhaustible and limitless unlike specific pieces of jade ore or tree trunk. However, to continue the metaphor, one could carve or sculpt as many dragons, phoenixes, birds and cabbages from the Great Uncarved, yet "the artisan" could continue to carve endlessly many more, even other than dragons, phoenixes, birds, and cabbages. However, whatever the image might be, it is intended to convey the view that the Dao is inexhaustible, all-encompassing and limitless unlike the specific, particularistic *daos* which are limited and finite.

The Metaphysical and the Empirical/Scientific

Specific *daos*, such as *qidao*, *tiandao*, and *didao* do have empirical content, whereas the Dao is a *metaphysical* concept. This then raises an issue which has to be addressed: what is the relationship between the metaphysical on the one hand and the empirical/scientific on the other? We start to explore the relationship by looking at it from the standpoint of modern Western philosophy.

The mainstream in this tradition proclaims that metaphysics and empirical/scientific matters are mutually exclusive, they do not mix. However, this view is nothing but an uncritical reflection of positivist philosophy, which has decreed from Auguste Comte (1794–1859 CE) onward, if not before, starting with Thomas Hobbes (1588–1679 CE), that humankind historically passed through three distinct stages of thought, the mythological, the metaphysical and finally the scientific, which constitutes the Age of Modernity and Progress. These three modes are, indeed, attempts to explain the world and its phenomena which we can observe. We know what positivism means by the mythological type of explanation—for instance, in Greek mythology, storms at sea were explained in terms of Neptune's anger; summer and winter were explained in terms of the story of Demeter, the goddess in charge of good harvest, her daughter Persephone, and Hades, the god of the underworld. Hades fell in love with the beautiful Persephone, taking her with him to the underworld. This distressed her mother so much that she began to neglect her duties which in turn worried Zeus. With a lot of diplomatic maneuvring between these various deities, finally it was settled that Persephone would stay with Hades for six months of the year and with her mother Demeter for the other six months. It is obvious that the lives, likes, and dislikes of gods and goddesses were invoked to explain natural phenomena.

People grew out of that mode and moved on to the metaphysical mode at least in the history of Western Europe, when Aristotelianism was established by the Middle Ages. This mode explained by invoking four causes, the material, efficient, formal and final causes. Take a statue of Churchill—it is made of marble/bronze (material), by a sculptor (efficient), in the likeness of Winston Churchill, an image of which could be carried in the head of the artist as he sculpted (formal), and it has been commissioned after the Second World War by the British government/people to commemorate the great War leader (final). Positivism considered this to be an improvement on the mythological mode but it is not good enough, as it relied on four causes when two would have been sufficient—the material and the efficient causes alone suffice, the other two are not only dispensable but also obscurantist when these are applied in the context of naturally-occurring phenomena. Take the law of acceleration—when an object is dropped from say the window of the top floor of a skyscraper, it falls faster and faster. Why? The Aristotelian explanatory framework says that every object has its own natural home—as fire tends to rise, the sky above is its natural home. The natural home of heavy objects is the ground. Just as a human, at the thought of going home, may walk faster and faster because she feels happier at the prospect of seeing her family or eating the meal already prepared and waiting, in the same way, the stone falls faster and faster as it feels happier and happier as it gets closer to its natural home, the ground. The scientific mode cuts through all such nonsense and endorses only the material and the efficient. Appealing to the emotions, desires and intentions of stones seems as futile as appealing to the emotions, desires and intentions of supernatural deities called gods and goddesses. The alternative ploy used by those who deployed the metaphysical mode was not much better when it invoked essences to explain natural phenomena—for instance, why does opium send one to sleep? Answer: its essence is to be sleep-inducing. Resorting to essences only makes the explanation an empty one, a tautology as it tells you no more than that opium sends you to sleep because it sends you to sleep. Molière, the great seventeenth-century French playwright (1622–1673 CE) satirized this enterprise by giving the essence of opium a high-sounding Latin name, *vis dormitiva*.

In other words, the metaphysical mode of explanation was a con. As a result, the term "metaphysical" at the hands of the positivists and those who follow them (whether wittingly or unwittingly) became an abusive, unflattering one.[33] The scientific mode of explanation did and does its best to distance itself from anything which even vaguely smacks(-ed) of the metaphysical. After all, science confines itself solely to the domain of what is empirically ascertainable, verifiable and most of all quantifiable. What one can say intelligibly and usefully about the law of acceleration is that the rate of fall is 22 feet per second; it is not possible without falling into tautologies or outright gibberish to ask the "why" question. Science should not and must not be tainted by metaphysics, as *ex hypothesi*, the metaphysical domain is beyond science and any dabbling in it would lead one to talk if not total nonsense, at least, to engage in pseudo-science.[34] Science should only ask "how" questions. However, the whole tenor of this book as well as its companion, 2012b, is to argue that any science and its activities presuppose a particular philosophical framework—of which metaphysics is an important component—in which they are embedded and within which only then do they make sense. The spirit of positivist science should not get away with monopolising the term "metaphysics" as a term of philosophical abuse. If this is so, then metaphysics and science cannot be separated by impermeable walls or boundaries and that at least a corridor of communication must remain between them. What then is this corridor?

Surprisingly, upon careful examination, not even the mythological mode of explanation is totally devoid of empirical content. Take the Persephone myth—there may be minimal empirical content but it is there. The ancient Greeks had observed that summer followed winter, and winter followed summer, that there was a regularity to be found with the cyclical succession of the seasons from year to year. Is this not sound observation? Their explanation in terms of the love life of their goddess and god might not be very illuminating but one could detach ultimately the unhelpful myth from the empirical observation upon which the myth was based.

One could say the same also of a Chinese myth from which we can "excavate" some sound astronomical information. Like other cultures in ancient times, the Chinese looking up at the skies would see up there what today we would call stars and planets. They saw a star (in Western astronomical terms called Vega but which the ancient Chinese called The Weaver Maiden Star/织女星/*zhinüxing*; they saw another star, Altair, which they called the Cowherd Star/ 牵牛 星/*qianniuxing*. (Admittedly the ancient Chinese did not distinguish so clearly between stars and planets as we do today.) They then used their imagination to spin a story about these two heavenly bodies which ran as follows: the cowherd (Altair) and the weaving maiden (Vega) fell in love but such romantic relationships were forbidden by the rules of Heaven enforced by the Heavenly Emperor and his court. When the Heavenly Empress got to hear about such a transgression which involved her own grand-daughter, she was furious and banished Altair, sending him down to Earth to become a mere mortal, while her grand-daughter, Vega, was ordained to weave non-stop forevermore up in the sky. Hence Vega is called the Weaver Maiden star. The Weaver Maiden wove the clouds with her magical silk threads on her loom, *in different colors depending on the time of day and season of the year*. Thus the young couple was separated until one day the Heavenly Empress permitted her grand-daughter to visit Earth when she accidentally encountered her old lover, now living the life of farmer and cowherd. (Hence Altair was known as the Cowherd star.) They recognised each other, married, had two children and nearly lived happily ever after but for the wrath of the Heavenly Empress when she found out what they had done behind her back. She transported the cowherd and their two children back to Heaven; the wife and mother followed desperately and just as she got close enough to be reunited with her family, their fate was decided by the vengeful Heavenly Empress, who with the wave of her hairpin, *created a galaxy (the Milky Way) to separate them for eternity*. However, eventually, the cruel Empress relented when all the gods and fairies in the Heavenly palace cried out for pity on their behalf—as a result, she permitted them to meet but_*only once a year, on the seventh day of the seventh moon. On that day, countless magpies would appear to form a bridge to reunite the couple and* *their children*. The Chinese people celebrated and still do celebrate that day, calling it the Qixi Festival (七夕节—literally, this means the festival of the seventh evening).

In this myth, the parts italicized above by the author, contain information as to what the ancient myth-creating Chinese knew about astronomical matters, that is to say, empirical knowledge about the phenomena which they observed in the sky. One could elicit the following nuggets:

1. Clouds of different colors, shapes and forms could be observed, varying according to the time of day and season of the year.
2. The Milky Way (the Chinese call it *Yinhe* 银河, Silvery River) could be observed in the sky.
3. And so could the two stars, Vega and Altair, which were distantly situated in the night sky—Vega is the brightest star in the constellation, Lyra, while Altair is the brightest star in the constellation, Aquila.[35]
4. The Milky Way (which is the galaxy to which our Sun belongs) is in between, separating them. This galaxy is visible throughout the year in the night sky but in Summer it is even more obvious, looking very much like a river. Hence in many ancient cultures, it is seen as some sort of celestial river—to the Egyptians it was like their Nile, acting as a waterway to the next life; the Osage Indians in America thought that it was the way for souls of the departed to go in search of a suitable star to dwell upon; the Chinese, like the Egyptians, also thought of it as a river, the *tian he*, the celestial counterpart of their Yellow River.
5. The ancient Chinese also observed a connection between the Milky Way and the seasonal rains—in the winter which was their dry season, they noticed that the Milky Way was thinner, looking less dense in the sky. In the Summer, the rainy season, the Milky Way was much wider, looking like a swollen river.
6. The seventh day of the seventh lunar month would fall usually in August (the eighth month of the Gregorian calendar) which is the end of the rainy season as well as the beginning of Autumn. The day of the festival, therefore, takes place when the Milky Way is high above the sky, and Vega (seen at its best at 9:00 p.m. on the evening of the seventh day of the seventh lunar month) and Altair are clearly visible.[36]

Is such a mode of explanation as worthless and as detached from the empirical domain as modern Western philosophy, by and large, had made it out to be? It definitely is not scientific when judged against the imprimatur of positivist science, but is it necessarily devoid of sense and must be cast into the rubbish hold-all called "metaphysics?" Perhaps only when metaphysics is presented in the manner which positivism has chosen to do in terms of empty essences or anthropomorphism (the stone feeling happy as it knows it is on its way home). Those who adhere to the positivist line are mistaken in implying that this version of metaphysics exhausts the subject called metaphysics, thereby throwing the baby out with the bath water. It bears repeating the point that every science (be this European medieval or European modern, be it Newtonian within the family of European modern or post-Newtonian such as quantum or relativity physics, be it ancient Chinese, based on concepts of the *Yijing*, the *Laozi*, the *Zhuangzi*) presupposes its own particular kind of metaphysics, including ontology, which lays down the philosophical framework within which alone the science could/would take place—Lee, 2012b, argues that the ontological *volte face* of transforming the naturally-occurring to become the artefactual, of which the machine is paradigmatic, dictates how Modern Medicine is theorized and practiced. The relationship between the metaphysical in particular/the philosophical in general, on the one hand, and the empirical/scientific, on the other, is profound as well as intricately entwined. Without grasping the role played by Materialism, Cartesian Mind/Body dualism, Reductionism, and many other metaphysical concepts, one would not be able to see, for instance, why anatomy played such a crucial role in the history of medical education and training in Modern Medicine, why surgery is so highly regarded, why lab experiments are considered to be methodologically superior to other forms of investigation (leading to epidemiology being perceived as playing the "Cinderella" role to bacteriology), to name only a few areas of impact.

We would like to argue in this context that a conception of the relationship between the metaphysical and the empirical/scientific, different from that espoused by mainstream modern Western philosophy, can be found in Chinese *philosophy* which perceives it to be one of fruitful exchange. Let us first turn to the distinction in the *Laozi* between *wu*/无 and *you*/有. Where would the *Laozi* have remotely got this distinction from? Once we rule out a mythological source, a supernatural/sacred source, a source from oracles (such as the Delphic oracle), or a dream or hallucinatory/drug source, then the only source which remained would be the observational source. What sort of observation could have prompted the author(s) of the *Laozi* to postulate the distinction between *wu* and *you*? The *Laozi* gave some instances of the distinction. In chapter Eleven, we find this passage: 三十辐, 共一 毂, 当其无, 有车之用。埏埴以为器, 当其无, 有器之用。凿户以为室, 当其无, 有室之用。故有之以为 利, 无之以为用。Feng & English, 1989 translate as:

Thirty spokes share the wheel's hub;
It is the centre hole that makes it useful.
Shape clay into a vessel;
It is the space within that makes it useful.

Cut door and windows for a room;
It is the hole which makes it useful.
Therefore benefit comes from what is there;
Usefulness from what is not there.

Three examples are mentioned above: (a) spokes/wheel/hole in the center for the axle; (b) vessel/clay; (c) doors and windows/room. Note that they are examples based on observation of people making and doing things rather than on observation of natural phenomena per se. The concept of a wheel rests on a round rim held together by spokes (just a round wooden rim would not be strong enough for a wheel); a wheel in a cart cannot turn and the cart cannot move unless an axle links the two wheels; yet an axle cannot connect the two wheels unless a hole is created in the center which holds all the spokes permitting the axle to be slotted through it. A construction identical to it, but without the hole in the center of the spokes, would, at best, be a decorative object, not a functional one. The wheel rim, the spokes, the axle are all material things, they have the two sets of properties identified in the last chapter that matter must possess as they have shape, size, as well as impenetrability, solidity, stability, and weight which belong to the domain of *xingerxia*, to the domain of being/*you*. Yet paradoxically, *xingerxia* and *you* on their own in the context of wheels attached to a cart are not enough; one must complement them with the domain of *wu*. It is obvious that here *you* and *wu* can neither be understood nor separated from each other—one cannot just create a hole without its boundaries being determined by things which are not holes. Hence *you* on its own cannot lead to *wu*, no more than *wu* on its own can lead to *you*. The two seeming polarities are therefore complementary, not mutually exclusive. This in turn leads the *Laozi* and other related texts to advocate a very distinctive type of *logic* which would be explored further in Chapter Nine, their implicit rejection of the principle of excluded middle and of two-valued logic, principles of reasoning so characteristic of, and deeply embedded in Western thought. Is this not a clear demonstration of how from observing something very concrete, very specific, such as wheel-making, could lead one to higher and higher levels of abstraction, to *metaphysics*, even *logic*?

It is also paradoxical then that to be of use to us humans, in this context of creating artifacts, it is *wu* which turns out to be eminently relevant. The same is true of the other two examples. A vessel, such as a cup or a bucket, can serve as such only given the empty space in the middle, *wu* being bounded by *you* (being as matter in this kind of context). A room is normally for living in, for storing things in, hence there must be designed into the concept as well as into the construction of a room, a door or window for entry and exit. Here, the *you* in question (being as matter) must be punctuated by *wu* (in this context, it stands for emptiness). This kind of room is unlike a tomb which is designed not to be disturbed after burial, hence a tomb must be permanently and carefully sealed. In this context, one could say that the *Laozi*'s notion of *wu* can be likened to the Aristotelian notions of formal and final cause—we need to know the purpose of the object under design before we can know how to design it properly. Modern Western philosophy, as already noted, has dispensed with these two causes, claiming that they are obscurantist if not outright unintelligible. Yet at least in the context of designing and making artifacts, it is not obvious that one can dispense with these two notions. The ancient Chinese, through their distinction of *wu/you* tried in their own distinctive manner to grapple with a similar set of issues.

What else did the ancient Chinese observe, but this time, not in the context of making artefacts but of observing *Ziran* processes and phenomena? The *Laozi* also gives some examples, the most powerful of which comes from observing how water behaves. In chapter 8 is the following:上善若水。水善利万物而不争, 处众人之所恶, 故几于道。。。Feng and English, 1989 translate as:

> The highest good is like water,
> Water gives life to the ten thousand things and does
> not strive.
> It flows in places men reject and so is like the Dao. . .

A passage in chapter 43 reads: 天下之至柔, 驰骋天下之至坚。。。Feng and English, 1989 translate as:

> "The softest thing in the universe/ Overcomes the hardest thing in the universe."

This quotation when read in conjunction with passage from chapter 8 could be interpreted to refer to water, as water must be considered as one of the softest things in the world; yet it is one of the most powerful, as not only does it nourish *Wanwu* (in the narrow sense of the term), but it erodes (over time) some of the hardest things in the world, such as granite; it can penetrate all nooks and corners as it needs only a hairline crack on a surface for its potency to be realised. In chapter 78, a passage reads: 天下莫柔弱於

水，而攻堅強者莫之能勝，其無以易之。弱之勝強，柔之勝剛，天下莫不知，莫能行 which is rendered by this author as:

> "Nothing in the world is softer and weaker than water, and yet nothing can surpass it in subduing the firm and the strong. (Paradoxically), the weak triumphs over the strong, the soft over the hard—everyone knows this, yet no-one is able to carry out this piece of wisdom in practice."

In this sense, how water works may be seen as a fitting analogy of how the Dao works, although it is true that while water is in the domain of *you*, the Dao is in the domain of *wu*. However, the Dao is more powerful than water because of this difference as the Dao can go even to places where water cannot go, where there is no crevice or hairline—in other words, the Dao is everywhere as it is above *xingerxia* and even *xingershang*, although both the Dao and water act *via wuwei*/无为 (happenings in accordance with the Dao, which in sinological discourse is translated literally as "non-action"[37]). One knows therefore the benefits of following *wuwei*. This interpretation is captured by the line which follows that cited above from chapter 43 which reads: 无有入无间，吾是以知无为之益。。。 This rendering is compatible with what chapter 37 says: 道常无为而无不为。。。which Feng and English, 1989 translate as: "Dao abides in non-action/ Yet nothing is left undone. . ."

The real purpose of rendering the passages cited above in this particular way is to show that the *metaphysical* concept of the Dao and its related concepts such as *wu/you* and *wuwei* do have an empirical base. In other words, metaphysical concepts, contrary to what positivist philosophy says, cannot entirely be divorced from scientific observations, no matter how humble and lowly these discoveries and findings might seem to our modern sensibility. Human consciousness is unique, as no other animals have evolved to the level of language with such a wide and distinctive range of uses as human language, including that of abstraction, extrapolation and generalization. In the light of such empirical/scientific findings, this peculiar kind of consciousness proceeded to extrapolate from a concrete situation to a higher, more abstract level, even to the level of *metaphysics* even *logic*, which in turn inform the way we think and act. From observing the artisan at work, constructing a wheel/a vessel/a room in a house, from observing how the heavenly bodies appear and (appear to) move during the passage of the day and of the seasons in the year, how water behaves and so on, the philosopher/*philosopher* in us human beings, dating back to ancient times, rose to the occasion, leading us to construct an abstract framework within which we could attempt to explain what we have observed and discovered. The specific *daos* lead to the Dao rising over and beyond them, in particular, rising above the empirical level to the level of *metaphysics*—from the specific, limited, particular *dao* of water to the Dao which no longer is simply part of the domain of *you*, but enters that of *wu*, as well as to generate the relationship between *wu* and *you*; from the specific, limited, particular *you* of the rim of the wheel, its spokes, its axle to the *wu* of the specific, limited, particular *wu* of the hole through which the axle could be inserted to make the wheels move the cart, the Dao rises above that empirical context to the *metaphysical* level of *wu* and *you*. It is the specific, particular *wu*, of the cup, for example, which had inspired the *Laozi* to the higher plane of *philosophical* abstraction—this is born out in Chapter 4 which reads: 道冲而用之或不盈。渊兮似万物之宗。。。Feng & English, 1989 translate as: "The Dao is an empty vessel; / it is used, but never filled. Oh, unfathomable source of the ten thousand things!"

We have attempted to establish that there is a passage from the empirical to the *metaphysical*—but is there an analogous link from the *metaphysical* to the empirical level? Yes, there is. In the previous chapter, we showed that the *Laozi*'s account of cosmology could be spelt out as follows (with the arrow → standing for the notion of engendering):

Dao (*wu*) → One (*you*: Original *qi*) → Two (*Yin qi* & *Yang qi*) → Three (co-operation, mutual response and interaction of *Yinyang*) → *Wanwu*

In other words, the Dao as the *metaphysical* concept of *wu* can ultimately lead to phenomena which are in principle observable—first the Dao engendered *Yuanqi*/Original *qi* which in turn engendered *yin qi* and *yang qi* which all belonged to the domain of *you*/being. When the author(s) of the *Laozi* and other related texts postulated the existence of *Yuanqi*, the notion looked then as a purely *metaphysical* entailment of the Dao, as it appeared then to have no empirical implication of any kind which could be tested or observed. However, it remained true, that even if it were merely a *metaphysical* implicate of the Dao, it in turn engendered, yielded, implied two types of *qi*, *yin qi* and *yang qi*, which did have testable consequences, as we shall go on to argue in chapter 6 which looks into how these two observable forms of *Yuanqi* lay the foundation of the *Yi* and in turn of the account of the diagnosis as well as therapeutic interventions of illnesses in CCM.

However, for the moment, let us return to the notion of *Yuanqi* which at the time of its postulation seemed incapable of summoning up any empirical evidence in its support. To say of a notion X that it at the time of postulation had no empirical evidence which could be cited in its favor, is not tantamount to saying that X is in principle incapable of having observable consequences. Part of the reason might lie in the fact that the technology available at a certain moment in time was just not available to be used in ascertaining it. The history of modern Western science offers many instances of such delayed empirical support—we have already mentioned one example regarding Einstein's $E = mc^2$, postulated in 1905 but had to wait for three decades or thereabouts before experimental evidence was forthcoming to support it. The work of Peter Higgs and others in the 1960s led to the postulation of the existence of a particle called the Higgs boson for which no empirical evidence was available. To get evidence one way or the other involved building the Large Hadron Collider underneath the city of Geneva; the Atlas machine did not become satisfactorily operational until mid-2012, after numerous false starts and millions of euros plus several hundreds if not thousands of some of the (reputedly) best scientific brains in the world serving the LHC and its vociferous needs and demands. Finally in July 2012, some evidence had emerged. The popular press and some scientists in the field proclaimed with confident jubilation that the particle had been found;[38] yet their more sober colleagues, who had kept a cooler head, maintain that further work must be done before one could be sure that it had. However, as things turned out, the Nobel Committee in the autumn of 2013 had awarded the Nobel Prize in physics to François Englert and Peter Higgs.[39]

When the ancient Chinese postulated the hypothesis that at the beginning of the universe, *Yuanqi* emerged, not only was there no empirical evidence in its support, there was no high tech either naturally. For more than two and a half thousand years, no high tech existed in the world which could conceivably have looked for the evidence which might support or undermine the hypothesis that *Yuanqi* came into existence in the early days of the universe. However, some evidence today does exist which accords with the *Yuanqi* account, although the evidence was neither collated nor designed to test it, naturally. The theory, today, in modern cosmology about the origin of the universe in general (and of our Solar system in particular) as well as the evidence amassed on their behalf, appear to support the *Yuanqi* theory. The modern cosmological theory in brief goes as follows: about 1.38 billion years ago, the so-called Big Bang[40] occurred, which involved a roiling soup of energy. When things cooled somewhat, the energy condensed into the first particles, although for the first few hundred million years, the universe was simply a huge cloud of hydrogen and helium gases. Our Solar system thus began life as an enormous cloud of gas and dust, as a star-forming nebula. Our Sun came into existence as gravity caused part of the cloud to collapse into a swirling disk of gas, from which our Sun, a star began to grow. The Sun, as it grew in strength, began to blast high-energy radiation into the disk—this solar wind then pushed the gases, namely hydrogen and helium (the lighter elements) to the edge of the disk, while the heavier elements remained nearer the center, forming a dusty band. From this, the rocky planets were formed (Mercury, Venus, Earth, and Mars containing mainly rock and metal, with high densities, slow rotation, and solid surfaces), while the outer planets, such as Jupiter, Saturn, Uranus and Neptune became gaseous ones (containing mainly hydrogen and helium, have low densities, rapid rotation, deep atmospheres).[41] Well, one can see that the Big Bang account and the ancient Chinese account are not at odds with each other—the latter relying on the Dao (*metaphysical* concept) engendering *Yuanqi* turned out in the end to be capable of empirical support, even if it had to wait more than two millennia before the evidence became forthcoming.

The cosmology set out in the *Laozi* and other related texts also postulate an intimate causal relationship between the *yin qi* and the *yang qi* (which by and large are empirical concepts in the domain of *you*) leading to a new *metaphysical* concept, *Yinyang*, which in turn leads to the engendering of *Wanwu* in the domain of *you*. As the book develops, all these notions and relationships will be further explored.

In the light of this analysis given above, it looks as if that ancient Chinese *philosophy* as developed in the *Laozi* and other related texts was not shy of interweaving the empirical with the *metaphysical*; they did not perceive that the two levels or domains were mutually exclusive, that is to say, to do *science* one must exclude doing *philosophy*. Instead, they could be inferred to say that to do *science* one must do *philosophy* at the same time; that the former could not be articulated or carried out unless its theory and practice were conducted within a framework provided by the latter.

At this point of the discussion, it may be helpful here to introduce a distinction between the context of hypothesis-generation which may be metaphysically-inspired and the context of finding empirical support for the implications of such generation.[42] The relationship between these two contexts may be displayed as follows, where → stands for "leading to" or "generating," depending on the context:

ES (1): empirical support/base →
EGN (1): broader empirical notion →
MGC (1): *metaphysical* concept (at high level of abstraction) →
ES (2): empirical support for MGC (1) →
MGC (2): *metaphysical* concept at another level of abstraction) →
ES (3) . . .

An example of the above re-constructed chain of reasoning is as follows:

ES1→ broader empirical concepts (EGN1): observations of heavenly bodies and how they behaved in the course of day and night as well as in the course of a year generated specific, particular *daos*, the *dao* of Heaven and the *dao* of Earth *via Laws of Nature* such as the *zhouye jielü*, *sishi jielü* and *zhou er fu shi* (for which see chapters 4 and 2).

EGN1 → MGC1: specific, particular *daos* (EGN1) generated the notion of the *metaphysical* Dao (MGC1)

MGC1 → EC2 and EC3: the Dao (MGC1) generated the empirical concept of *Yuanqi* (EGN2) on the one hand and the two specific types of *qi*, *yin qi*, and *yang qi* (EGN3) on the other.

EGN2 → ES2: the empirical evidence for *Yuanqi* (ES2), as a matter of fact, took a very long time to be forthcoming.

EGN3 → ES3: empirical evidence for *yin qi* and *yang qi* (EC3) was immediately forthcoming in terms of observations such as the heat of Summer, the cold of Winter, the growth/development of plants and animals in Spring and Summer, the maturity/dieback during the dormant stages in the lives of plants and animals in Autumn and Winter.

EGN2 and EGN3 → MGC2: *Yuanqi* (EC2) as well as *yin qi* and *yang qi* (EC3) generated the *metaphysical* concept of *Yinyang* (MGC2).

MGC2 → ES4: *Yinyang* (MGC2), for instance, in the context of CCM finds empirical support (ES4) in the diagnosis and treatment of illnesses (to be explored in detail in Lee [forthcoming].

MGC1 → MGC2: the *metaphysical* Dao (MGC1) in turn led to the postulation of *Ziran*/autopoiesis (MGC2).

MGC2 → MGC3: *Ziran*/autopoiesis (MGC2) led to the concept of process-ontology (MGC3), to be explored in chapter 8, where it would, in turn, be shown to imply consequences which are ultimately observable (ES5).

MGC2 → EC4: *Ziran*/autopoiesis (MGC2) leads to the notion of *Wanwu* (EC4) whose domain is that of *you*, covering both the abiotic and the biotic.

Another example of the re-constructed chain of reasoning:

ES1 → MGC1: cup and clay/door and room/spokes of wheel and hole for axel which are artifacts (ES1) in the world of particular *you* (the walls in the room, for example) and of particular *wu* (the breach in the wall to create the door) lead to the *metaphysical* concept of *youwu* (MGC1).

MGC1 → MGC2: *youwu* (MGC1) leads to the higher-level *metaphysical* concept of the Dao (MGC2).

MGC2 → MGC2.1: the Dao (MGC2) generates *Ziran* (MGC2.1) and so on.

Conclusion

The main conclusions which may be drawn from the interpretation of the *Laozi* (and other related texts) are:

1. It proposes that the concept of *Ziran* be conveniently translated as "autopoiesis" provided the term is understood only and simply in its literal meaning as derived from its Greek etymology.

2. The primary meaning of *Ziran* implies process-ontology, and not substance/thing-ontology—this constitutes a fundamental difference between Western philosophy and Chinese *philosophy* as chapter 8 argues.
3. However, its derivative meaning in terms of "Nature," is, by and large correct as *Ziran* processes are precisely what are at work in nature/Nature, standing for the biotic and the abiotic domains found on Earth and in the universe.
4. The *metaphysical* concept of the Dao and what it stands for must accord with *Ziran*; the two should be understood hand in hand.
5. The Dao and *Ziran* as *metaphysical* concepts, nevertheless, are not adrift from the empirical world as in ancient Chinese *philosophy*, such concepts looked both backward to the context of their emergence resting on empirical findings and observations as well as forward to the context of finding further support for them *via* their consequences which are, in principle, observable. In this, too, it differs profoundly from the mainstream of modern Western philosophy which holds that metaphysics (philosophy in general) and the empirical/scientific level of investigation are mutually exclusive.
6. This chapter has significantly left out the key issue of the relationship between Humans (*ren*) on the one hand and Heaven, Earth, the Dao and *Ziran* on the other, a theme to be explored in chapters 10 and 11.
7. In case some readers are still suspicious of the postulated link between the levels of the *metaphysical* and the empirical, let us finish this chapter by reminding them that such a link can be found in the history of Western philosophy itself. For instance, take Aristotle's notions of the four causes. Where would Aristotle have got them from? Aristotle himself as good as told us via his use of artifacts to illustrate them, just as the *Laozi* author(s) did to illuminate the distinction between the particular *you* and the particular *wu*, and were thus inspired to abstract from them to the *metaphysical* level, the concept of *wuyou* (or *youwu*). Take the concept of Materialism. Where would philosophers have got it from? By observing particular things such as trees, rocks, and so on and their various properties (such as shape, size, solidity, and impenetrability) and in turn extrapolating and abstracting from them to the metaphysical level of Materialism. In turn, Materialism involves consequences which are empirically ascertainable. Suppose someone says that a strange-looking being is lurking at the bottom of the garden. Given today's high tech, we can set up CCTV cameras to photograph this being; to mount crude or even sophisticated traps to capture this being, to use sophisticated devices such as infrared heat to work out

the surface area of such being and so on. But if none of these measures show up anything, we can then infer that the being is not what one would call a material being, but very probably, it is an hallucinatory figure of the person who persistently claims to see such a being—this entire set of procedures for getting empirical evidence for/against the claim would be in accordance with the metaphysics of Materialism.

Notes

1. The *Xunzi*, in this respect, is no different from the *Laozi* and the *Zhuangzi*.

2. The title has been variously translated but in the Needham version, it reads: *Discourses Weighed in the Balance*.

The chapter in the text challenging the said degeneration is called "物势" ("The power inherent in things"). It repeatedly made the point that the engendering of *Wanwu* is a process which had nothing to do with human manipulation and desire (and by implication nothing to do with divine intervention or creation). The key phrases in this chapter expressing this theme are: 万物 生天地之间, 皆一实也/ "The myriad things are engendered by the interaction between the *qi* of Heaven and that of Earth, all from the One (that is, the Dao);" 天地和气, 物偶自生矣/ "The *qi* of Heaven and Earth harmoniously combine, engendering *Wanwu* as a result." (Renderings are provided by the author.)

3. An example to make this distinction clear: in biotechnology today, it is possible to insert a gene from a jellyfish into the tomato plant in order to render the latter immune from frost, and thereby to save the tomato-growing industry from economic loss incurred through frost damage. The jellyfish lives in the depth of the ocean, in very cold waters. The long history of evolution of life in the ocean has ensured that it comes to possess a gene which can resist the cold. In biology, the jellyfish is classified as belonging to the animal kingdom, the tomato to the plant kingdom. Evolutionary processes at work in *Wanwu* have ensured that there would be no gene transfer between the jellyfish and the tomato plant. However, with the advent of biotechnology based on the basic science of molecular genetics/biology, it is possible to transfer the gene for frost protection from the jellyfish to the tomato plant in a laboratory, to produce what is called a transgenic organism. (See Lee, 2005 for detailed philosophical discussion of biotechnology, the relationship between deep science and deep technology and the artefactual status of transgenic organisms.)

4. Modern scholarship has established that the names for these twenty four divisions (based on the solar year) were already in place toward the end of the Warring States Period and the beginning of the Han Dynasty; the earliest texts mentioning these divisions extant today are the《周髀算经》/*Zhou bi suan jing*/*The Arithmetical Classic of the Zhou Gnomon and the Circular Paths of the Heavens* (ca. 100 BCE–100 CE) and the《淮南子·时则训》*Huainanzi*—see *Liu, 2008: 431.

5. See **(The) Scorpio constellation*, 2013.

6. Another astronomical "map" which covers similar grounds as these Neolithic remains was found on a box in the tomb of the Marquis Yi of the state of Zeng (entombed ca 433 BCE during the Warring States Period); this box was excavated in 1978 in Hubei Province (湖北省擂鼓墩). This map also showed what Chinese astronomers called the Twenty Eight Mansions or Lodges (二十八宿 *ershiba xiu*) in which they grouped all the constellations of importance and known to them; such knowledge had matured by the Spring and Autumn Period. Furthermore, those constellations grouped together at four compass points (seven in each group) are given names of animals: Eastern group/Spring—the Blue Dragon/青龙; Southern group/Summer—the Red Bird/朱雀; Western group/Autumn—the White Tiger/白虎; Northern group/Winter—the Black Tortoise 玄武. For details, see *Liu, 2008: 432-434; a spectacular image can be found at the British Library's website.

7. See *Chinese astronomical record keeping*, 2013; see also Kelley & Milone, 2005.

8. Shaughnessy in Loewe and Shaughnessy, 1999.

9. For a brief, accessible read on this vast and complicated subject, see Lee, 2008.

10. For the deconstruction of specific words, this author relies, in the main, though not exclusively, on *Zhao, 2006; *Chen, 2006.

11. *Zhao, 2006: 347; *Chen, 2006: 600.

12. It is of relevance here to raise another aspect of the philological history of the word 寺*si*. Today it refers to a Buddhist temple, and indeed, had done so, since the Eastern Han Dynasty. However, it had earlier stood for a certain Han bureaucratic unit of government whose remit included ensuring the proper administration of laws and regulations, as well as looking after important guests of the realm. The emperor Mingdi明帝（57–75 CE）of the Eastern Han had a dream, after which he sent word to India requesting the Buddhist gospel to be brought to China. Naturally, when the first monks arrived from India, bearing their scriptures, they were handsomely looked after, and in the first instance were accommodated within such an administrative quarter called the鸿胪寺 /Honglu *si* in Luoyang, the capital. A year after, the emperor ordered a new dwelling to be built for them also in Luoyang and called it the 白马寺, in honor of the white horses upon which these missionaries rode to China from India. From then onward, the word 寺/*si*, slowly lost its old meaning of being a governmental bureau and acquired its new meaning of "Buddhist temple." See *Wu, D., 2006: 267–268; *Zhao, 2006: 373–374.

13. On the gnomon and other astronomical matters which follow, see Maspero, 1938: 183-370; Needham and Wang, 1956.

14. The word "分" refers to the equinoxes; "至" refers to the solstices; the word 启 refers to the (official) beginning of Spring and Summer while 闭refers to the (official) beginning of Autumn and Winter.

15. For the details of an account of how to measure and calculate the results as recorded by one called Liu Zhao/ 刘照 of the Liang dynasty (502-556 CE), in 《后汉书·律历下》/*Houhan shu:lüli xia*, see *Liu, 2008: 434–436.

16. Juxian was one of the centers of early Chinese civilization. Modern scholarship has now ascertained that the Yellow River Basin was not the only cradle. Similar wine vessels were found in Anhui, Zhejiang Province in the 1990s. See *Dawenkou writing*, 2013.

17. This would push back the history of Chinese writing by two thousand years. Though this sounds surprising, it might not be so, once we bear in mind that the Oracle Bone inscriptions discovered at the turn of the twentieth century covered the reigns of the last nine Shang kings from Wu Ding, but that the entire Shang Dynasty dated from the seventeenth or sixteenth century BCE. It is true that while so far no version of the script in the early part of the Shang Dynasty has been found, it remains also true that any ancient script would have taken a very long time to evolve and mature. As a result, it would be too simplistic to assume that the Oracle Bone Script arrived fully-fledged, like a mushroom, grown overnight. From this perspective, the Dawenkou forms of writing regarding certain words as found on their wine vessels could plausibly be seen as part of this long process of development which did not come to maturity until later in the Shang Dynasty. Professor Qiu Xigui/裘锡圭 of Beijing University concludes: "Even though the Dawenkou Culture type B symbols still cannot be definitively treated as primitive writing, nevertheless they are symbols which resemble most the ancient pictographic script discovered thus far in China. . . . They undoubtedly can be viewed as the forerunners of primitive writing." (裘锡圭, 《文字学概论》/*Wenzi xue gai lun*. For English translation, see Mattos and Norman, 2000: 11. On the other hand, Professor Qiu does not think that the symbols discovered between 1954–1957 in Banpo (dating from the fifth millennium BCE) and nearby at Jiangzhai, in Lintong County in Shaanxi Province (dating from the fourth millennium BCE) could constitute primitive writing, or even that they resemble script. Professor Qiu is more hospital to the Dawenkou symbols being the forerunners of primitive writing, as Dawenkou Culture was nearer in time (only earlier by 1,400 years) as well as in space to Shang culture. The Oracle Bone Script could then be considered to lead back to the Shandong Longshan Culture which in turn may have given rise to early Shang culture.

18. On these points, see *Chen, 2006: 330.

19. On these points, see *Chen, 2006: 255.

20. See *Liu, 2008: 432.

21. See Defoort, 1997.

22. See *Zhao, 2006: 267-268; *Chen, 2006: 244–247.

23. As China is in the northern hemisphere, the North is where the bitterly cold winds come from and the South is where the Sun and its warmth prevail more abundantly. In terms of architectural design, the door faces South, and when seated in a room, the most desirable position would then be the south-facing position. Formal social etiquette would demand that such a position be reserved for the guest; as the most important person in a realm was the king/emperor, he would always sit with the back to the North, facing South, as the expression 坐北朝南/*zuo bei chao nan*, says.

24. See *Chen, 2006: 452–454.

25. See *Chen, 2006: 387–388, 455–457.

26. In modern Chinese, the two words—土地*tudi*—are often used together thereby creating a new two-syllabic word—see Lee, 2008: Part II—to refer not only to cultivated fields but also to land or territory.

27. The number of words culled from the extant pieces of shells and blades amounts to over four thousand, of which scholars, so far, have successfully deciphered about half.

28. See *Wu, D., 2006: 165.

29. The word for "head" does exist in the Oracle Bone Script.

30. On this discussion regarding *xing*, *dao*, and *shou*, see *Chen, 2006: 279–281; *Wu, D., 2006: 165, 367; *Wu, Y., 2006: 60, 62, 95; *Zhao, 2006: 361.

31. For those who would like a more poetic rendering, see the *Legge translation of the Daodejing*, 2012. More recent translations include Feng and English, 1989.

32. See also Ziporyn, 2013.

33. The meaning of the term itself has a history. Aristotle simply called those lectures he was to give after the ones on physics "metaphysics," a merely factual business. Later, it acquired a philosophical meaning, to talk about concepts/issues which are over and beyond those discussed in physics/science but which physics/science presuppose. This meaning received bad press with the rise of philosophers of the positivist ilk (Comte and later the Logical Positivists). That battle cry has since quieted down with the decline in the fortunes of that strident philosophy.

34. See Lee, 1989a for the methodological implications of the philosophy of positivism for doing science.

35. Both constellations were first identified in the history of Western astronomy by Ptolemy in 2 CE. Today, astronomers draw an imaginary triangle, called the Summer Triangle, between Altair, Vega, and Deneb in the Cygnus constellation. In the Indian tradition, these three stars are considered to be the footprints of Vishnu, a prominent Hindu god.

36. See *Milky Way*, 2013 (for two images which make these points clear). The Milky Way passes through the Summer Triangle. Altair is the bright star in the lower right. Vega is the bright star in upper middle. The third star in the triangle is Deneb (lower left) in Cygnus.

37. Depending on the context, "Dao-informed action" may or may not require intervention or action on the part of the human agent. No action/interference/intervention would be required when the Dao is applied to understanding an ecosystem deemed to be entirely self-regulating or autopoietic, a situation which could be found plentifully in very early times in ancient China. In the context of agriculture, *wuwei* would require action/intervention but all the same, such action must be in accordance with the Dao, with *Ziran* processes—one must carry out agricultural and hunting activities observing carefully the two fundamental *Laws of Nature*, namely, the cyclic reversions of the day/night as well as the yearly four seasons sequences, and what they imply for plants and animals (including humankind). For

a brief discussion of how this term is understood in general in sinological literature, see Lai, 2006: 99–101.

38. See, for instance, Close, 2013.

39. For a brief account of the data following July 2012, see *Higgs' bosun*, 2013.

40. The theory rests on two theoretical legs: (a) Einstein's General Theory of Relativity as the new theory of gravity, (b) the Cosmological Principle which holds that the matter in the universe is by and large homogenous, that is roughly the same everywhere and in all directions—see *(The) Big bang theory*, 2013 (which shows that although evidence of an impressive kind occurs in its support, nevertheless, it is not without its critics).

41. Uranus and Neptune were only discovered in modern times, whereas Mercury, Venus, Mars, Jupiter and Saturn were known to ancient astronomers. The ancient Chinese call Jupiter *suixing*/ 岁星, Mars *yinghuo*/荧惑 , Saturn, *zhenxing*/镇星， Venus, *taibai*/太白, and Mercury, *chenxing*/辰星. The sequel given above would follow the commonly accepted *Wuxing*/五行 (Five Transformative Phases—see chapter 7 for discussion) as *Wood*, *Fire*, *Earth*, *Metal* and *Water*.

42. This author would have called it the context of discovery and the context of justification after Karl Popper. However, upon reflection, this would not be wise as Popper's preoccupations were not identical to those pursued here. Popper (and before him Reichenbach, 1938) made that distinction famous in *The Logic of Scientific Discovery* which was first published in German in the 1930s but not translated into English till after World War II, when the text began to have a major impact on the philosophy of science in the English speaking world. Furthermore, that distinction has over the last few decades collected too much of its own baggage in the debate between Popper/Popperians and Kuhn/Kuhnians to be of use in the context of discussion about the relationship between the metaphysical and the empirical in this book, although it is true that Popper, who did not subscribe to mainstream Western philosophy of the day, was hospital to metaphysics and the role it could play in science.

CHAPTER FIVE

The *Zhouyi/Yi*

Meanings and Significance

It bears repeating it is not an exaggeration to say that the oldest extant text in Chinese culture is also the most influential in its history, as it affects all aspects of its civilization, including theoretical discourses in subjects as far ranging as agriculture, architecture, calligraphy, ethics, *medicine*, military, management, music/painting/performing arts, *philosophy*, politics/government, *science*, technology, and so on. (This list is simply alphabetically arranged.)[1] The *Yijing* qualifies to be the oldest in existence because some of its contents, such as the names of its *gua* were already found in the Oracle Bone inscriptions (and that would be roughly three thousand five hundred, if not more, years ago). Anyone who wishes to come to grips with Chinese civilization must ultimately come to have some understanding of this text as well as its much later appendage, the *Ten Wings*, a work probably dating some six hundred years later. (Together, as earlier shown, these two parts make up the *Zhouyi* which matured as a text, probably during the early Han Dynasty.)

This, then, immediately raises a puzzle. We have already earlier observed that the *Yijing* began life without any shadow of doubt as a text in divination. Yet, as just observed, it seems to have become the *fons et origo* of Chinese cosmology and Chinese *philosophy*, permeating theory as well as practice throughout Chinese culture down the millennia. How can we explain such a *volte face*? There are two ways of accounting for its change in fate. The first is superficial—this is simply to say that Confucius, by lending his great prestige to it, ensured not only that the text survived when it could have been lost and forgotten like a good many other ancient texts in Chinese history, but also because his long lineage of disciples down the line about six hundred years later gave the text an interpretation turning it away from its origin in divination to the more intellectually respectable discourses of cosmology and *philosophy*. The Confucian tradition put the *Yi* even before the other four canonical texts, such as the *Analects*. This account is valid up to a point; Confucius was, indeed, so much addicted to the text that he wore out three copies, according to Sima Qian, the Grand Historian.[2] Furthermore, it is well accepted that Confucius was against soothsaying and all forms of superstition; hence it follows that it seemed unlikely that he was interested in the text for divinatory purpose. But what other purpose could the Sage have in mind?

However, even an initial attempt to answer this question would lead us to the less superficial answer to the question. Confucius's main goal was to construct a social/moral/political *philosophy* which would underpin Chinese society.[3] He realized that this project could not be carried out unless he grounded it within a larger theoretical framework. In this spirit, he turned to the *Yijing* for guidance and inspiration, as he (and other thinkers through the ages) had realized that this text, in spite of its divinatory origin, had appeared to have created an (embryonic) systemic framework, nevertheless, which they could borrow while trying to tease out some ideas in it which had implications for cosmology and *philosophy*. This important realization meant that the humanizing and secularizing strands in Chinese intellectual life could easily appropriate the text for their own project (be it *Rujia*/儒家/the Confucian School or the Daojia/道家, associated with the *Laozi* and the *Zhuangzi* as its foundational texts) leaving its original divinatory purpose far behind. This make-over leading to a variety of innovations and embellishments, ultimately altering the character of the original text, meant that the key concepts in cosmology/*philosophy* which self-consciously emerged provided the backbone for the development of theoretical discourses throughout Chinese civilization, down the millennia, and which continues to do so for, at least, two key discourses even today, namely, Chinese *Medicine*, and the *philosophy*/strategic thinking in matters relating to war (《孙子兵法》*Sunzi's Art of War*, a text of the Spring and Autumn Period) which are still alive and taken seriously by many people throughout the world today. Furthermore, as this book would show, these key concepts are by no means outmoded and irrelevant to scientific thinking today, especially in those new fields of scientific development beginning from the early twentieth century. However, this should not be taken to claim that the original purpose of the text as divinatory died a death following its appropriation by "rationalist" thinkers such as Confucius/Confucians and *Daojia*—for from it, it enjoys even today numerous adherents from around the world who study it seriously from the divinatory standpoint. In the main, the text enjoys two separate "incarnations" down the ages to the present day, one being pertinent to *philosophy* and *scientific* thinking and the other to divination.[4]

Deconstructing *Yi* to Reveal Its Meanings

To back up the interpretation given above to explain away the apparent puzzle, we begin by turning to the original meaning of 易. The single most crucial word in the *Yijing* is naturally the word 易/*yi*. How should this be deconstructed? Deconstruction, as we know, generally involves looking up what a word would look like in some ancient scripts. However, some sinologists even today imply that the word 易 does not exist in the oldest of such scripts, the Oracle Bone script—see Wang, 2012: 63. Instead, they pursue a view which is no longer, in the main, adhered to in modern philological scholarship. For instance, Wu, 2003: xvii—with whom Wang appears to concur (ibid[5])—without specifying which ancient script he has in mind, writes: "In ancient script, the character *yi* consists of two parts, the upper part being the character *ri* (日) , the sun, and the lower part being the character *yue* (月), the moon. In its present form the character *yi* (易) still retains the sun script, although the moon script has become slightly modified."

The account given by Wang and Wu, in so far as this author can track, appears to have come from Xu Shen's dictionary of the Han Dynasty. By Han times, as we now know, the Oracle Bone Script had long been lost to the Chinese peoples for more than a thousand years until the re-discovery of its existence at the very beginning of the twentieth century CE. So it should not surprise us today that Xu Shen had not deconstructed the word according to the Oracle Bone Script.[6] As a matter of fact, the two components do not refer to the Sun and the Moon respectively. This would become obvious when we look at the various scripts for the word (*yi*) known today in the history of Chinese writing.[7]

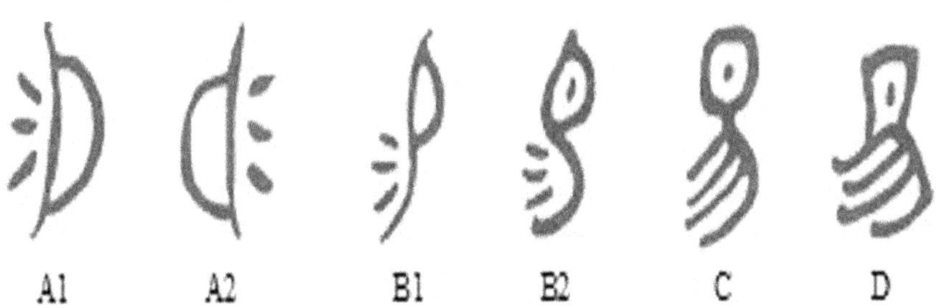

Figure 5.1. Character "yi" in various scripts

A1 and A2 are the Oracle Bone Script, being mirror images of each other. What do they stand for? They both stand for the Sun. They show the Sun (the bit which looks like a hump) being partially obscured by some clouds (the line drawn under the hump), with the three dots below the line representing shafts of sunlight which manage to break through the clouds. A slightly different deconstruction understands the three dots to stand for many clouds, as ancient Chinese quite often used "three" to stand for "many"; in this case, the Sun is simply partially hidden by clouds. The original meanings of 易 are: 乍晴乍阴/"suddenly fine, suddenly cloudy," 天明天暗/"the sky is bright, then it is dark," 经常变换/"changing regularly." The Oracle Bone Script inscriptions often referred to 易日 and 不其易日—the former may be rendered as "relatively fine day with some sun" and the latter "day with little or no sun." In other words, the ancient Chinese had observed, like other peoples, at other times, that the weather was variable, fine one day or one moment, not fine another day or another moment.

B1 and B2 are the same words but in the Bronze Script, although the forms above are taken from two different inscriptions found in two different bronze vessels. One thing of interest is that in B2 the sun component sports a dot, making the whole graph look like a bird; but actually the dot may have been an attempt to represent the occasional appearance of a dark spot in the sun which we today call "sunspot." The orthography of 易 in its present form has evolved from them, as can be seen in C (Lesser Seal Script) and D (Clerical Script) from which the Standard Script (still used today) is derived.

It is clear from this brief philological account that the word had nothing to do with the Sun and the Moon and their relationship to each other. Instead, it had much to do with variable weather conditions. However, if the ancient Chinese had simply noted this common meteorological phenomenon, the *Yijing* and indeed the entire *Zhouyi*, would never have emerged as a text. However, these observers of something as mundane as the weather were not content to stay at the level of mere weather watching. Instead, it appeared that they went beyond plain observation as well as the literal meaning of the word 易, in the first instance, to bestow a more conceptual meaning on it, and that meaning is "change." So in one obvious sense, then, the text, given the title *Yi*/《易》would naturally be a text about the concept of change. They further built on this level of abstraction and conceptualisation to formulate systematically a cosmology and hence also a *philosophy*, as well as pioneer (or consolidate) a mode of thinking which remained by and large unique to Chinese culture and civilization—various strands of this unique mode of thinking would be explored in greater detail in the chapters to follow. In other words, the authors of the *Yi*, just as the author(s) of the *Laozi*, as shown in chapter 4, moved from the observational, purely empirical level to a higher level of abstraction and conceptualisation until they reached the *philosophical* level of thought.

This process of evolving from the empirical to the *philosophical* level had definitely begun by the Han Dynasty, if not earlier. In Western Han times (206 BCE–9 CE), a work commonly referred to as《乾凿度 》/ *Qianzaodu* had emerged which distinguished between three senses of the term 易 *yi*: 易一名而含三义[8]—this author's rendering reads: "A single term but embodying three meanings." This work was very influential and was adopted by another scholar towards the end of the (Eastern) Han Dynasty (25–220 CE) who wrote: 易之为名也，一言而函三义：简易一也；变易二也；不易三也。This author's rendering reads: "The term is *yi*, but it contains three meanings—(1) Essence of *yi*简易/*jian yi*, (2) Change变易/ *bian yi*, (3) No Change不易/*bu yi*."[9] The scholar was Zheng Xuan郑玄(128–200 CE), a man of humble origin, noted not only for his great learning but also his laudable determination to resist the blandishments of high office.[10]

The text *Qianzaodu* elucidated the Essence of *yi* in the following terms: that the Dao as set out in the *Yi* accounted for astronomical knowledge concerning the Sun, Moon, the stars, and planets, the four seasons and the type of *qi* they stood for respectively, for the emergence and evolution of *Wanwu*. The text also held that the highest virtue consisted of following the Dao, of embracing *wuwei via* understanding the notions of movement (embodied in Pure Yang, *Qian*) and tranquillity (embodied in Pure *Yin*, *Kun*).[11] It elucidated the sense of Change in terms of *qi*; in astronomical/*scientific* terms, it referred to the orderly change of *qi* as the seasons advanced in the course of a year or in the course of day and night. Change, therefore, was the order of natural phenomena. Without change of *qi*, without intercourse between *yin qi* and *yang qi* standing in the right relationship to each other, growth and development would be arrested—similarly, in other domains such as the social and the political. The 否卦/*Pi gua* stood for such a situation. Why? In this hexagram, the top trigram is *Qian*, the bottom is *Kun*. The former stands for *yang qi*, which has the tendency to ascend, the latter for *yin qi* which has a tendency to descend. In this hexagram, the two types of *qi* are each going their separate ways and neither the twain would meet. But if they did not meet, there would be no interaction or exchange between them—without such intercourse, *Wanwu* would not be sustainable, growth/development as well as re-engendering would grind to a halt. That is why the text reads: 天地不变不能通气, which could be rendered as: "If Heaven (*yang qi*) and Earth (*yin qi*) were static or could not interact, there would be no possibility of a smooth passage and exchange of *qi*." Should such an unfortunate situation obtain, then not only would *Wanwu* not thrive, kingdoms would not either. Hence this model of non-interacting *qi* could be used to account for the fall and decay of states. The polar opposite of *Pi gua* (which stands for an inauspicious overall outcome) is *Tai gua*泰卦 which stands for an auspicious set of circumstances. In this hexagram, the top trigram is *Kun*, the bottom is *Qian*. The *yin qi* descends, the *yang qi* ascends, the twain would meet and interact, permitting intercourse of the two types of *qi* leading to healthy growth and regeneration.

The *Gua*: Beyond Divination to *Philosophy* and *Science*

The most striking feature of the *Yijing* is the *gua* themselves, whether they are in the form of trigrams (the *bagua*/八卦 or the *jinggua*/经卦) or hexagrams (the *liushisigua*/六十四卦 or the *biegua*/别卦). For want of a better term to describe them, they may be called diagrams, even drawings, just as architectural diagrams are drawings. Diagrams and drawings by their nature are intended to convey to the reader information in a graphic fashion without resorting to words. The ancient Chinese call this type of presenting thought *xiang*/ 象: 象也者, 像也 《周易 · 系辞下》/ *Treatise on The Appended Terms*, *Part II*. (This in turn has profound significance for *epistemology* and *scientific* methodology in the Chinese tradition of *philosophy* and *science*, as we shall see later, but for the moment, let us keep to the brief outline. The *Xiang* Mode of Thinking is explored in chapter 9.) The *Ten Wings* (*Part I*, *Treatise on the Appended Terms*) elaborates as follows: 书不尽言, 言不尽意 It also says: 圣人立象以尽意。。。 The gist of these short quotes may be summarized (by this author) as follows: the written word cannot entirely convey all that speech does, as the latter possesses sounds and intonation through which one can express emotions; speech in turn cannot convey in entirety and with absolute clarity all shades of meaning. Hence the sage uses the *xiang* (image/drawing/graph) to accomplish this; *xiang* (together with the written word) can convey more adequately what language is meant to convey.

The *bagua* look like this:

Table 5.1.

☰	☱	☲	☳	☴	☵	☶	☷
Qian	Dui	Li	Zhen	Xun	Kan	Gen	Kun

Each trigram consists of three *yaos* 爻 which this book prefers to leave untranslated. A *yao* is of two kinds: like this — (unbroken) or like this - - (broken); the former is a *yang yao*, the latter a *yin yao*. The former stands for *yang*, the latter for *yin* (the opposite of *yang*). As it is immediately obvious, every trigram contains three of these *yaos*, but the actual composition of each in terms of their respective components is different. Herein lie their commonality and their difference. However, *Qian* and *Kun* are unlike the other six in that *Qian* has only *yang yaos* and *Kun* only *yin yaos* (the former represents pure/undiluted *yang* and the latter pure/undiluted *yin*); the other six have at least one *yang yao* or one *yin yao*. For instance, *Dui* and *Xun* each have two *yang yaos*, but note that their respective positions are different—they are inverted images of each other. In the same way, *Zhen* and *Gen* each have two *yin yaos* but their respective positions are different; they, too, are the inverted images of each other.

Let us look briefly at the *gua* itself from two aspects: (a) how the internal components of the *gua* of the set of trigrams change both in quality (that is from *yang* to *yin* or *vice versa*) and position, whether the *yang yao* or the *yin yao* occupies the lower, middle, or upper position in the *gua* as a whole; (b) each *gua* (whether trigram or hexagram) is meant to stand for a particular state of affairs/phenomenon (also in terms of their properties) in the world.

How the *yao* in the trigram/hexagram changes follows certain rules of permutation; but as such technical procedures of derivation[12] are not absolutely essential to the main theme of this book, and with the lack of space as an excuse, only some general remarks in brief will be made here about the matter, sticking to trigrams for the purpose of exposition. *Qian* and *Kun* each may be said to have three movements as reflected in the shift of their *yaos*.[13] *Qian* (among other things) stands for Heaven or the sky which appears as layers of clouds; hence it is represented by three unbroken *yaos*. The *gua* changes in terms of *yao* changes in a trigram are as follows:

(a) When its bottom (first) *yao*[14] changes from *yang* to *yin*, the trigram becomes *Xun*; the natural phenomenon *Xun* represents is Wind/风/*feng*). In the West, one says that the trees move when the wind blows, rather than the wind is moving; but the *Yijing* sees Wind as the agent behind the moving trees, hence it is Wind which is the mover, and the moving trees are but a mere manifestation of its movement.

(b) When middle (second) *yao* changes from *yang* to *yin*, the trigram becomes *Li*; the natural phenomenon *Li* represents is Fire (火 *huo*). Fire goes upward, as if going even beyond the lower layers of clouds; hence it is fitting that one uses the change in the second *yao* to stand for it. (Note, too, that this trigram is a *xiang* for how to prevent a fire from spreading, by creating a fire gap, which is represented by the *yin yao* between the two *yang yaos*.)

(c) When top (third) *yao* changes from *yang* to *yin*, the trigram becomes *Dui*. The natural phenomenon *Dui* stands for is the changes really high up in the sky. The only way in which ancient peoples could observe what was happening so high up was to look at the reflection of the sky in a pool of water (that is, before the invention of bronze and of the bronze mirror); hence pool/pond/marsh/泽/*ze* is used to stand for this phenomenon.

Kun can stand for Earth/soil which appears as three broken *yaos*. This is because, *Kun*, unlike *Qian*, is broken up, when plants germinate, breaking through the soil (or when humans plough up the land in order to plant, when farmers break up the soil before they can put a seed or seedling in the soil).

(a) When its bottom *yao* changes from *yin* to *yang*, the trigram becomes *Zhen*; the natural phenomenon it represents is Thunder or Quake (*lei*/雷). Earthquakes and volcanic eruptions come from deep under, the bowels of Earth; hence it is fitting that *Kun* should change its bottom *yao* to a *yang* one, as *yang* stands for Motion/Movement while *yin* stands for Rest/Tranquility.

(b) When its middle *yao* changes from *yin* to *yang*, the trigram becomes *Kan*; the natural phenomenon it represents is Water. Now water, as underground water is beneath the soil and so may be considered to occupy the middle space between the surface of Earth and its deep innards. (It may be of interest to note that the character for "water"/水/*shui*, is simply the *Kan* trigram rotated 180 degrees.)

(c) When its top *yao* changes from *yin* to *yang*, the trigram becomes *Gen*; the natural phenomenon it represents is Mountain (*shan*/山). Mountains are formed when Earth's crust is pushed upward (in today's scientific terms, we say that the tectonic plates push up against one another); hence it is fitting that the phenomenon of mountains and orogenesis (mountain formation process) should involve the top *yao*.

There are two main trigrams configurations, one called the *Former Heaven* (*xiantiantu*/先天图), the other, the *Later Heaven* (*houtiantu*/后天图).[15] The *Former Heaven* configuration—see image below—illustrates clearly a certain notion at work, namely, that of complementary opposites—*Qian* and *Kun*; *Li* and *Kan*; Zhen and *Xun*; *Dui* and *Gen*. (This configuration is in accordance with *wu*/无, the domain of great openness and is in accordance with *Tianren-heyi*/*Tianren-xiangying*.) At the same time, this configuration also implies dynamic change, which was pointed out by Shao Yong[16] (邵雍—1011–1077 CE—a noted Song scholar in what today is called *yilogy*, the academic study of the *Yijing*): clockwise from *Zhen*, through *Li* and *Dui* to *Qian*, the trigrams represent what has already been generated in the world (*yisheng* 已生), while the remaining four trigrams from *Xun* through *Kan* and *Gen* to *Kun* are concerned with what is yet to be generated (*weisheng*/未生)—these two divisions are an attempt to understand the past, the present, and the future.[17] These *gua* are also related to time; time for the ancient Chinese is marked primarily in terms of the passing of natural phenomena such as the four seasons, the interaction between *yin* and *yang* as the seasons change in the course of a year or a day. This is how the *Zhouyi* understands the concept of time as shown below.

The characteristics associated with each trigram based on this configuration are set out below (table 5.2):

The *Later Heaven* Configuration (*Houtiantu*)—below—illustrates the phenomenon of periodicity, that is, the cyclic nature of natural phenomena, as well as its understanding of the concept of space. The trigram for Fire (*Li*) is now in the South.[18]

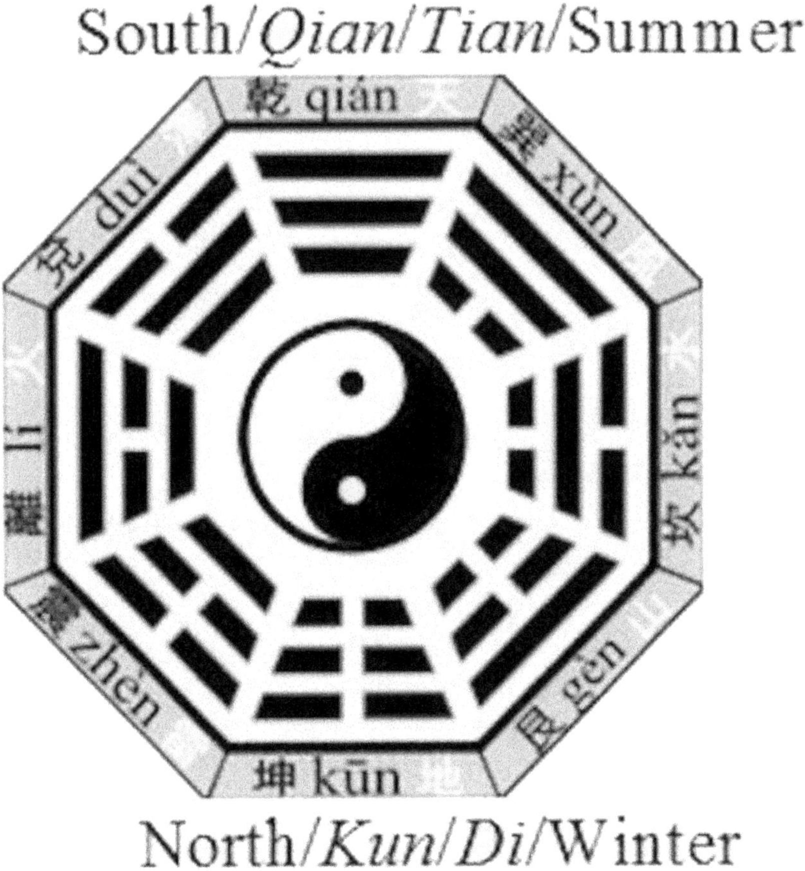

Figure 5.2. Xiantiantu

Table 5.2.

	Compass	*Natural Phenomena*	*Season*	Yinyang
Qian	South	Heaven	Summer	*Taiyang*
Dui	Southeast	Marsh	Mid-Spring/Summer Beginning/Li Xia/立夏	
Li	East	Fire	Spring	*Shaoyin*
Zhen	Northeast	Thunder	Mid-winter/Spring Beginning/Li Chun/立春	
Xun	Southwest	Wind	Mid-summer Autumn Beginning/ Li Qiu立秋	*Shaoyang*
Kan	West	Water	Autumn	
Gen	Northwest	Mountain	Mid-autumn/Winter Beginning/ Li Dong/立冬	*Taiyin*
Kun	North	Earth	Winter	

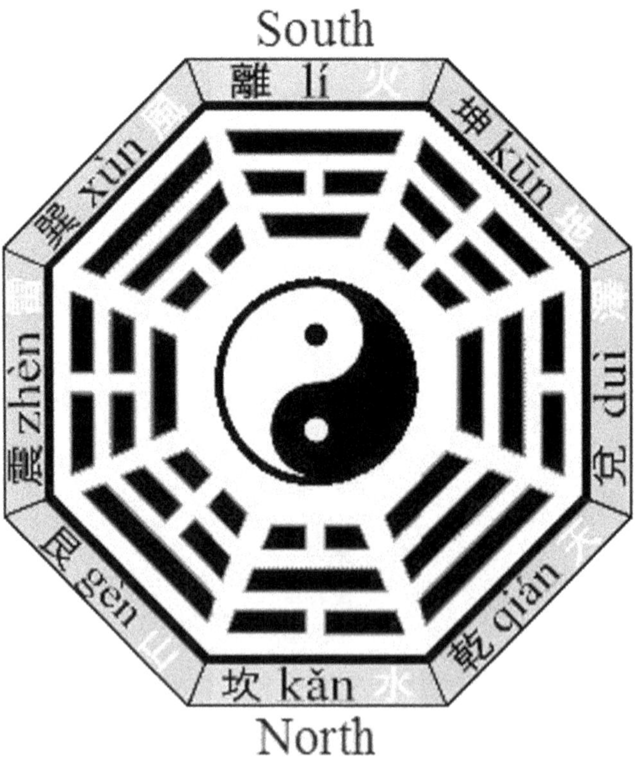

Figure 5.3. Houtiantu

The characteristics of each trigram presented in this configuration could be inferred from the diagram and/or are found in the Eighth Treatise of the *Ten Wings*.[19] This arrangement starts with *Zhen*, working clockwise until it ends with *Gen*—see table 5.3 below where the trigrams are associated with their phenomenal correlations.

Together, the two configurations touch upon the notions of Time and Space, but as this is not the right place for their detailed examination, we simply signpost them here for an exploration of the Chinese conception of Timespace in chapter 10. We conclude these initial remarks about the trigrams and their relationship with cosmological understanding with a brief account of the endowments or movements associated with each of them, as shown in table 5.4.[20]

So far we have been talking in the main about the trigrams. Let us next take a quick look at the hexagrams. As already observed, a hexagram consists of two trigrams, one stacked upon the other. Each trigram is a unit or *Whole*; hence a hexagram is itself a *Whole* made up of two sub-*Wholes*. It also follows that it has six *yaos*. Two hexagrams may stand for very different things even should they share the same two trigrams in their composition, as the

Table 5.3.

Trigrams	*Compass*	*Season*	*Stages of Changes of Development of* Wanwu *in a Year*
Zhen	East	Spring	Where & when *Wanwu*[1] start to stir into life
Xun	Southeast	Spring/Summer	Where & when *Wanwu* enjoy "equality" in the sense that each kind in developing is true to itself
Li	South	Summer	Bringing light–*Wanwu* is visible[2]
Kun	Earth/Center	Summer/Autumn	Nourishing/Supporting *Wanwu*
Dui	West	Autumn	Where & when *Wanwu* find joy/pleasure and achieve harmonious state
Qian	Northwest	Autumn/Winter	Where & when *Wanwu* compete for *Qian*, as *yin* increases at the expense of *yang*
Kan	North	Winter	Where & when *Wanwu* return to rest
Gen	Northeast	Winter/Spring	Where & when *Wanwu* start and finish, where they complete their course (but waiting to begin anew when Zhen comes round again)

[1]*Wanwu* is also best left untranslated—its literal meaning is "ten thousands things", the term standing for all things but in some contexts for all living things (as the human being is an organism) especially in the *Neijing*.
[2]For this trigram, the passage makes reference to its political associations which are ignored for now in this specific context.

Table 5.4.

Trigrams	*Characteristic Associated With Each Trigram*
Qia	Strength/健
Kun	Compliance/顺
Zhen	Motion/Quake/Stirring/动
Xun	Penetration/入
Kan	Falling into, Entrapment/陷
Li	Radiance/丽
Gen	Stopping/止
Dui	Joy, Pleasure/悦

position of each component trigram may differ—in the first hexagram, one trigram may occupy the bottom position but in the second, the same trigram may occupy the top position. An example of this kind of arrangement would be Hexagram 37 *Jiaren gua*/家人卦 (Family), and Hexagram 50 *Ding gua*/鼎卦 (Cauldron). The former has the trigram *Li* at the bottom and *Xun* above it, whereas the latter has *Li* above and *Xun* at the bottom—see table 5.5 to follow. The kind of relationship represented by these two hexagrams is characterized as one of inversion. Hexagram 37 is focused on females, as both its constituent trigrams are said to relate to that gender. Hexagram 50 invokes a symbol, a ceremonial cooking pot called the *ding*, a symbol of political power in Chinese culture. While the former hexagram pertains to the family and its affairs (that is the private or inner domain of life), the latter pertains to the public domain of governance and political power.[21]

Having now completed a severely brief and limited outline of the trigrams and hexagrams, what immediate outstanding conclusion could one draw from it? First and foremost, each *gua* is to be understood as a *Whole* on its own, standing apart from the other *Wholes*, with all eight forming a series of *Wholes*, which in turn may be said to form a larger *Whole* (and likewise with each hexagram, with all sixty-four forming a series of *Wholes*, constituting a larger *Whole*). Putting it this way would, perhaps, make some readers think of a so-called new approach to the study of complex phenomena, such as chaos theory, control theory, cybernetics, ecological theory, and many others, all based on "systems thinking and systems practice"[22] which have become "fashionable" in the last four decades or so. Systems thinking is a form of Wholist thinking (about which this book has to lot to say later). Here is one account according to Ackoff, 1981: 64–65:[23]

A system is a set of two or more elements that satisfies the following three conditions:

1. The behavior of each has an effect on the behaviour of the whole . . .
2. The behavior of the elements and their effects on the whole are interdependent . . .
3. However subgroups of the elements are formed, each has an effect on the behavior of the whole and none has an independent effect on it . . .

   A system, therefore, is a whole that cannot be divided into independent parts. . . . The essential properties of a system taken as a whole derive from the interaction of its parts.

The second quotation is from Checkland, 1981: 3: "The central concept 'system' embodies the idea of a set of elements connected together which form a whole, this showing properties which are properties of the whole, rather than the properties of its component parts."

We can now turn our attention to testing the claim that the *Yi* mode of thinking amounts to systems thinking. Well, it seems to satisfy the following requirements:

(a) Two or more elements are involved, as each trigram involves three *yaos* (and each hexagram six *yaos*).
(b) The behavior of each component *yao* affects the behavior of the *Whole*—when a *yao* alters, the *Whole* alters.
(c) It follows from (b) that the behaviour of the component *yaos* and their effects on the *Whole* are interdependent;
(d) It follows from (b) and (c) that the relationship between any sub-group of the elements and the *Whole* is one not of independence but inter-dependence—see especially in the case of the hexagram;
(e) The properties of a system (the *Whole*) derive from the interactions of its parts—the *gua* itself stands for a very different state of affairs and has very different properties possessed by its component three (or six) *yaos*. In the case of the hexagrams, it is obvious that the different position of exactly the same trigrams alters the meaning of the entire *gua*.

The mode of systems thinking in the history of Western philosophy and Western science is said to be in direct contrast to the more mainstream mode of thinking which has held sway since the beginning of Modernity from the seventeenth century in Western Europe; it is an aspect of scientific investigation ignored or excluded by the framework of Newtonian science which dominated scientific thinking for at least three hundred years in the West. This mainstream Western mode of thinking is called *Reductionist thinking* together with its companion, *linear thinking*.[24] It is true that Reductionist and linear thinking have brought with them great achievements in Modern Science and later, Modern

Technology, although it remains true that they cannot do justice to really complex phenomena such as those studied by the new sciences just mentioned above, and which thinkers by the middle of the last century (or earlier) have struggled to accommodate by pioneering an alternative mode of thinking to try to make sense of them. In contrast, Chinese thinking, ever since the *Yijing*, has not strayed from the systems thinking (*Wholism*) embedded in it; its hegemonic presence, in theory and practice over every domain of activity that one can think of, was only challenged when missionaries in the form of Jesuits first appeared on the Chinese scene bringing salvation for Chinese souls by tempting them with the fruit of Western scientific and technological labours, and later when gunboats appeared, followed by the carving up of parts of China under European jurisdiction in the nineteenth century. Reductionist/linear thinking, today, as part of the globalization of knowledge poses, as we shall see, the most severe challenge in particular to that conception of Chinese *Medicine* which this book refers to as CCM. However, as the above account shows, all may not be doom and gloom from the standpoint of the traditional Chinese mode of thinking, as Western thinking itself appears to be moving nearer and nearer to the Chinese model from the last half of the last century into the beginning of the twenty-first century. Some writers on the subject of systems thinking have been knowledgeable and generous enough to mention the existence of such a tradition of thinking in Chinese culture and history. For instance, Hejazi, 2013 writes:

> 11. Have there been cultures that have wholistic systems thinking?
>
> Yes, there are. In Chinese culture everything is comprehended within the conceptual frame of Yin and Yang that is a holistic system. Yin and Yang are counterparts for negative and positive or female and male. Yin and yang are co-dependent. Within such a system, the notion of absolute independence makes no sense. A human relationship is also a state of interdependence; both extreme dependence and independence are seen as dysfunctional. Yin and yang also complete each other; neither is fully realized without the other. For humans, full individuality is realized in the context of the other. And when yin and yang are combined together, we get the Tao, a synergistic emergence and co-creation; something new emerges that transcends the parts.

This book will also later show that other areas of Modern Science such as quantum physics, since the beginning of the twentieth century, has been moving closer to the *Yinyang* model of complementarity, when it looks at the work of Niels Bohr (chapter 8). This book would have been far harder to write in the past because there would be no easy analogues that one could find in the history of Modern Science to render remotely intelligible the

Chinese *weltanschaung* to those steeped exclusively in the modern world-view of Reductionist/linear thinking. There is an adage about fashions which seems appropriate to describe this situation: in fashions, it is said, if one stood still for long enough, fashions would come back in style. Long skirts may this season be abominably démodé, but five seasons later, they are likely to be in fashion again. The Chinese did not change for more than three millenia; it looks, today, as if their traditional type of thinking may have, at last, found favor with some of the world's advanced scholars working at the cutting edge of knowledge.

With this brief examination of systems thinking in the context of both traditional Chinese and contemporary world-views in place, let us go back to the initial puzzle about how a divinatory text could turn out eventually to be about a version of systems thinking, to use a contemporary analogue. First, let us go back to early Chinese dynastic history, to a dynasty for which today exists a fair amount of direct information based on the accidental discovery of the Oracle Bone Script in 1899 near Anyang, Henan Province, the capital of the late Shang Dynasty.[25] The Shang people not only practiced life burial of servants or household slaves to accompany their departed nobles, they also believed in a god or gods, transcendent beings whom they honored and with whom they attempted to communicate via shamans. Like many other peoples down the ages, they were anxious about their future, which was necessarily open and uncertain. Hence, they resorted to divination. Their divination records, such as those which survived, show a wide range of problems for which divination was sought, whether it would be auspicious to go to battle against another tribe, to hunt, to marry, or even to have a tooth extracted, and so on. It appeared that they used at least two methods, although from the surviving records of divination, they appeared to have relied heavily on the first, but this could just simply be because some material were more fragile than others and so had failed to survive.

The first method (which continued even to the early part of the succeeding Zhou Dynasty), as already mentioned in an earlier chapter, is *bu* 卜, of reading the cracks produced in burning specially prepared tortoise shells or ox shoulder blades for the purpose of divination. Often these lines literally looked like this 卜, and hence that pattern was conveniently taken over as the word to stand for this particular method of divination. This practice is sometimes called *guibu* 龟卜, which literally means "tortoise shell divination" but which covers the use of ox shoulder blade as well. The method involved is 观象/*guan xiang* literally meaning "looking at the image." The second major method was *zhan*占, conducted within the framework of the *gua* 卦 (that is the eight trigrams and the sixty four hexagrams of the *Yijing*), using yarrow stalks *shi*/蓍to set up the *gua* which was relevant to the situation in hand for which a divinatory outcome was sought. The method (based on 数/ numbers) consists in the first instance of counting the number of stalks left in the hand, starting with 49, before drawing the *gua*.[26] However, as the yarrow stalks turned out to be difficult to obtain and also were fragile, easily damaged, people began to use bamboo strips instead, written as 筮, but also pronounced *shi*. Hence there are two equivalent expressions: *zhanshi*/占蓍, *zhanshi*/占筮. The *Yijing* only dealt with this method and had nothing to do with *guibu*/龟卜.[27]

For the purpose of understanding why the ancient Chinese, especially from the Warring States Period onward, turned to the second rather than the first method, one should straightaway realize that the first method left little or no room for development and innovation in terms of what (in today's language from Western science) we call *systems thinking*, whereas the second did. The Oracle Bone method simply permitted two outcomes logically to the divinatory exercise, auspicious *ji*/吉 or inauspicious *xiong*/凶, whereas the *zhanshi* method permitted more room for subtle interpretation, given that a hexagram has six *yaos*. Furthermore, a *yao*, as we have seen can either look like this (a) — or like this (b) - -. (Originally what happened was that one yarrow stalk was broken into two pieces, which then came to be represented as a pair of shorter pieces (b), whereas the unbroken stalk was represented by (a).) In the original text, simply as a divinatory text, they were just noted down as presented here, as the *gua* was being constructed. The diviners or the archivists in charge of divination would record whether a particular *gua* was generally auspicious or inauspicious as well as whether a particular *yao* was auspicious or inauspicious. From this, it would have been a small step to introducing the concept of numbers or numerology into the divination practice—the ancient diviners called this — *ji* /奇 or九, the number nine and this - - is called *ou*偶 or六, the number six. (Later on, in the history of this subject, the former was referred to as奇数/*jishu* [sic] meaning odd number(s) while the latter was referred to as偶数/*oushu*, meaning even number(s).[28])

At the end of each divination, the person in charge would note down what the diviner would have said about the *gua* and its *yao* (卦爻辞/*guayaoci*); at the end of the year such persons/archivists would go through the drawers containing these records. What we see as the *guayaoci* in the *Yijing* would have passed through the hands of many such editors over the long period of time taken for the text to emerge, pared down from archives-full of such records. We have already seen the diverse range of problems for which divination was sought; hence, too in the days (before the make-over of the text by later intellectuals starting even from the Spring and Autumn Period), the names of the *gua* or the properties associated with it probably arose from the very nature of the specific problem raised in a particular divinatory exercise—for instance, the *gua* looking like this ≡ ≡ was associated with the mare as well as the characteristic of compliance (顺), and probably arose because a mare went missing; the diviner delivered an auspicious prognostication that the mare would soon return or be found nearby on the grounds that the nature of a mare, compared to a stallion, would be much less impetuous/ spirited/ adventurous. Contemporary scholarship tends not to read profundity or mystery into the *gua*, but adopts a mundane approach, regarding them as an immense depository of information about the Neolithic, the late Shang and the early Zhou periods of Chinese society and their times, and that the *Yijing*, standing as a bare text, was no more than the work of diviners and their methods, of the archivists in charge of those divination records over the long centuries before its emergence.[29]

In spite of its obvious divinatory origin, it transpired that the long line of archivists/officials in charge of divinatory matters, had probably, in tidying up the material, unwittingly created an embryonic form of what today we call systems thinking. Their tidying up and paring down of material eventually led them to create the images of the *gua* as well as presenting them in the sequence the text eventually displayed. When we peer beneath the surface, we would soon detect that there is a logic implied in these arrangements. Take the eight trigrams—each was created, as observed above, out of the two kinds of *yao*, the odd number and the even number *yao*. Odd and even as concepts are what may be called "polar opposites." The eight trigrams form four such polar opposite pairs, as follows: Qian/Kun; *Li*/Kan; Dui/*Gen*; Zhen/ Xun. Regarding the sixty-four hexagrams, they can be divided into eight contrasting sub-sets in terms of their *gua* images and into thirty-two sets of polar contrasting pairs. In terms of the sequence of these *guas*, they are ordered in terms of pairs of polar contrasting pairs.[30] We have already cited earlier an example of a pair of hexagrams which stand as inverted to each other, namely, *Jiaren gua* and the *Ding gua*. But the former also stands in other relations with other *guas* in the sixty-four *gua* arrangement,[31] a small set of examples are out below (table 5.5).

Table 5.5.

Hexagram 37 *Jiaren* 家人 Bottom *Li*; Top *Xun*	Inverted	Hexagram 50 *Ding* 鼎 Bottom *Xun*; Top *Li*
	Complementary	Hexagram 40 *Jie* 解 Bottom *Kan*; Top *Zhen*
	Anti-parallel	Hexagram 38 *Kui* 睽 Bottom *Dui*; Top *Li*
	Derived	Hexagram 64 *Weiji* 未济 Bottom *Kan*: Top *Li*

Such an arrangement implies a version of systems thinking; but it also sets out one of the most crucial concept in Chinese *philosophy*, namely, that of polar opposites, of which *yin* and *yang* are its most famous paradigm, a detailed discussion of which would be given in chapter 6.

Unlike other peoples, the ancient Chinese, or at least the elites amongst them, rather early in their history, abandoned the belief in a transcendent being which had created and controlled the world, including the fate of humans. This erosion in supernatural religious belief took place sometime after the demise of the Shang Dynasty during the succeeding Zhou Dynasty. Certainly, by the time of the Spring and Autumn Period, leading intellectuals such as Confucius and others had long frowned on what they called "superstitious" beliefs. In the *Analects*, there are two passages[32] which records Confucius's attitude toward divination. The first reads: 不占而已矣 which could be said to convey bluntly the message "Don't bother with divination altogether, that's all" to a query posed by one of his disciples regarding a problem in the divinatory domain. The second passage reads: 加我数年，五十以学易，可以无大过矣《论语·述而》, which loosely translated (by this author) reads:

> If additional years were given to me [that is if I were able to live my life again][33], I would have studied the *Yi* when I was fifty and I would not have committed too many mistakes.

Another lengthier passage which claimed to attest to the Sage's attitude to divination may be found in one of the Mawangdui fragments of the *Zhouyi*; the relevant passage reads:

> 吾求其德而已，吾与史巫同途而殊归者也。君子德行焉求福故祭祀而寡也；仁义焉求吉，故卜筮而希也。祝巫卜筮其后乎！（马王堆帛书《周易 要》第八章）.[34]

Loosely rendered (by this author), it states:

> I, Confucius, was interested in it in order to grasp *de*/德/virtue and *yi*/义/right conduct; I, the historian and the shaman are all students of the text but all the same, at the end of the journey, our respective destinations are different. For the *junzi*/君子, one who seeks virtue, attaining spiritual/ethical enrichment would for him constitute blessings, and hence he would rarely participate in ceremonies to ask the gods for their protection. It is also the case that he would attempt to achieve an auspicious outcome through benevolent and just conduct; as a result, he would rarely engage in divination.

The right approach to the *Zhouyi* is to regard its divinatory aspects as secondary, rather than primary.

We see then that Confucius immersed himself in the study of the *Yijing* in order to advance his own ethical/political ideas and ideals, and in particular to inculcate them in the minds of the ruling classes of his time. However, to achieve this grand objective, he must first demolish the idea that human beings could not be held responsible for the consequences of their actions as these were beyond the domain of human agency, being controlled by a god/gods, whose intentions were to be gauged by divination, to find out if they had consequences which would be auspicious or inauspicious for us, humans. The *Shiji* recorded that the last Shang king, Zhou/纣, attributed his fate in life to God, thereby absolving himself (and human beings in general) from responsibility to change or alter circumstances in his life: 我生不有命在天《史记·殷本纪》. In contrast, by even early Zhou times, the *Zuozhuan* recorded passages like this: 黄天无亲，唯德是辅 (《左传》僖公五年)[35]; loosely rendered, it reads: "One cannot rely on the Heavens, as we humans have no "special relations" with it; hence we could only rely on our own virtuous conduct. We, humans, must, therefore, assume responsibility for our actions and strive hard to improve ourselves." This constituted a fundamental difference between Shang and Zhou cultures, a difference which had and continue to have a long-lasting influence in more than two and a half thousand years of Chinese civilization.

For Confucius and his followers, the future, too, might be uncertain, open, and therefore worrying, but all the same, *zhanshi* 占筮 was not the way forward to resolve this uncertainty. Instead, Zhou culture, through the representative figure of Confucius, appeared to have seen an alternative way of interpreting/exploiting the divinatory text, by implying that although a divinatory outcome might not be auspicious, nevertheless, it was possible for the human agent to work hard to alter the present circumstances he found himself in, in order to bring about a better outcome in the future. We human beings could be held responsible for our conduct because, unlike other animals, we are capable of grasping that any event or state of affairs in the present is part of a network of events/states of affairs which have preceded in time; if one were to study it, one would find clues as to how things get to the present. Analogously, we can reason, that there may be clues here and now which can guide decisions regarding the future, as we possess the ability to foresee some, even if not all the consequences of our actions. In other words, a *gua* as well as the set of *guas* (whether trigrams or hexagrams) could be understood as an image of this network of related events/states of affair, between past, present, and future. This image of a network lent itself to analyzing an outcome in terms of stages (the six *yaos* of the *gua* in a hexagram). One could schematically read each *yao* as a step in the process—always starting from the bottom of a *gua*, the first *yao* could be said to be the first stage. Between the stages are changes (when a *yao* in a *gua* alters, the *gua* becomes a different *gua*, as already mentioned). An inauspicious outcome might no longer be so, if one were to work hard to change it at an earlier stage. (This could be one source of inspiration in CCM that the most brilliant physician is the one who practices preventive medicine.)

Given such an early tendency to turn away from the supernatural to the natural, it is easy to see how intellectuals such as Confucius, Confucians and others would put a rationalistic twist to the early contents of the *Yijing* by introducing the ethical dimension into *Yi* discourse. We have observed above that they appropriated the divinatory text, making use of its strengths, in terms of its systemic framework, and bringing out certain other implied concepts in such an arrangement, but yet subverting it ultimately to promote their own goals. However, the humanists were not the only intellectuals to exploit the text—one other very important group could be labeled the "naturalistic" tradition as represented by the *Laozi* (early parts were probably earlier than the *Zhuangzi* and the *Chuci/《楚辞》/Songs of Chu*, but the bulk was sometime in the fourth century BCE, making it, by and large, a Warring States text)[36] and the *Zhuangzi* (a Warring States text).[37] The secularizing tendency in terms of naturalistic thinking increased and gathered greater momentum by the time of the Warring States. However, this does not mean that in the developing discourse about the *Yijing*, the two tendencies did not talk to each other. For instance, the Confucian humanistic outlook was not narrowly nor exclusively interpreted to refer only to the ethical ideas of the Sage—its culmination in the *Ten Wings* showed that the Confucian thinkers were capable of appreciating and embracing the insights of the naturalistic tendency. This is primarily because, as already mentioned, both tendencies embraced the teaching of *Yinyang philosophy* as purveyed by the *Yinyang* School especially during the Warring States Period.

This more generous spirit in general was also evidenced in the *philosophy* of Xunzi/荀子. Although considered a leading Confucian thinker, yet his thoughts also embraced the so-called naturalistic perspective. For Xunzi, it turns out that his humanism could be said to rest on a strand of naturalism. He offered naturalistic explanations for untoward or strange happenings in the world; the following is a typical passage which can be found in the chapter of the *Xunzi*, called "Discourse on Heaven:"

> 星队木鸣,国人皆恐。曰:是何也? 曰: 无何也! 是天地之变, 阴阳之化, 物之罕至者也。怪之, 可也; 而畏之, 非也。夫日月之有食, 风雨之不时, 怪星之党见, 是无世而不常有之。 。。。物之罕至者也; 怪之, 可也; 而畏之, 非也《荀子·天论》,

which loosely rendered by this author reads:

> Stars fall and singing ensues from wood. People are afraid and ask: what can these mean? They mean nothing, as they are no more than natural changes, owing to the mutually transforming effect of *Yinyang*. With regard to such rare phenomena, we do find them strange and puzzling, of course, but it would not be appropriate to be frightened by them. Eclipses of the sun and moon, unseasonal winds and rain do occur; a strange heavenly body appearing in the sky, all such things do happen. . . . such not infrequent phenomena are indeed strange and puzzling, but one need not be filled with fear because of them. Eclipses or earthquakes were just phenomena which sometimes happened, and should not be interpreted as omens sent by some god or gods. They were perfectly capable of a naturalistic explanation. No amount of dancing, offering sacrifices to appease the gods, such as in a rain dance during a drought, would make any difference to the outcome. We sacrificed, we danced under such stressful times, primarily for psychological/social reasons, not because in truth, such activities could make the world of spirits (if it existed) have pity on us and send us rain. Furthermore, disasters such as floods, famines were not things sent by the god/gods to punish evil rulers or as a sign of ending their mandate to rule. In fact, it would be a mistake to regard such disasters as "natural," as they were usually caused by an irresponsible ruler who had forsaken his duties to his people which required him to manage carefully the system of dykes and other devices as part of an effective flood control system, or to store grain when the harvests were good in order to release it to feed the people when the harvests were bad.[38]

Xunzi appeared to be passionate about demystification, and about celebrating the role of the rational faculty in humankind. Xunzi was eager to point out that *Tian* (standing for Nature) has its own laws/regularities/patterns of functioning which have nothing to do with the political fortunes of the realm, whether it was being ruled by a benevolent philosopher-king or by the most vicious, corrupt villain. The opening line from the discourse cited just now reads: 天行有常, 不为尧存, 不为桀 亡《荀子·天论》, which may be rendered (by this author) as:

> Natural phenomena following the *Laws of Nature* are entirely independent of the domain of political phenomena. These *Laws of Nature* would continue to obtain, whether a benevolent sage-king such as Yao (one of the early sage kings) reigned or whether a wicked, corrupt tyrant such as Jie (one of the early rulers in Chinese history who was regarded as the embodiment of wickedness) sat on the throne.

His variety of Confucian ethical thought did not exclude the contribution of the naturalistic outlook, and in this respect is very close to *Daojia* thinking.

That tradition in the developing discourse of the *Yijing* may be summarized briefly here as follows (with further details to be spelt out later in the book):

1. One should get back to the original meaning of the word 易 which we have already deconstructed; it means乍晴乍阴 ("suddenly fine, suddenly cloudy"). This meaning would have been available to scholars even with the loss of the Oracle Bone Script itself after the demise of the late Shang Dynasty, as Xu Shen recorded that same meaning for the word in his dictionary. This would lend itself very readily to interpreting the text, should one so wish, within a naturalistic framework, to make it stand for natural phenomena, such as meteorological conditions. Variability of weather apart, one could also incorporate other natural phenomena such as the seasons (*sishi jielü*), the daily day/night rhythm (*zhouye jielü*), the relationships between the Sun and the Moon, the Sun, the Moon, the Earth, the movements of the other heavenly bodies with regard to the four seasons, such as the asterism which the Chinese called the *Beidouxing*/the Great Bear and so on. As earlier shown, the Chinese even in Neolithic times had been keen and knowledgeable about such matters—that an interest in astronomy had run long and deep in the history of Chinese civilization. The Chinese were also interested in exploring the three meanings of *yi* not merely in the context of divination but beyond to other domains of theory and praxis.
2. We have already observed that the two basic *yaos* in a *gua* (*yang* or *yin yao*) and that the former was later called an odd number and the latter an even number. The next development for the naturalistic tendency consisted of creating the equivalences set out below.

   This set up a series of pairs of polar contrasting terms, the most important of which is the *Yinyang* pairing, as already observed. The naturalistic tendency as represented by the *Laozi* and the *Zhuangzi* (*Daojia* texts, although the *Laozi* was also adopted later as a *Daojiao* text) did not themselves invent this most important pairing, as the

Table 5.6.

Unbroken yang yao	*Broken* yin yao
Yang 阳—the Sun/sunlight/brightness/warmth/Summer	*Yin* 阴—the Moon/moonlight/darkness/cold/Winter
动 *dong* Moving or motion	静 *jing* Being still or rest/tranquillity
Qian 乾—Tian 天 Heaven/Male	*Kun* 坤—Di 地 Earth/Female
Gang 刚 hard (such as rock)	*Rou* 柔 soft (such as water)

concept of *Yinyang* came from the *Yinyang* School which had existed by the second half of the Zhou Dynasty and soon became common intellectual property. It is obvious that the pairing was also central and foundational in the *Yijing* itself. The naturalistic tendency would incline toward explicating the third meaning of *yi*, 简易/*jian yi*, the Essential *Yi* in terms of the *Yinyang* pairing, and of the notion behind it of two forces in Nature, so to speak, which caused change in natural phenomena, namely, *yang qi*/阳气 and *yin qi*/阴气. However, these points can only be raised but not pursued here in detail.

3. Although the above schema of developments in *Yi* discourse was heavily influenced by the naturalistic tendency, nevertheless, as already observed, it was hospitably accepted by the Confucian scholars who were responsible for constructing the treatises in the *Ten Wings*. However, in spite of their commonality, they differed in one very important respect. The humanistic tendency, given its own specific ideological agendum of providing a cosmological/*philosophical* underpinning for its conception of the good society in terms of feudalism, though a feudalism informed deeply by ethical concepts, tended, as we shall see later, to favor a particular way of understanding the series of pairs of polar contrasting terms noted in 2 above. The naturalistic/*Daojia* tendency confined itself, in the main, to considering them as a form of what this book intends to call "dyadic thinking"; the humanistic tendency found it relevant to its own ideological goal to interpret the pairs of polar contrasts in the direction of dualist thinking especially with the contribution of Confucian scholarship during the early Han Dynasty, a form of thinking which is very familiar in Western philosophy, after its initiation by Descartes in the seventeenth century. Very briefly summarized, their difference lies crucially in this—dyadism simply notes their contrastive character, which from the naturalistic perspective, can also at the same time be regarded to complement each other—in other words, there is not only co-existence but they are also capable of mutually helping each other to achieve a certain effect or outcome. Together they form a *Whole* whereas dualism, on the other hand, reads into these polar contrasting terms, the notion of superiority or inferiority, one member of the pair being privileged over the other. That is why the later humanistic/Confucian tendency would add to the schema above, the following associations. Spelled out, its fuller schema would now look as shown below (dualistic terms or their implications are presented in bold font in table 5.7).

Table 5.7.

Unbroken *yang yao*	Broken *yin yao*
Yang 阳—the Sun/sunlight/brightness/ warmth/Summer	*Yin* 阴—the Moon/moonlight/darkness/ cold/Winter
Qian 乾—*Tian* 天 Heaven/**Male/Ruler/ Superior Man**	*Kun* 坤—*Di* 地 Earth/**Female/the Ruled/ the Common Man**
Gang 刚 hard (such as rock/**Ruler/Husband**)	*Rou* 柔 soft (such as water/**Official/Wife**)
Jian 健strong (**Ruler/Husband**)	*Shun* 顺 compliant (**Ruled/Wife**)

As one can see, a new set of social relationships of a specific kind or a new interpretation of an extant pairing had been mapped on to the original series of pairings. The profound differences between dyadic and dualistic thinking will be examined in greater detail in chapter 9 when this schema will be again invoked to explore more explicitly the humanistic/Confucian distortion (by early Han times) of the Contextual-dyadic Mode of thinking.

Conclusion

1. The《易经》/*Yijing*, without a shadow of doubt, began its life as a divinatory text, the handiwork crafted in the main by generations of those in charge of recording and sorting out records of divinatory outcomes.
2. Perhaps unwittingly, this skillful crafting created an early version of Wholism/*Wholism*, of which today's systems thinking is an instantiation. Another way of making this point but in a more general fashion is to say that such skillful crafting led in the end to the emergence of the *Yi* as a set of generalized analytical tools which could be understood independently of the divinatory context altogether (though arising from it) and which could be applied to many other different domains, historically, covering as a matter of fact, all areas of intellectual activities in Chinese culture and civilization, from rulership, to the military, the martial arts, music, calligraphy/painting, to architecture, *medicine*.
3. Such a kind of systematic *gua* arrangement lent itself to be exploited by rationalist thinkers whether of the humanistic Confucian tendency or the naturalistic/*Daojia* tendency, thereby ultimately subverting its original nature. The former introduced the ethical dimension into social/political life in its attempt to give a powerful underpinning to feudalism; the latter in the end provided a cosmological/*philosophical* dimension (but also very importantly incorporated the ethical dimension), hospital to the investigation of phenomena from the *scientific* standpoint as well as to providing a foundation for human conduct in terms of *wuwei*.[39]

4. These two tendencies in the *Yi*, between them, provided the theoretical unifying framework to embrace nearly every aspect of the cultural/intellectual life in the history of Chinese civilization. That is why before one can begin to understand CCM, one must try to understand, as best one can, the impact of the *Zhouyi* upon it. It is in this spirit that this chapter has been written, even though it is obvious that it can deal with a very few and limited aspects only, given the limitation of space, not to mention the limitations of its author's scholarship about this intriguing text.

Notes

1. The *Yi* is comparable to other texts in other cultures, such as the *Bible* or the *Koran*, except for this important difference. The *Yi* is not sacred scripture; those who study it have very different pre-occupations, from seekers of virtue/wisdom, to seekers of assurance and re-assurance. Each finds in it what satisfies his/her respective needs; it is multi-faceted, like a prism, refracting the different kinds of light in the spectrum. The Confucian dictum 仁者见仁, 智者见智, 各得欲见, 各取所需 (*renzhe jian ren, zhizhe jian zhi, ge de yu jian, ge qu suo xu*) as well as the expression 世间万象 /*shi jian wan xiang* could be suitably applied to it.

2. According to Sima Qian, Confucius studied it with great enthusiasm in his later years: 孔子晚而喜易《史记·孔子世家》.

3. Confucius lived during the Spring and Autumn Period, a very troubled time indeed. The Zhou Dynasty was in decline, and as power at the centre weakened, the rulers of feudal states (themselves originally created by the Zhou Dynasty) initiated a vigorous and vicious campaign against one another to gain hegemonic control. Given such a context, it was not a surprise that his *philosophy* and social vision fell on deaf ears in spite of his "hard sell," doing the round of these states to persuade their rulers that his path was the true "dao." It was not until the Han Dynasty (under Han Wudi) that his ideas finally attained political fruition.

4. Even this could be said to be an over-simplification as some scholars also devote efforts to showing what must be the Spacetime (or Timespace as this author prefers—see chapter 10) framework which renders the *Yijing* method of divination intelligible and *scientific*—see Olshin, 2005.

5. Wang, 2012 also appears to have misread Xu Shen's entry on the word *yi*易. Xu Shen's entry used the Lesser Seal Script, the approved script of his day. Although the older Oracle Bone Script was not available to Xu Shen, the meaning of the word *yi*/易 in the Lesser Seal Script which he relied on had the same meaning as that in the Oracle Bone Script. In other words, the meaning was not lost but only the form of the word as it had appeared in the older script. The word *xiyi*/蜥易 (in today's dictionaries, it appears as 蜥蜴) which Wang mentions has nothing to do with the meaning of the word *yi*易 in the context of the *Yijing*, which is our concern here.

6. Nor should the remark be interpreted to mean that what Xu Shen said was wrong or implausible.

7. For what follows, see *Chen, 2006: 557.

8. See *Zhu, 2005: Vol. 1, 179-181.

9. *See Mou, 1998: 37-38.

10. See *Zheng Xuan*, 2013.

11. This is the author's rendering of the cited passage which is found in *Zhu, 2005: Vol.1, 179.

12. See, for instance, Wu, 2003: li-lx; for a very detailed account, see *Pan, 2012: Vol. 1.

13. See *Zeng, 2010.

14. The sequence in a trigram (or hexagram) is always read from the bottom upward; the hexagram continues after the third with the fourth, through the fifth to the sixth *yao*.

15. All Chinese diagrams in this book follow the Chinese tradition of South being on top and North at the bottom; hence East is left and West is right. The compass points are presented in the following sequence: East-South-West-North /东南西北.

16. See Smith, 2008: 46.

17. See Smith, 2008: 46.

18. See Wu, 2003 for an explanation how this change of geographical space takes place.

19. The Chinese text regarding the Later Heaven trigram configuration reads: 万物出乎震，震，东方也。齐乎巽，巽，南方也。齐也者，言万物之絜齐也。离也者，明也,万物皆相见，南方之卦也；圣人南面而听天下，向明而治，盖取诸此也。坤也者,地也,万物皆致养焉，故曰致役乎坤。兑，正秋也，万物之所说也，故曰说言乎兑。战乎乾，乾，西北之卦也，言阴阳相薄也。坎者，水也，正北方之卦也，劳卦也，万物之所归也，故曰劳乎坎。艮，东北之卦也，万物之所成终，而所成始也，故曰成言乎艮。'《说卦》(*Discourses on the Trigrams*). This passage has not been translated by this author but the account given is based on the author's understanding of it. See Wu, 2003: 87 for a translation as well as comments.

20. The passage, on which this summary sketch is based, reads, in the original, as follows: '乾，健也；坤，顺也；震，动也；巽，入也；坎，陷也；离，丽也；艮，止也；兑，说（悦）也。雷以动之，风以散之，日以烜之，艮以止之，兑以说（悦）之。。。'《说卦》(*Discourses on the Trigrams*).

21. The relationship between trigrams and trigrams within hexagrams, between hexagram and other hexagrams are an immensely complicated matter—see, for instance, Wu, 2003; *Zhu, 2005: 18.

22. This interpretation and understanding of the text and of ancient Chinese thought is set out admirably in *Liu, 2008.

23. For a very user-friendly general account, see The Open University, T551. Ackoff's account is intended for readers involved with business and its organization; for one geared to ecological pre-occupations, see Meadows, 2009.

24. On the subject of the relationship between modern philosophy and Modern Science; the implications of the former for the latter in the Western tradition; as well as the concepts of Reductionist and linear thinking, see Lee, 2012b.

25. For a quick read, see Lee, 2008.

26. There is an account of the procedure of setting up a *gua* in Part I, Treatise of the Appended Terms—see original text as cited in *Zhu, 2005: Vol. 1, 6; *Pan, 2013: Vol. 1, 78-89. For a version in English, see Wu, 2003: 22-23.

27. See Wang, 2012: 29 for an alternative account, but which according to this book is mistaken.

28. *Zhu, 2005: Vol. 1, 18.

29. *Zhu, 2005: Vol. 1, chapter 1.

30. *Zhu, 2005: Vol. 1, 18.

31. Wu, 2003: 341.

32. *Zhu, 2005: Vol. 1, 35.

33. This author has added what is within the square brackets in order to render the sentence intelligible in English as far as its logic is concerned.

34. See also Rutt, 1999.

35. As cited by *Zhu, 2005: Vol. 1, 21.

36. See Chan, 2014.

37. See Roth, 2014; this aspect has already been covered in chapter 2.

38. See also chapter 17 on 天*Tian* in the *Xunzi*. For a brief but succinct account of the *Xunzi*, see Robins, 2014.

39. After all, it is not for no good reason that the *Laozi* also goes under the title, *Daodejing*—to put matters simplistically, as chapter 4 has already shown, one ought to follow the Dao in our behavior to others. In other words, the "ethical" cannot be understood apart from *Ziran*, the "Natural", the Dao.

CHAPTER SIX

The *Yi*

Yin Qi, Yang Qi, Yinyang, *and the* Yao-gua *Model*

Deconstructing the Words *Yin* and *Yang*

A pair of concepts which are integral to the cosmology/*philosophy* of the *Yijing*, although not directly mentioned by the text, is *yin*/阴and *yang*/阳. Some sinologists appear to think that these words do not exist either in the Oracle Bone Script or even in the Bronze Script,[1] but they do. *Yang*/阳looks like this (Version I).

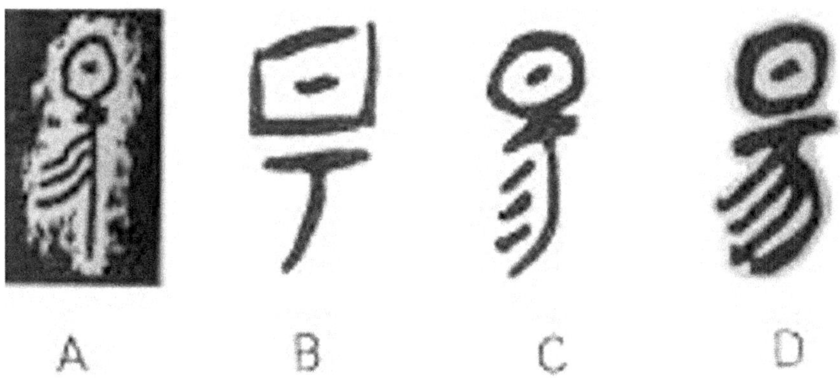

Figure 6.1. Version I of "yang"

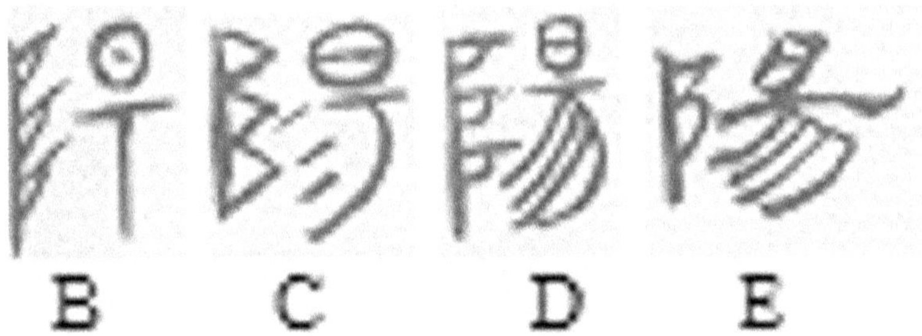

Figure 6.2. Version II of "yang"

or like this (Version II).

In *fanti* which is the unmodified form of the Standard Script used in Taiwan today, the word for *yang* looks like this: 陽. A in Version I is the very earliest form of writing the word; one of its components shows a round sun on top of what looks like a pole to which some fluttering streamers have been tied—a scholar in the Tang dynasty said that it was pronounced as *yang*. This first form is even older than the Oracle Bone Script as by the late Shang Dynasty, it had evolved to look like B (Versions I and II), which, indeed, is the Oracle Bone Script version of the word. Carving with a knife on shell/bone meant that the scribe found it difficult to create circles and curvy lines—hence the circle became square (or at least squarish) and the streamers in Version I were dispensed with. C is the Bronze Script (in both versions), where the change to clay from shell/bone made it feasible for the scribe to restore the circle and the streamers. D is the Lesser Seal Script version, looking very much like the word 昜 which occurs in the text, the *Yijing*, in Version I. E is the Clerical Script.[2]

Below are the various versions of the word for *yin*, the counter-part of *yang*.

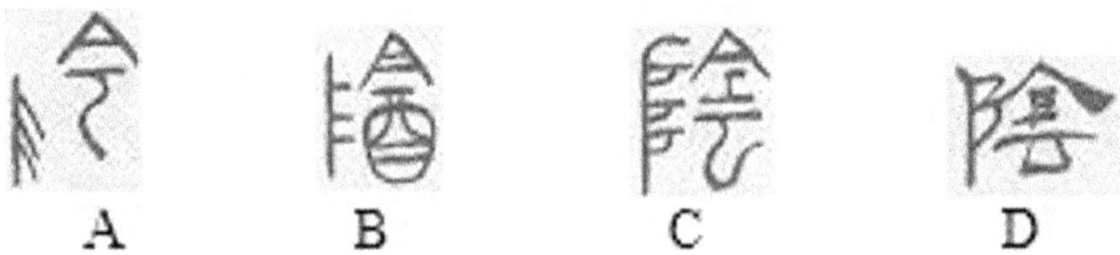

Figure 6.3. Character "yin" in various scripts

A is the Oracle Bone Script; the right component stands for dark clouds, masking the sun, as well as donating its sound to the whole word. B is the Bronze, C the Lesser Seal, and D the Clerical Script which is no different from today's unmodified *fanti*, looking like this 陰.[3]

A careful study shows that the left hand component of the different forms of these two words for *yin* and *yang*, is 阝, which the word 阜/*fu* takes when it acts as a radical/部首/*bushou* for another word; one of its meanings is hill or mountain (if one were to rotate 阝 ninety degrees counter-clockwise, with the vertical stroke becoming the horizontal base, with the "bumps" standing for peaks, then that component could be said to represent a mountain range). This then alerts one to the possible meanings of the words, *yin* and *yang*. To appreciate this, one must turn again to that indissoluble link between astronomy and geography in Chinese thought, as they had to do with the relationship between the Sun casting its light as well as its shade during the day/year on certain specific geographical locations. China is in the northern hemisphere; its physical geography is such that its major geological features stretch from West to East (certainly its large rivers flow in such a direction). Under such circumstances, when the Sun shines, its light falls mainly on the southern slopes of a mountain, rarely on the northern slope; that face which enjoys sunlight/sunshine is the *yang*/southern side and that which is outside the sunshine zone is the *yin*/northern side. Locations and even different states in Chinese history would be divided into two types, *yang* and *yin*. For instance, the ancient state of 鲁/Lu was to the south of 泰山 *Taishan*, while the state of 齐/Qi was to the north; hence in the *Shiji*, we find that these two states were referred to in the following terms: 泰山之阳则鲁，其阴则齐 (《史记·货殖传》) which may be translated (by this author) as: "The state which is on the *yang* (that is, the southern) slope of Taishan is called Lu, while that which is on the *yin* (that is the northern) slope of the mountain is called Qi." Xu Shen, the Han lexicographer, primarily referred to this meaning of *yang*. Several towns in China incorporate this character in their names, such as 衡阳/Hengyang which indicates that the town is on the southern slope of the Heng Mountain.

As far as sunlight and its relationship with rivers are concerned, the ancient Chinese observed that sunlight fell on the northern bank of the river, while the southern bank remained in the shade. Hence the southern bank was *yin*; examples of place names in China abound such as 华阴/Huayin, the shady/southern bank of the Hua River, 淮阴/Huaiyin, the shady/southern bank of the Huai River. In the same spirit, there is a place called 渭阳/Weiyang (whose name could be found in as early a text as the *Shijing* (poems dating from the eleventh to the eighth century BCE) which was on the northern bank of the Wei River. This means that from knowledge of a place name, whether the place mentioned contains a mountain or a river, one can infer its location, whether it is to be found on the southern or northern bank of a river or slope of a mountain. *Yang* comes to stand, in general, for the Sun, for the sunny southern slope of a mountain but the sunny northern bank of a river/lake; *mutatis mutandis*, *yin* stands for the Moon (which is not itself the source of light and heat), the shady northern slope of a mountain but the southern bank of a river/lake.

Derived from these correlations between sunlight and geographical locations are expressions that call any position in the shade *yin*, such as the shade under a tree (树阴/*shuyin*), drying something in the shade (阴干/*yingan*) and so on. Other kinds of derivation involve associating *yin* with being damp, as a spot which gets no sun would be damp, with anything hidden, not in the public gaze, or something concave in shape. It is obvious also why the Chinese call a day when the sun is hidden behind clouds 阴天/*yin tian*, while an atmosphere which is sombre and heavy is called 阴沉/*yinchen*; and a person with bad intentions or evil ideas 阴险/*yinxian*.

The *Zhouli kaokong ji*/《周礼·考工记· 轮人》(a Warring States text which constitutes a manual of the various crafts) has something interesting to tell us about how the ancient Chinese appreciated the implications of *yin qi* and *yang qi* in terms of sunlight or its absence as far as plant growth is concerned. It says that one ought carefully to mark, on a tree just felled, which side faced the sun, as the fibers on that side were denser, and hence stronger, whereas that side in shadow would not be as strong, such that before use, one ought to expose it to heat in order to strengthen it. This is not to say that the ancient Chinese had articulated the theory of photosynthesis, but it clearly showed that they were not unaware that heat and the light of the Sun do have a great influence on plant growth and the quality of such growth. Such knowledge could ultimately have influenced the *philosophical* meaning of *yang* in the polar yet complementary pair of notions called *yin* and *yang*. But this is already jumping too far ahead, as we shall be returning to this distinctive theme in Chinese cosmology and *philosophy* as well as Chinese *science* and its methodology.

The brief philological exploration above illustrates yet again that the ancient Chinese were close observers of their environment, of where exactly sunlight fell, and where the shady areas of a landscape were. They also had observed that sunlight hours were longest in Summer, shortest in Winter, that the Sun was strongest in Summer and weakest in Winter, that when the Sun disappeared below the horizon or set in the West, darkness fell, that when the Sun rose in the East above the horizon, brightness appeared. It is obvious that ancient peoples throughout world history would have noticed what the ancient Chinese had noticed. However, the ancient Chinese appeared more dedicated than most to constructing a systematic theoretical structure resting upon such mundane empirical data. For instance, the above account showed that from such a lowly observational basis, they then proceeded to another level of observation, the link between the quality of wood with its exposure to either the sunny or shady side of the tree as it stood before it was felled. This level of association implied an embryonic understanding of the power of the Sun in terms of its heat and light on the quality of plant growth.

Constructing the *Gua* out of *Yin Qi* and *Yang Qi*

It bears repeating that the *Yijing* began its existence as a divinatory text; it also bears repeating that credit must be given to those, whoever they might have been, who crafted the trigrams by basing it on the *yao*爻, either as *yang yao* or as *yin yao*, as a theoretical way forward in order to bring order, coherence and economy into the vast empirical data yielded by using the *Yijing* method of divination. This process of going beyond merely the empirical to the theoretical level of representation was clearly an attempt at systematization, although it is also obviously correct to note that the *gua* model of systematization, did not conform to the model endorsed by Western philosophy and science in terms of axiomatization. In the Western tradition, ever since Euclid's *Elements*, the highest form of systematization is axiomatization; consequently any other model which falls short of this standard could/would be judged to be defective as science, or even as falling outside the domain of science altogether. Leaving aside this thesis of misjudged "high-mindedness," let us here simply focus on the *gua* model as an alternative model of systematization which should be given a serious hearing. In the philosophy of science as understood today, it is respectable to judge a theory in terms of methodological criteria such as unity, economy, and explanatory scope.[4] One wishes to argue here that the *gua* model satisfies them.

The term "science" could and should be understood in the wider sense of *wissenschaft*, and not merely in the narrower Anglo-Saxon, Baconian understanding of the term. *Wissenschaft* means systematic knowledge, and systematic knowledge in turn implies that the theory in question provides a unifying framework. So if the *gua* model is an attempt at systematization, then it would obviously satisfy the criterion of unity. (As a *gua* consists of three *yaos*, it may be more appropriate to call the model the *Yao-gua* Model.)

The criterion of economy or parsimony is also called Ockham's Razor,[5] although William of Ockham/Occam (1287?–1347), a late medieval monk and philosopher was not the only person in the history of philosophy to have used or implied the principle. His is sometimes formulated as the idea that entities should not be multiplied unnecessarily. There are several versions and interpretations of this principle.[6] One interpretation reads as follows: of two competing theories, choose that which invokes fewer (theoretical) entities over one which invokes more in explaining broadly the same range of data. Another reads: when there are two competing theories that make the same predictions, the simpler one is the better one. In the history of Western astronomy, the case of Copernican heliocentrism and Ptolemaic geocentrism[7] could perhaps be cited as an illustration—put simplistically, to render the latter capable of accounting for certain key astronomical data based on observation, its defenders were forced to add additional terms such as *deferent* and *epicycle* into the main theory, whereas the former had no need for such terms and what they stood for. Hence heliocentrism is said to be preferable to geocentrism.

However, the reader must immediately be reminded of a distinction between what the author of a text had written and the formulations extracted from the text by later scholars—in reality, the formulation usually attributed to William of Ockham (entities should not be multiplied unnecessarily) cannot be found in his writing, although in spirit it does not depart totally from what the author meant. The formulation, as it stands, is taken out of the general philosophical context in which William of Ockham's thoughts are embedded.[8] It is perhaps best to use the formulation as a methodological guideline rather than a methodological entailment of William of Ockham's specific philosophy of nominalism. With these qualifications, let us proceed to assess in what sense the *Yao-gua* Model could be said to satisfy Ockham's Razor as a methodological requirement. Even at first glance, it looks very economical in the theoretical terms it invokes. At the most fundamental level, we have already seen what the model invoked in chapters 3 and 4 via that famous passage found in chapter 42 of the *Laozi*: The Dao engenders one, one engenders two, two engenders three, three engenders *Wanwu*. As already observed, Chinese scholarship equated "one" with *Taiji* 太极 of the *Yi*. "Two" is understood to refer to the two types of *qi*, namely, *yin qi* and *yang qi*. The meaning of "three" is understood to refer to that peculiar relationship and interaction between these types of *qi* (of which more exploration will be made later), pointing to the concept of *Yinyang*. "Three engenders *Wanwu*" is understood to refer to *Yinyang* accounting for the emergence of *Wanwu* (the universe, in its widest meaning).

In *Part I, Treatise on the Appended Terms* of the *Ten Wings* of the *Zhouyi*, a passage reads: 易有太极，是生两仪，两仪生四象，四象生八卦。《周易·系辞上》. This author renders it as: "The notion of change presupposes that of *Taiji* while *Taiji* manifests itself as *yin* and *yang*, *yin* and *yang* in turn engender four images which between them engender *bagua*/eight trigrams." This could be read as an expansion of the *Laozi* passage. If one studies the two passages closely, one would notice that while the *Laozi* focuses on cosmology, the *Ten Wings* focuses on the construction of the *gua* to account for such a cosmology. In the *Yao-gua* Model, the terms introduced are intended as images (*xiang*) to encapsulate the cosmology as articulated in the *Laozi*.[9]

At **Level 1**, T*aiji* as *wu*/the Dao/the Nebulous Void is represented by the image or symbol, the outline of a circle.

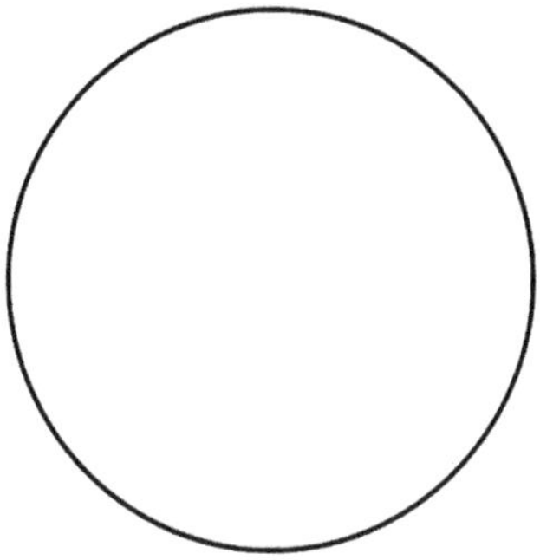

Figure 6.4. Wuji/Taiji

At **Level 2**, when *Taiji* manifests itself as *yin qi* and *yang qi*, the image takes the familiar form;[10] strictly speaking it should not be called the *Taiji* symbol but more accurately perhaps as the *Yinyang-Taiji* symbol (or *Liangyitaijitu*/两仪太极图).

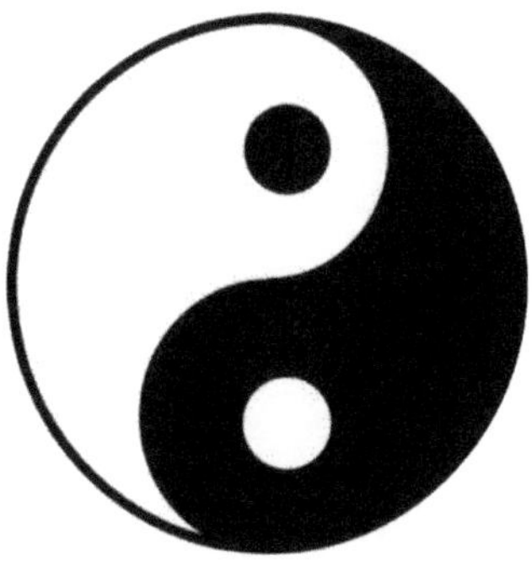

Figure 6.5. Liangyitaijitu

In *Yao-gua* Model the *yin* and *yang* (*liangyi*两仪) are thus represented: — 阳 爻/*yangyao*， - - 阴爻/*yinyao*.

Level 3 of *yin* and *yang* engendering the four images (*liangyi sheng sixiang*/两仪生四象) is represented in table 6.1 below.

Table 6.1.

taiyang **太阳** (Greater Yang) ⚌	*taiyin* **太阴** (Greater Yin) ⚏
shaoyang **少阳** (Lesser Yang) ⚎	*shaoyin* **少阴** (Lesser Yin) ⚍

The introduction of an image with two *yaos* at Level 2 delivers four possibilities, permitting a degree of complexity not available at Level 2.

Level 4 of engendering permits even greater complexity as it involves three *yaos* leading to the formation of the familiar eight trigrams which stand for eight different kinds of natural phenomena or states of affairs in the world.

The introduction of three *yaos* (in order to create a trigram) is not arbitrary. Chapter 1 shows that they stand for Heaven, Earth and Humans, the three powers/*sancai*—the top *yao* represents Heaven, the bottom *yao* Earth, and the middle *yao* Humans. This ordering was itself based on the observation that while humans lived on the surface of Earth, the sky (Heaven) was above Earth and therefore Humans on Earth. As observed in that chapter, the three *yaos* constitute the identity of a trigram which encapsulates for Chinese culture and civilization true wisdom, the wisdom that comes from grasping the Dao which, in turn, comes from knowing the specific *daos* of Heaven, Earth and Humans, as well as the relationship between them.

Below shows what the *Yao-gua* Model of the trigrams looks like.[11]

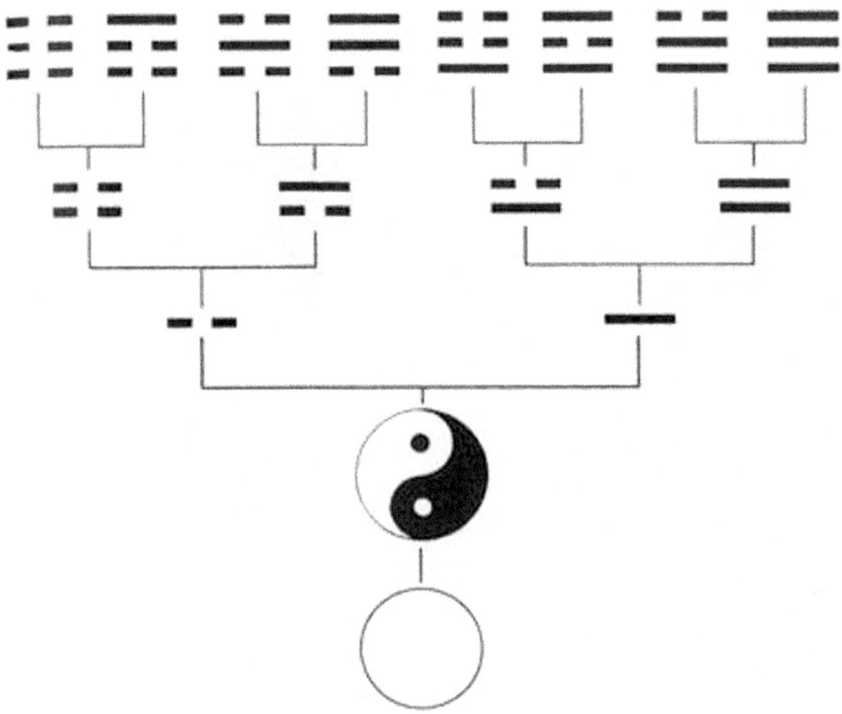

Figure 6.6. ***The* Yao-gua *Model of the trigrams***

Observe that ultimately only one basic term is required by the *Yao-gua* Model, namely, *Taiji*. If the *Laozi* account of the Dao were to be read in conjunction with the Ten Wings, then *Taiji* could be construed as *wu* (the domain of great openness), with *Yuanqi* as well as *yin qi* and *yang qi* as *you*, with *wu* engendering *you*. In this sense, it is plausible to argue that the *Yao-gua* Model satisfies the criterion of economy, when compared to another model which might invoke several different theoretical entities, each entity attempting to account for a particular phenomenon represented by each of the eight trigrams, such as a god of thunder (*Zhen*), a god of fire (*Li*), a god of water (*Kan*) and so on.

Thus set up, the *Yao-gua* Model can be read as a set of analytical tools for ordering a vast range of material in whatever domain one wants to be explore, be it astronomy (or *science* in general), martial arts, military matters, *medicine*, or politics. As an instance of this fruitful methodological flexibility, go back to the example of the impact of *yin* and *yang qi* on plant growth and fiber density. In modern biology today, one studies annual rings. But what are annual rings but the impact of the passage of the two types of *qi* in the course of the four seasons of a year—in other words, the annual rings are nothing but the ecological imprint of *yin qi* and *yang qi*. In Spring, cells in the organism grow big, even bigger in Summer; in Autumn they become smaller and smaller still in Winter. The bigger cells are lighter in color and the smaller ones darker. The study of annual rings in trees, today, is called dendrochronology;[12] scientists by studying them can obtain information about the weather conditions of the seasons of each year, whether they were normal for the time of year, or too wet, too dry. Such scientists are studying no more than the marks left by *yin qi* and *yang qi* during years gone by. Similarly one can study the teeth of horses to determine their ages, as *yin* and *yang* have also left their imprints on their teeth. One can also tell the age of a tortoise by counting the seasonal/annual rings on its shell. So accurate are these rings in an organism that we can tell the actual age of the tree or the tortoise. There is a fish called *huanghuayu*/黄花鱼 or *shishouyu*/石首鱼[13] with two big bones in its head. By making thin slices of these bones and putting them under powerful microscopes, scientists can study not merely the annual growth rings but also its monthly, not to mention its daily rings. If the fish had found plenty of nutrition that day and it had perhaps happily mated, then the mark would be light but on a bad day, the mark would be darker.[14]

The methodological criterion of explanatory scope when assessed against the *Yao-gua* Model may be said to be satisfied, as it has, indeed, evolved into a general set of analytical tools which can usefully be deployed in numerous different domains of activities both at the theoretical as well as practical levels. However what is important to grasp is that even as a generalized analytical tool, it is not content-free (in the way Western formal logic is content-free)—the model never departs from *yin* and *yang* (and hence *Taiji*), although its various applications may be understood in somewhat different ways depending on the context in which they are invoked (we shall be exploring this feature later). In this way, the model, nevertheless, permits a whole range of otherwise disparate material to be brought within its explanatory scope.

To grasp these points better, let us look again at the following schema which we have already offered in table 5.1. Each trigram invokes a particular compass point (geography/location/Space), a particular season or sub-season in the course of a year or even a day (astronomy/Time), a particular natural phenomenon (meteorology and geography), a particular reflection of the relation between *yin* and *yang* (as *Yinyang*, a concept in *philosophy*) at a specific moment of time in the year. In other words, one can say that the *Yua-gua* Model offered a Timespace framework which will be explored in greater depth in chapter 10. (Note that this framework is called "Timespace" and not "Spacetime" in order to mark a striking difference between the ancient Chinese conception and that endorsed in modern physics and contemporary Western philosophy since Einstein's theories of relativity.)

The foregoing discussion may have then made a case for saying that the *Yao-gua* Model can be meaningfully assessed in terms of the methodological criteria of unity, economy, and explanatory scope, tests which the model could be said to have passed. However, what it has failed to address is the concept of *Yinyang* itself which goes beyond the concepts of *yin* and *yang* to the inter-active relationships between them. This will be done in the following chapter (chapter 7) when it would be examined in association with another concept, namely, that of *Wuxing*/五行—an exploration of *Yinyang-Wuxing*/阴阳五行 will show even more clearly that the *Yao-gua* Model rises above any one specific domain of enquiry, be this divination, astronomy and is, indeed, a set of analytical/methodological tools for any domain of activity which involves theory and praxis.

Doing *Science*: the *Yao-gua* Model and the Three Meanings of *Yi*

The above section has commented upon the *Yao-gua* Model for doing *science* as *wissenschaft*; we next need to explore further the relation between such a model and the three meanings of *yi* of which a brief account has been given in chapter 5.

How could the relationship among these three meanings be articulated? Look first at the relationship between the first and second meanings of 简易 and变易. 简易/*jianyi* should not be translated literally as "easy/not difficult" in the sense of readily grasped by someone not very bright. *Jianyi* is to be understood as the Essence of *Yi*, which one comes to grasp by investigating the nature of 变易/*bianyi*, making explicit what is already implicit in it. According to *Xici* 系辞 (one of the Treatises in the *Ten Wings*), *jianyi* arises from the significance of the two *guas*, *Qian* and *Kun*, which together embody the Essence of *Yi*. And what do these two trigrams/hexagrams themselves embody or refer to? They respectively refer to *yang* and *yin*. *Yin* and *yang* refer in turn to two types of *qi* which stand as polar extremes of each other; at the same time, they are, nevertheless, inter-related, as they mutually inter-act to produce change. This is the relationship between *jianyi* and *bianyi*—the former arises from the latter. Everything in the universe is the product of processes of change but these processes of change come about because of the intrinsic character of *yi*, of *Qiankun*/乾坤, of *Yinyang*. It says more or less what the *Laozi* (chapter 48) has said: 为学日益, 为道日损/*wei xue ri yi, wei dao ri sun* which may be rendered (by this author) as: "One attains the heights of knowledge by adding to it day by day (*you*); on the contrary, one gets to the *Dao* by paring down all that is absolutely unnecessary in arriving at understanding the world." For instance, a painter who adds more and more colors to create a painting is operating on the level of *wei xue ri yi*; the less colors the painter uses, and the lighter the colour s/he chooses, the more does the painting get closer to the ideal of *wei dao ri sun*. In the case of grasping *yi*, it would involve getting to the *fons et origo* of all existence (*Metaphysics*) and knowledge (*Epistemology*), that is, of *yin* and *yang*, of *Qian* and *Kun* as well as the relationship between the polarities in each pair. It is in this sense that the Dao is simple, and that the Essence of *Yi* is simple; it also implies that the Dao once grasped and understood could be readily applied to any situation to help us analyze it and to find a solution for whatever problem arising from such a state of affairs.[15]

We next look at a possible relationship between the second and third meanings of the term *yi*, namely, 变易/Change/*bianyi* and No Change/不易/*buyi*. As already observed, the basic meaning of *yi* is change which could be observed at the empirical level in terms of an intercourse between *yin qi* and *yang qi* and their resulting consequences. The ancient Chinese also had a habit of pushing a term beyond its initial empirical reference to another level, more abstract and theoretical. It may then seem plausible to argue that the concept of change (having extrapolated itself from empirical observation of meteorological variability) in turn would imply the concept of constancy, as behind the pattern of change at a more superficial level stands constancy at a deeper level—if it is a *Law of Nature* that everything is constantly changing, then it in turn implies a meta-law of No Change. Discussion in chapter 4 shows that the Chinese mode of thinking always seeks to establish a partner-concept which stands behind another concept to form a pairing—in the

Laozi, for instance, we have discussed the *you/wu* pairing. That same tendency obtains here—behind change would stand a partner-concept but which is the polar opposite of change, and that is, no change. In other words, to grasp the concept of Change, one must grasp at the same time that of No Change, just as to grasp the concept of *you*, one must grasp that of *wu*. One must bear in mind that Chinese *philosophy* understands such polar contrasts very differently from Western philosophy; the former understands them in terms of complementarity whereas the latter in terms of mutual exclusivity. This fundamental difference will be clarified and explained in chapter 9.[16]

To help readers only familiar with the Western mode of thinking to more easily grasp the relationship between Change and its polar opposite, No Change, we would like to draw attention to a slightly more familiar problem in Western philosophy, namely, the relationship between inductive logic and the principle/notion of the Uniformity of Nature. Inductive logic tells us that we may extrapolate from repeated and widespread observation of two things, A and B (such as A is a swan and B is its white color), associated with each other to the generalization "All As (swans) are B (white)" (I). Historically, we had great confidence in this generalisation until Captain Cook by a twist of fortune landed in Western Australia, and saw birds swimming in the river, looking and behaving exactly like the white swans, but their color happened to be black. As a result of such encounters, we now have revised our earlier generalization (I) to a new more modest and nuanced claim "Some swans (those in the northern hemisphere) are white, some swans are black (those in the southern hemisphere)" (II).[17] (I) cannot accommodate variability but (II) can. However, conceding that variability exists in Nature does not necessarily mean that standing behind the variations is not a principle at work which may be called the Uniformity of Nature. In other words, it is a principle which we assume to be correct in order to make sense of variability. Another way of putting it is to say that we, the observers (that is, Western Europeans, or people living in the northern hemisphere), had made a mistake about Nature in arriving at generalization (I) which turned out to be unreliable—our evidence for saying that all swans were white was not comprehensive enough, our knowledge base of the subject matter was too limited. After all, we came to that conclusion when we had never been to the Southern continents or even known of their existence and what life forms we might find there. In the light of Cook's observation, we then came to know that Nature exhibits variation in the color of swans. We are right to revise our knowledge claim about swans (epistemology) but we need not doubt that Nature is constant. We can with confidence predict that the next native swan we see in Western Australia would be black, not white, and that the next native swan we see in the Northern hemisphere would be white, not black. We do not doubt that Nature stays constant or uniform, because patterns in Nature repeat themselves. Without this axiom of constancy, no science (whether modern Western or ancient Chinese) is possible. In other words, behind Change is No Change, as the *Yi* and the *Laozi* appeared to imply.

Scientific methodology as understood today includes the critical methodological requirement of Repeatability. This is to say that we can have confidence in the results of an experiment only if the same experiment (under similar conditions) carried out by other teams of scientists elsewhere, preferably spread over different geographical regions would yield the same results. "Good" science demands this degree of epistemological caution. That is fair; however, does this methodological requirement itself make sense without presupposing the Principle of the Uniformity of Nature or constancy in Nature? If the world were not assumed to remain constant, the demand for Repeatability would itself be unintelligible. Not only would there be no "good" science, there would be no science at all. Indeed, even normal, humble, ordinary daily activities could not meaningfully be carried out. We need to eat, to breathe, to drink, to keep ourselves alive. But why eat bread or rice, drink water, if we do not hold that such things would remain constant and therefore continue to nourish and sustain us? We do not allow empirical observations to undermine this Principle, as we have already seen in the case of Cook and the black swans. We do not give it up; instead, we simply revise our database (epistemology). For this reason, it may be fitting to call such a principle a metaphysical principle, in the derived "Aristotelian" sense of "metaphysics" as that domain of investigation which is "over"/ "beyond"/"above" physics. It is what makes physics (and therefore other sciences) possible and intelligible.[18]

Another way of elucidating the meanings of *yi* in terms of No Change standing behind Change, which people today brought up in the tradition of Modern Science may find easier to grasp, is to say that "the laws of physics remain unchanged with time." As Cox and Forshaw, 2012: 118, put it: "That statement (that the laws of physics remain unchanged with time) does not mean that things do not happen, which would obviously be silly. Instead it means that if Maxwell's equations hold true today, then they ought also to hold true tomorrow. You can replace 'Maxwell's equations' with any fundamental law of physics . . . "

Yet another way to illustrate the meanings of *yi* as Change and No Change is to see the past as exemplifying the latter, as the past is not something one could change, the present or now could be said to be poised between Change and No Change, while the future contains potential for change and/or no change. Chapter 7 will look at yet another possibility of understanding the polar contrasting pair.

A perfect concrete example to illustrate the three meanings of *yi* is in terms of that well-known artefact called the chopsticks. Chopsticks operate as a pair, one of which is held firm and still while the other is flexible and movable. They form polar contrasts, yet they harmoniously form a functioning *Whole*. The rigid one (No Change) is the *yin* component, the movable one (Change) is the *yang* component—in the absence of the *yang* chopstick, the *yin* becomes irrelevant; *mutatis mutandis*, in the absence of the *yin* chopstick, the *yang* becomes irrelevant. Together as a harmonious functioning *Whole*, they manifest the *essential yi/jianyi* which embodies the notion of simplicity itself. With a pair of chopsticks, one can pick or lift up any food (thing) which is solid (semi-solid), one can use it even to cook with; it is a multi-purpose tool yet it is easy to carry about, convenient to use. It may be said to be an embodiment of the Dao in action at the level of artifacts/technology. If one had to nominate an iconic symbol of Chinese culture and civilization, it would be hard to ignore the chopstick, as it embodies not only *Yinyang* but also so brilliantly the three meanings of *yi* in the *Yijing*. Furthermore, it brings out an aspect of simplicity in the notion of *jianyi*, that is, beauty as simplicity. Indeed, it is the perfect marriage of utility, beauty, and simplicity. In this context, one cannot help but be reminded of William Morris (1834–96), the Marxist/socialist political philosopher *cum* designer (amongst his many faceted talents) who had written: "If you want a golden rule that will fit everybody, this is it: Have nothing in your houses that you do not know to be useful, or believe to be beautiful;" "Simplicity of life, even the barest, is not a misery, but the very foundation of refinement . . ."[19] Morris turned out to be a follower of the *Laozi* without knowing it himself. With regard to holding the chopsticks, that which stays rigid is *yin* and that which moves is *yang*.

Sun-driven Cosmology, *Yinyang* metaphysics

From the preceding sections and chapters, it is plausible to infer that Chinese cosmology and the *philosophy* based on it may be said to be a Sun-driven one. This claim is to be distinguished from that of heliocentrism, which is generally acknowledged to have ushered in modern astronomy, and indeed, even Modern Science, by Copernicus. The ancient Chinese were not so concerned with the exact location of the Sun and Earth in what today we call our Solar System;[20] rather they were more pre-occupied with the relationship between Earth and Sun with regard to the notion of *Qi*. We have argued that *Qi* is the fundamental ontological category in Chinese *philosophy*; furthermore, that *Qi* exists in two modes, *Qi*-in-dissipating and *Qi*-in-concentrating modes. Chapter 3 also argues that the mutual transformation of the one into the other could be said to be an analogue of thermodynamics (at least of the First Law of Thermodynamics). *Qi* is also distinguished in terms of *yang qi* and *yin qi*. These two kinds of *qi* have an empirical base (we can feel the former, typically, in Summer, at noon and the latter in Winter, in the middle of the night), although it is also correct to observe that they went beyond empiricism to acquire abstract/theoretical status, as *Yinyang*. At the empirical level, the ancient Chinese knew that *yang qi* as a force in the world could/would come only from the Sun, that *yin qi* would be found when *yang qi* declined, progressively retreating as the season changed from Autumn to Winter or as twilight turned into the depth of night. In their language, Spring was the time when *yin qi* began its retreat and *yang qi* reappeared at Earth's surface, that the increase of *yang qi* was what brought forth new growth in plants, renewed reproductive activities on the parts of animals. From this, they inferred that, *au fond*, *Wanwu* on Earth came into existence and could sustainably maintain themselves because of *yang qi*. However, they inferred that *yang qi* was only a necessary condition of Life on Earth, and were careful not to infer that it was both a necessary and sufficient condition—on the contrary, they inferred that *Wanwu* was only possible because both *tian qi* (*yang qi*) and *di qi* (*yin qi*) were both present and interacted harmoniously in a complementary manner as *Yinyang*. Their empirical observations, in other words, generated their *metaphysics*, but in turn their *metaphysics* did not abandon the empirical base. Hence, they held that *yin* and *yang*, though existing as polar contrasts, were not mutually exclusive but complementary to each other—indeed, the one cannot endure without the other, as pure *yin* and pure *yang* were, so to speak, only ideal types but which empirically did not and could not exist, that, therefore, within *yin* was *yang* and within *yang* was *yin*, even when *yin* and *yang* were each at their respective maximum—look again at the *yinyang liangyitu*.

While Chinese cosmology is Sun-driven, its *metaphysics* is not, as the latter transcended the empirical base in articulating a world-view which is not a dualistic, but a dyadic one—Chapter 9 which explores this in depth argues that the fundamental Chinese mode of thinking is what may be called the Contextual-dyadic Mode. However, at the cosmological/empirical level, it remains correct to say that it is *yang qi* which makes it possible (but only as a necessary condition) for *Wanwu* to emerge and to thrive. Without *yang qi*, there would only be *yin qi* in whose presence alone, *Wanwu* would not have emerged and/or thrived (not a sufficient condition), no more than *Wanwu* would have emerged and/or thrived in the presence alone of *yang qi*. Empirically, *Wanwu* required the conjoint presence of *yin qi* and *yang qi* to evolve, survive, and thrive just as metaphysically, it is *Yinyang* alone which could account for the existence and flourishing of *Wanwu*. However, in terms of *thermodynamics*/thermodynamics, it is *yang qi* (as solar energy) which provides the force which drives the cycle of birth/growth/maturity/death for *Wanwu* in the biotic domain—in this and only in this limited sense, one may say that *yang* is *primus inter pares* [21] in the relationship between *yin qi* and *yang qi* at the empirical level. Metaphysically, *yang* does not occupy such a status, as the concept, *Yinyang*, within the Contextual-dyadic Mode of thinking obviously makes clear.

In empirical terms, in the domain of astronomy, amongst all the heavenly bodies known to the ancient Chinese, three were singled out for special attention—these are Sun, Earth and Earth's Moon and the relationship between them. The main relationship was between Sun and Earth, as it was this set of relationships which led them to discover three fundamental *Laws of Nature*, namely *zhouye jielü* (the daily rhythm of change between the two *qis*), *sishi jielü* (the annual rhythm of change) and *zhou er fu shi*/Cyclic Reversion which in turn led them to formulate their *philosophy* of *Yinyang* as well as process-ontology. (On *Yinyang*/*Yinyang-Wuxing*, see chapter 7, on process-ontology, chapter 8 for further exploration.) The *xiang* (for details about this mode of thinking, see chapter 9) as shown in the figure below brilliantly captures both the cosmological (empirical) aspect of physical reality as well as the *metaphysical* aspect of *philosophical* reality as understood by the ancient Chinese. What follows (figure 6.7) shows *yin qi* and *yang qi* in terms of the *Sixiang* (see table 6.1) and their relationship with Sun and Earth at different seasons of the year and different times of the day.

The details of this *xiang* will be explained in chapter 7.

What follows is a cartoonish *xiang* of the empirical relationship among Sun, Earth and Moon as presented in today's astronomical maps.

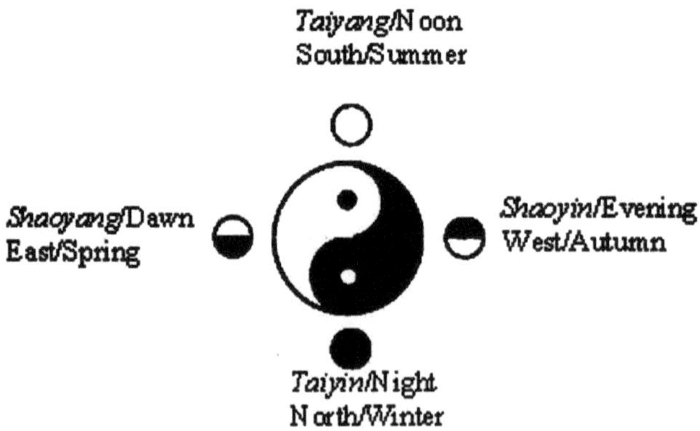

Figure 6.7. Yin qi and yang qi in terms of the Liangyitaijitu showing the relationship of Sun and Earth at different seasons of the year and different times of the day.

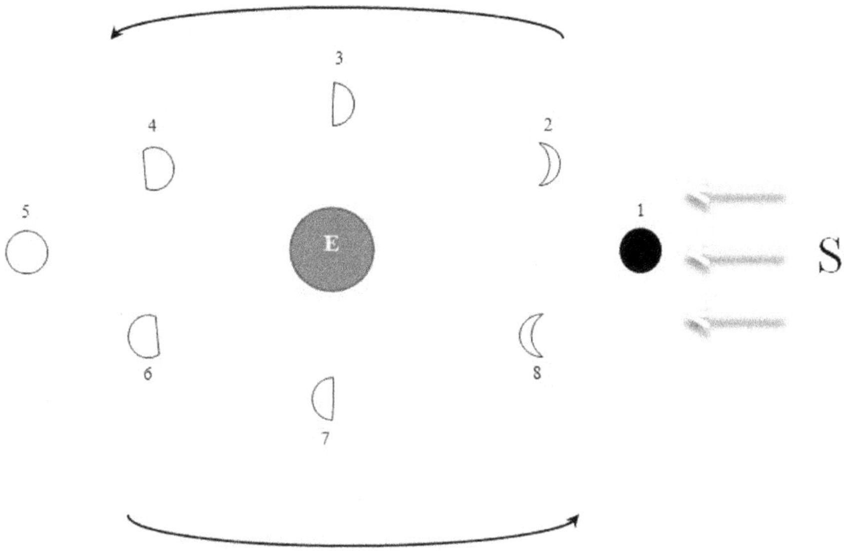

Figure 6.8. Relationship between Sunk Earth, Moon.

In the figure above:

S = Sun; E = Earth.

1: New Moon; 2: Crescent Moon; 3: Quarter Moon; 4: Gibbous Moon; 5: Full Moon; 6: Gibbous Moon; 7: Quarter Moon; 8: Crescent Moon.

On the waxing/waning cycles, the phases show only those parts visible to us on the surface of Earth.

As for the empirical relationship among Sun, Earth and Moon, for the ancient Chinese, the most important two moments lie with the New Moon and the Full Moon. The former was referred to as 朔日/*shuori* (1 in figure above); it occurred on the first day of the Chinese (lunar)[22] month, when Moon got in between Earth and Sun, and hence, could not be observed from Earth's surface. The latter was called望日/*wangri* (5 in figure above) which occurred on the fifteenth (or sixteenth) day of the lunar month, when the Moon was aligned in such a way with Sun that a whole face of it could be observed from Earth's surface. Another two aspects which were significant are the Waxing half of the Lunar Cycle (the upper arrow in figure above from right to left) and the Waning half (the lower arrow from left to right).

The *raison d'être* for this more limited focus lies as follows: *shuori* stands for the maximum of *yin qi*; *wangri* stands for the maximum of *yang qi*; the waxing half of the Lunar Cycle from after 1, through 2 to 5 for the gradual decline of *yin qi* with corresponding increase of *yang qi*; the waning half from after 5, through 6 to 1 stands for the gradual decline of *yang qi* with corresponding increase of *yin qi*. This is analogous to the "waxing" half of the *sishi jielü* (from after Winter Solstice through Spring Equinox to Summer Solstice) as well as of the *zhouye jielü* (*zishi*/子时, striding between 11:00 p.m. to 1:00 a.m. of the following day). The "waning" half of the *sishi jielü* begins just after the Summer Solstice and that of the *zhouye jielü* just after twelve noon. The waning half is, therefore, associated with *yin qi*, and the waxing half of the cycle with *yang qi*. Hence in terms of CCM, during *shuori* only, according to the *Neijing*, one should "tonify" (补/*bu*)[23] *qi* and blood 气血/*qixue* (*qi*-blood); during *wangri*, one should refrain from doing so. This is because one should only use the technique of *bu* when *yin qi* predominates, and *yang qi* is insufficient. The ancient Chinese, however, found that this three-body relationship (Sun/Earth/Moon) to be just as compelling as the two-body relationship (Sun/Earth) in providing them with the basis for generating their *metaphysics* of *Yinyang* and *Yinyang-Wuxing*.

From the above discussion, it seems plausible to conclude that for the ancient Chinese, the empirical and the metaphysical are not mutually exclusive, and hence that their *science* was not exclusive of their *metaphysics* in the way that modern Western science makes it axiomatic that the empirical must not be tainted by the metaphysical. Their cosmology was Sun-driven; however, their *metaphysics* embraced both Sun (brightness and visibility/warmth and light/*yang qi*/*Tian qi*/Fire/movement/growth/development) and Earth (shadiness, darkness and hiddenness/cold/*yin qi*/*Di qi*/Water/tranquillity/maturity/decay). The processes of change in *Wanwu* involved both birth and growth, on the one hand, and maturity and eventual decline/death, on the other; in other words these processes must be understood within a framework of *Yinyang Wholist metaphysics*.

Conclusion

The main points emerging from this chapter are:

1. Paring down to the Essentials of *Yi* means that one would have grasped that standing behind Change is No Change, which could be said to constitute a *Law of Nature*—we shall have occasion later in the book to explore the notion of cyclic reversion in the Chinese mode of thought. Here we mention a quick example to make the point—Winter goes, Spring comes, Summer overtakes Spring as does Autumn Summer, and Winter itself overtakes Autumn (*sishi jielü*). Day follows Night, and Night follows Day (*zhouye jielü*). The changes of the seasons in the year, the changes of brightness and darkness in daily life follow a pat-

tern which we could detect. When one cycle of change ends, another cycle of change begins (*zhou er fu shi*)—therefore, beyond Change stands No Change. This is the Dao from which follows the specific *dao* of Heaven, of Earth; the *Laozi* says humankind must follow the Dao, and that Dao itself follows *Ziran* (of which more later in chapter 7).

2. However, the ancient Chinese did not merely see it as a *Law of Nature* but also went beyond the empirical base to articulate a piece of metaphysics, namely, that a term which appeared to stand for a polar extreme implied its own polar contrast—hence standing behind Change/*bianyi* is No Change/*buyi* or constancy.
3. The *Yao-gua* Model discussed in relation with the three meanings of *yi* reinforces the point which this book focuses on—the *Yi* has evolved beyond being a mere divination text, beyond even merely a text to account for astronomical and geographical phenomena to become a set of analytical tools which could account for phenomena in nearly every domain of activity whether this be biology/ecology, *medicine*, military affairs, martial arts, the fine and performing arts, rulership, and technology in general at the levels of theory and praxis. In other words, the model provided the framework for doing *science* in the sense of *wissenschaft*.
4. This limited discussion of the various meanings of *yi* here and in chapter 5 already signals an absolutely crucial feature of ancient Chinese cosmology/*philosophy* which underpins its account of *science* and *scientific* methodology—the notion of change implies processes at its core, rather than substance, functional rather than structural relationships. This book intends to explore in detail this theme of process-ontology in chapter 8.
5. It has also attempted further to clarify the relationship between Chinese cosmology and Chinese *philosophy*, between the empirical and the metaphysical, a discussion of which, with regard to another related theme, was initiated in chapter 4.

Notes

1. Wang, 2012: 22.

2. This book follows *Chen, 2006: 558–59 and *Zhao, 2006: 459–460 in their attempts at deconstructing the word. A point worth commenting upon is that the word in today's *jianti* looks like this 阳. Some readers may be surprised to know that this version had existed from the Song and Yuan dynasties, and so had an existence of nearly a thousand years before it became officially co-opted since the 1950s into

jianti—for a brief account of the convoluted relationship between *jianti* and *fanti*, see Lee, 2008.

3. This account follows *Zhao, 2006: 470–471.

4. However, one must immediately point out that standard philosophy of science today, by and large, considers these criteria to be secondary, rather than primary; Popper's thesis of falsifiability as a demarcation between science and pseudo-science is principally relied on.

5. See Thorburn , 1915, 1918.

6. See Gibbs and Hiroshi, 1997.

7. For details of the Ptolemaic system, see Van Helden, 1996; see also *Geocentric and heliocentric systems*, 2013.

8. See Spade, 2011 for one brief account of his philosophy in full.

9. For an account of the astronomy upon which the *Taiji* symbol was created, see Tsai, 2013. However, readers beware that Tsai's account of the meaning of *yi*, according to this author, is incorrect.

10. Note that the actual emergence of the *Taiji* symbols itself was late in the history of the *Yi*—in the Song Dynasty.

11. This figure has been adapted from *Pan, 2012: Vol.1: 43.

12. Interestingly, a dendrochronologist is defined as "a scientist who uses tree rings to answer questions about the natural world and the place of humans in its functioning"—see *Tree rings*, 2013.This definition sits snugly within the framework of the *Yao-gua* Model and *Yinyang philosophy*.

13. It belongs to the Sciaenidae, a family of fish which includes drums, croakers or hardheads.

14. See *Hao, 2011.

15. Zhuge Liang诸葛亮 (181–234 CE), considered by many Chinese (at the popular level) to be the most famous strategist in Chinese military history, was reputed to be able to divine so accurately because he understood so well the principles of change involved in the *Yi*: He was said to be able to do so，like a god, using only his five fingers: 掐指神算, 料事如神.

16. This author has been able to trace one work by an analytical philosopher who appeas to have invoked the spirit of the *Laozi* (without presumably having come across it, unlike Bohr who had). This is Haack, 1993, in which she proposes that an adequate epistemology requires both Foundationalism and Coherentism, complementing each other (instead of being regarded as mutually exclusive)—she calls it "Foundherentism".

17. There are other philosophical moves that one could make, but as this is not germane to the context at hand, we shall not raise them here. For the curious, see Lee, 2012b.

18. Besides the Principle of the Uniformity of Nature, there are also other metaphysical principles which render science intelligible, such as Every Event has a Cause.

19. These quotations are from "The Beauty of Life", a lecture delivered in 1880—see Morris, 1882.

20. As a matter of fact, the ancient Chinese knew that Earth moved—see chapter 4 for supporting quotations from the *Shangshu and* the *Neijing*; yet they let that fact lie on the table, so to speak.

21. The Latin phrase *Primus inter pares*, is generally used to refer to the lead role played by a member in a group of peers, as the expression literally means "first among equals".

22. As short hand, this is correct, but from the point of view of *science*/science, the so-called lunar calendar is best understood as a luni-solar calendar.

23. *Bu* does not mean "tonify" as that word in English understands the notion; hence the word is put within quotation marks.

CHAPTER SEVEN

Yinyang-Wuxing

This chapter extends the discussion of *Yinyang*, introduces a new notion, that of *Wuxing*, and explores the relationship between them, showing that their twinning provides a distinctive foundation for Chinese *philosophy* and Chinese *science* from the Han Dynasty onward, if not before.

Yinyang

The last two chapters established that the ancient Chinese abstracted and extrapolated from the empirical level of *yin qi* and *yang qi* to the more theoretical level of *yin* and *yang*. Ultimately, this process of abstraction led to the highest level, the inter-relationship between *yin* and *yang* (functioning as polar opposites) as the concept of *Yinyang* itself. This section will look in some detail at this development.

The basic meaning of *yi* in the *Yijing* is the notion of Change (*bianyi*). Chapter 6 has argued the point that Change implies No Change (as constancy) standing behind it. However, it may be possible to give another gloss to the relationship between *bianyi* and *buyi*. That everything in the universe is subject to change implies that the only thing which will not change, remaining constant (*buyi*), is Change itself, *bianyi*. This means that even if some object or state of affairs looks very stable, enduring, and permanent, if we study and analyze it closely, we will see that appearance notwithstanding, vast changes are taking place, though at a pace and scale that we, humans, do not immediately detect. What could be more solid than Mount Everest, yet Mount Everest has changed, changes and will change over time, so that much further in the geological future, that mighty mountain might become a rump of a hillock. Even our Sun, that brilliant star in our Solar system would one day become extinct. Our own bodies change, all the time, without our knowing that it does; the cells in us have to replace themselves. Red blood cells live about four months, white ones on average more than a year, colon cells die off after only four days, skin cells last about two or three weeks while sperm cells survive about three days. To use today's language, one could say that change is the default mode; or to use more traditional Western philosophical vocabulary, we say that behind the Appearance of stability (no change) is the Reality of change. Behind No Change/constancy stands Change, just as behind Change stands No Change/constancy, as set out in the context of chapter 6. This indicates that at the core of ancient Chinese *philosophy* is the view that the polar contrasting terms in a pair of such terms mutually relate to each other in a complex, intricate manner, embodying a unique perspective which will be explored further in chapter 9.

What drives this incessant change, according to the *Yi*? The impetus does not come merely from a force from without but also from forces within, namely, that of *yin* and *yang*, and the relationship between them.

According to the *Yi* and the *Laozi*, there is at work a *Law of Nature* which says that when a situation/state of affairs reaches its highest limit, it will start to change direction, from ascent, it will turn to descent, from growth and maturity to decline, from heat to cold. It is obvious that for the ancient Chinese this *Law of Nature* came from direct observation—they noticed that an organism started off its existence by being small, a mere shoot or fledgling, then overtime, it grew to become strong and big, reaching its height of maturity when it could reproduce, and after that, it would decline in vigor in its powers until decay and eventually death would set in. The same thing is true with the four seasons in the year—Spring brings the first warmth and light of the Sun (when plants start to bring forth shoots and leaves, animals come out of hibernation and their young are born), the temperature increases with each day that goes by until the height of Summer (solstice), after which the temperature progressively decreases through Autumn, ending up with the extreme cold of Winter. In the course of a day, dawn brings the first glimmer of light and warmth from the Sun, the temperature increases as the Sun rises above the horizon, at noon the Sun is at its zenith after which, it starts to "come down" from the sky above until eventually it dips below the horizon in the evening, bringing a drop of temperature, weaker light until the darkness and the cold of night descend.

The ancient Chinese knew that light and heat were related to and dependent on the Sun and its (apparent) movements in the Heaven above. The word for "sun" in Chinese is 日*ri* or 太阳*taiyang*. As shown in chapter 6, the

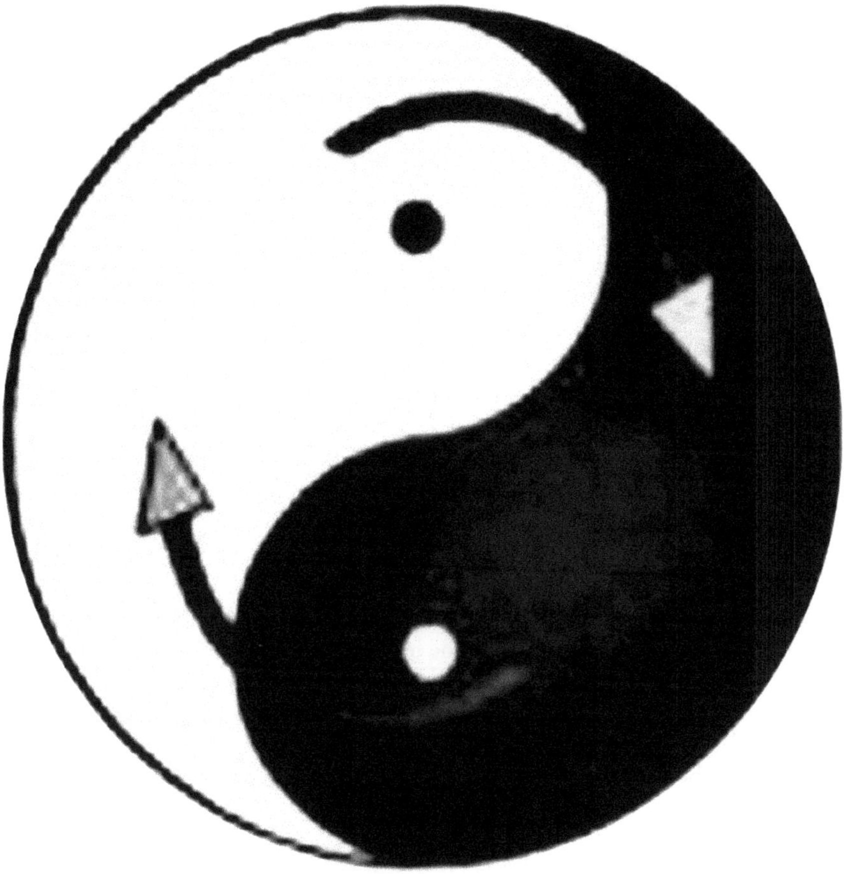

Figure 7.1. "Yin" and "Yang" as internal forces

latter term means Greater Yang and refers to one of the four images/*xiang* in the generation of the *Yao-gua* Model. The ancient Chinese held that it was in the nature of *yang (qi)* to ascend and of *yin (qi)* to descend. This circular movement represents clockwise the ascent of *yang qi* to its maximum on the left, the descent and diminution of *yang qi* (with corresponding increase of *yin qi* on the right). This is because in the Chinese representation of the compass points, East is to the left, West to the right, South to the top and North to the bottom. East is where the Sun rises, West where the Sun sets; East is therefore a fitting starting point for Spring as the temperature rises and daylight hours increase as Winter is left behind. South stands for where the Sun is strongest (as China is in the northern hemisphere); the Sun only "travels" as far north by the Summer solstice as the Tropic of Cancer, before it "turns back again to move" towards the Equator and ultimately to the Tropic of Capricorn when the northern Winter (Winter solstice) is at its coldest and its darkest. Such a characterisation makes clear the the temporal and spatial correlations with *yin* and *yang qi* as well as the changes in *Yinyang* during the traditional Chinese twelve hours/our modern twenty four hours clock systems. Figures 7.2, 7.3, and 7.4 shown respectively below encapsulate the information just given above.

The characterisation and the three figures may be said to embed a *Law of Nature* which are caught in the following sets of quotations and phrases:

(1)《黄帝内经·灵枢·论疾诊尺》: 四时之变, 寒暑之胜, 重阴必阳, 重阳必阴, 故阴主寒, 阳主热, 故寒甚则热, 热甚则寒, 故曰: 寒生热, 热生寒, 此阴阳之变也 /*Lingshu*, *Neijing*, chapter 74 which this author renders as: "(One observes) the changes of the four seasons, with their ascendance of either cold or hot, that when *yang* reaches its maximum, *yin* is bound to follow, when *yin* reaches its maximum, *yang* is bound to follow. Based on such observations, one says that *yin* is the foundation of cold and *yang* of hot, and hence that when cold reaches its maximum, hot will follow, when hot reaches its height, cold will inevitably follow. In this sense, one can say that cold engenders hot, hot engenders cold—this encapsulates the invariable change from *yin* to *yang* and *yang* to *yin*."

(2)《素问·阴阳应象大论》: 寒极生热, 热极生寒/*Suwen*, *Neijing*: Chapter 5 which this author renders as: "When cold reaches its extreme limit, it engenders hot; when hot reaches its extreme limit, it engenders cold."

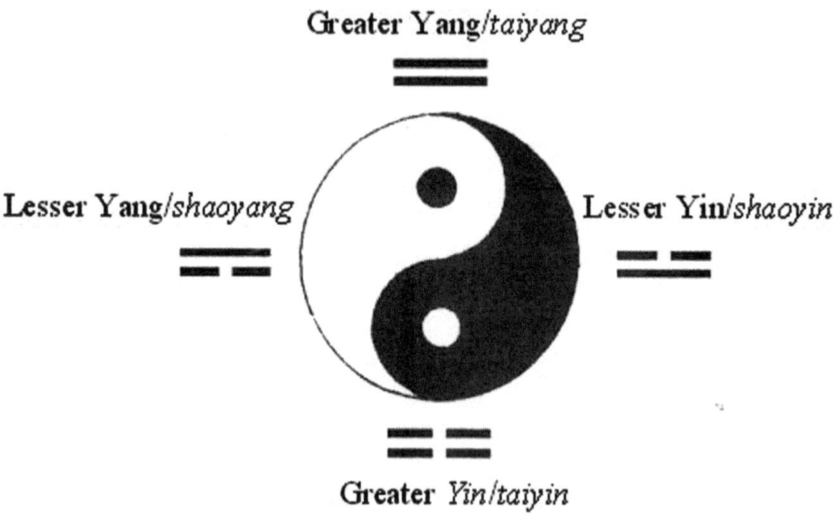

Figure 7.2. Sixiangtu

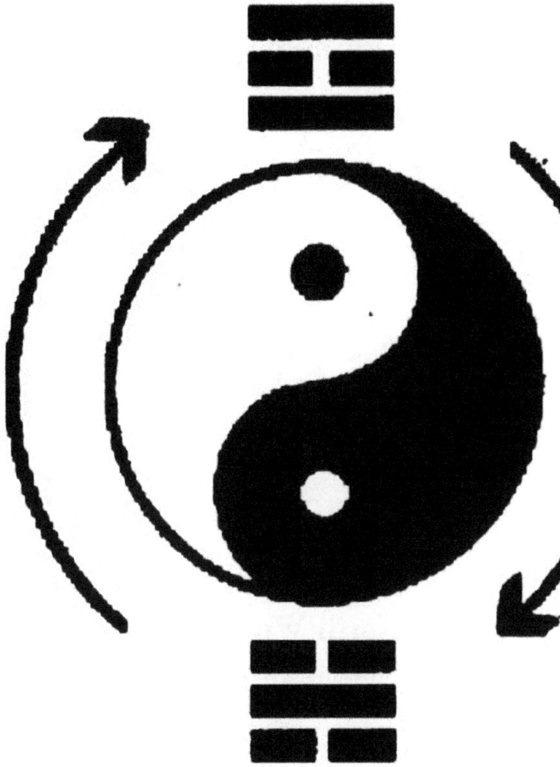

Figure 7.3. Ascent of yang qi on the left, descent of yang qi on the right

(3)《素问·六元正纪大论》：动复则静，阳极反阴。Author's own rendering of this passage from *Suwen, Neijing:* chapter 71 reads: "Extreme movement inevitably leads to stillness; *yang* at its extreme limit provokes its polar contrast *yin*."

(4)《太极图说》: 无极而太极, 太极动而生阳, 动极而静, 静而生阴, 静极复动, 一动一静, 互为其根, 分阴分阳, 两仪立焉。。。Author's rendering of this passage from the *Taijitu shuo*[1] reads: "The Nebulous Void (the One of the *Laozi*) leads to *Taiji* (the Two of the *Laozi*); *Taiji* moves, engendering *yang*; extreme movement inevitably leads to stillness; stillness engenders *yin*, extreme stillness inevitably leads to the return of movement. (The processes of change, therefore) involves two contrasting modes, movement and stillness, which mutually interact and can be called *yin* and *yang* which are the two manifestations of *Taiji*, the foundation of all change."

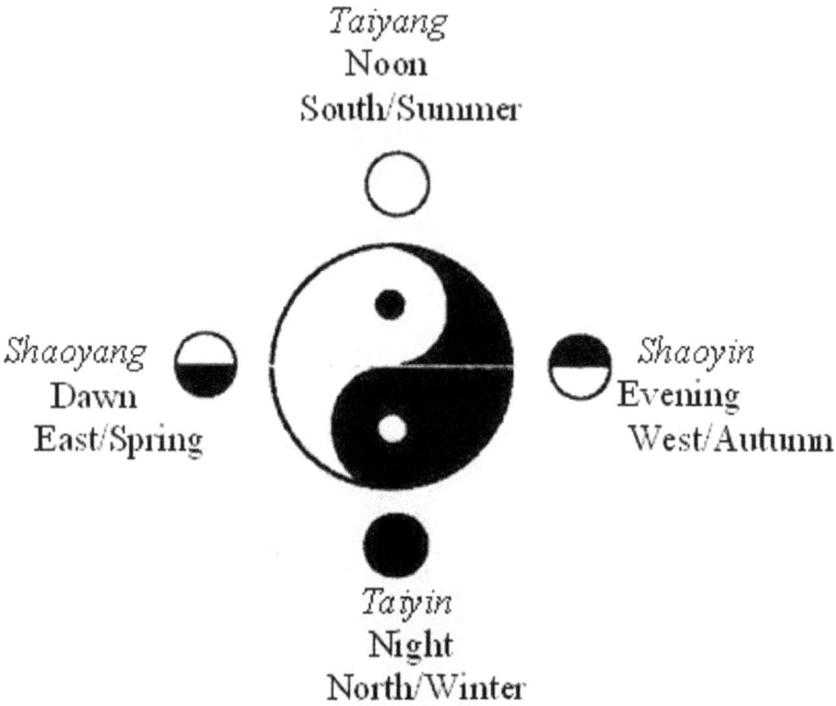

Figure 7.4. Temporal and spatial correlations with yin and yang qi

(5) 《周易·系辞下传》: 易穷则变， 变则通， 通则久. This passage from the *Zhouyi* (*Ten Wings/Treatise on the Appended Words, Part II*) is rendered by this author as: "When change has reached its limits, it would change, when change occurs, there will be through passage and when there is no blockage, the processes (of change) would endure." (In other words, because of change, evolution/development can take place in states of affairs—whether natural or social—without blockage.)

(6) 《周易·系辞上传》: 往来不穷谓之通. This phrase from the *Zhouyi* (*Ten Wings/Treatise on the Appended Words, Part I*) rendered by this author reads: "When there is endless "to-ing" and "fro-ing," through passage would be secured and no blockage ensured."

In other words, the last two quotations are also a way of referring to the concept of cyclic reversion, guaranteeing endurance/sustainability, which we have raised *en passant* in chapter 6.

Let us return to the Former Heaven (*xiantian*) Configuration already shown in chapter 5 in order this time to comment on the inter-active changes between *yin* and *yang* *via* the changes in the *yaos* of the eight trigrams. On the ascending left arm of the cycle, you will notice that *Kun* stands at the bottom, at North; its three *yin yaos* represent the limit which *yin* has reached. As *yin* has reached its maximum, it would be en route to turning into *yang*. Hence the next trigram *Zhen* on the ascending arm has its bottom *yin yao* replaced by a *yang yao*. (Remember that when a *gua* changes, the change starts with the bottom *yao*; as the *guas* are arranged in a hexagonal form, the *yaos* should be read from the inner toward the outer and the same holds true in the circular form.) *Zhen* is succeeded by *Li* with two *yang yaos* between one *yin yao*. *Li* in turn is succeeded by *Dui*, also with one *yin yao* but this time, it is above two *yang yaos*—recall that the difference between one trigram and another is not simply the number of *yin yaos* and *yang yaos* each possesses but the actual positioning of them. In the case of *Dui*, the topmost *yao* is the *yin yao* which is significant as its successor trigram is *Qian* which has three *yang yaos* just as its polar contrast, *Kun* has the maximum of three *yin yaos*. From this we can infer that the ascending arm of increasing *yang* has reached its limit, and therefore, the descending arm of *yang* will commence. *Xun* represents the first trigram in the descending arm with the bottom most *yang yao* of *Qian* being replaced by a *yin yao*. *Kan* follows with a *yang yao* between two *yin yaos*. *Gen* carries the descent further with two *yin yaos* below and the *yang yao* uppermost. And finally the descending arm of the trigrams is completed when *Kun* is reached, and the cycle of ascending *yang* from *yin*, from *Kun* to *Qian* followed by the descending of *yang* to *yin* to *Kun* begins all over again (Cyclic Reversion).

We have already observed that the impetus for change between *yin* and *yang* are internal to *Yinyang*. A common expression is 阳中有阴、阴中有阳 which can be rendered as: "In *yin* there is *yang*, and in *yang* there is *yin*," the one mode contains the potential/seeds of the other which then manifests itself when the circumstances are ripe. The Chinese commonly say that the symbol is made up of two fishes, the white fish on the left stands for *yang* while the black fish on the right stands for *yin*. However, the white fish has a black eye while the black fish has a white eye—the black eye in the former represents *yin* while the white eye in the latter represents *yang*. In other words, *yang* embraces *yin* and *yin* embraces *yang* as shown by the *Yinyang Liangyitu*, as shown in chapter 6.

All in all, one may conclude this section by saying that the *Yijing* lays the foundation for the *philosophy* of *Yinyang*. Later scholars having extrapolated that concept embodied in it, though not articulated by it, developed it explicitly, so much so that there was even a *Yinyang* School of *philosophy* whose texts have however been lost to posterity.[2] The *Laozi* appeared to have continued the tradition implicitly even though it itself only mentioned the concept once in chapter 42—see below for the quotation. However, it is difficult to understand the *Laozi* without referring back to the *Yijing* even if it itself did not mention the latter by name. The *Ten Wings* of the *Zhouyi* appeared to have absorbed both the *Yijing* and the *Laozi* as shown in this phrase: 一阴一阳之谓道 which may be rendered as: "The Dao is nothing more than the two modes of *yin* and *yang*, interacting with each other." A passage from chapter 42 of the *Laozi* reads: 万物负阴而抱阳, 冲气以为和 which is rendered by Feng and English, 1989 as: "The ten thousand things carry yin and embrace yang. They achieve harmony by combing these forces." Furthermore, the *Laozi* and the *Zhouyi* share another set of contrasting terms, 刚柔 (hard/soft) which the *Laozi* made great play of. (chapter 4 has commented on an aspect of it.) The *Zhouyi* as shown in chapter 5 identified *yang* with the *Qian gua*, equating *Qian* with hard; it identified *yin* with the *Kun gua*, equating *yin* with soft. For the processes of change to occur smoothly without hindrance so that they can be enduring, the *Yinyang* interaction, as well as its accompanying operational modes in terms of hard and soft, must take place—*yin* and *yang* each on its own would not thrive, just as hard and soft each on its own would not work properly. *Yin* and *yang* must work together as a harmonious *Whole* as *Yinyang* (and so must hard and soft). The *Wholism* of *Yinyang*, as we shall see in detail in the sequel to this volume (Lee, forthcoming) how it plays a key role in CCM, in which the conception of good health is understood as balance between *yin* and *yang*, and its polar contrast of illness as imbalance between the two.

The Roots and Stages of Development of *Wuxing*

Wuxing 五行[3] is today often translated as "Five Phases," although in sinological literature, the term "Five Elements" is still found; some scholars also use "five phase element system"—see Fruehauf, 2009. One might venture to say that although the first is a better fit than the second, none is a perfect fit. One could try "Five types of *qi* and their interactive processes at work." This, though more accurate, is not pithy; perhaps one should say "Five Qi Transformative Phases." Hence, all told, this author would prefer not to translate the term and simply let its meaning, significance and implications emerge from a detailed account of this concept. It is important to emphasise that *Wuxing* has to do with *Qi*, which chapter 3 shows exists in two modes; that this in turn, chapter 8 argues is a significant basis for claiming that Chinese *philosophy* involves process-ontology, not thing-ontology.

Wuxing refers to *Wood* 木, *Fire*火, *Earth*土, *Metal* 金, and *Water* 水. Confronted by these, it was, in a sense natural that the early sinologists translated it as "Five Elements," as to them trained in the Classical Greek tradition of philosophy, the concept appeared to bear a remarkable resemblance to the

Greek schema in terms of Fire, Earth, Water, and Air, which Empedocles from Sicily (c 504–433 BCE) was said to have put forward as the ultimate constituents of matter; these in turn were linked to four fundamental qualities and to four humors. Variations and changes in all things were to be explained in terms of different mixtures of the four elements. However, in spite of a certain superficial similarity, we shall show in due course that *Wuxing* differs profoundly from the Greek concept of the Four Elements.

What could *Wuxing* possibly refer to or mean? Let us first deconstruct the two characters constituting the term itself. These are *wu*/五 and *xing*/行. The former simply means "five" and the latter refers to movement/motion/moving. Hence the term *Wuxing*, one might say, could literally be translated as "five types of movement/motion/moving." This would not be entirely inaccurate but is too simplistic and would require filling in a lot of detailed background in order to give a more adequate understanding of what the concept stands for and entails but it would be a start.

Chapter 4 shows that even the Neolithic peoples of China were interested in and knowledgeable about astronomy and had a concept of cosmology. There is a Neolithic jade engraved as a cosmological map, found in Hanshan/含山 County. Experts have dated it to around 3000 BCE. It is roughly five thousand years old.[4] The engraving shows two circles, the inner smaller circle within an outer larger circle; at the center of the inner circle is a small square and the outer circle is within a large square. It also shows four arrows pointing to the four corners of the large square; eight arrows within the large circle also point outward at the large square. What cosmological themes could be read into this carving?

1. The four large arrows pointing at each of the four corners of the large square would indicate the four main compass points; the eight smaller arrows would stand for the eight compass points.
2. The smaller square within the smaller circle would stand for the Center, while the four large compass arrows for what surrounded the Center.
3. Even by Neolithic times, Chinese cosmology had developed the concept of *tianyuan-difang*/ 天圆地方 which literally means "Heaven is round and Earth is square." This was conveniently represented in this kind of cosmological iconography as circle and square and had persisted since Neolithic times down the ages of the history of Chinese culture and civilization. For instance, a bronze vessel of Shang and Zhou times is called *gui* 簋, which is a perfect embodiment of this cosmological iconography.[5]

A word of caution should be entered. It is, at times, taken to mean that the ancient Chinese literally believed that while Heaven was round, Earth was square. However, this could be too simplistic an account of what the belief really was. The word 圆/*yuan* not only could refer to something round in shape, such as a circle, but given the astronomical/cosmological context, it referred to 圆满 *yuanman*, a term which could describe the (apparent) movement of the Sun in the course of a day (from sunrise to sunset to sunrise . . .) and in the course of a year (from Winter to Spring, to Summer, to Autumn, to Winter, and back to Spring again . . .). In other words, it has nothing to do with the shape of the sky but the (apparent) movement of the Sun and the concept of Time in terms of cyclic reversion. In the same spirit, Earth was square should not be understood literally (chapter 4 has already cited evidence that the ancient Chinese did have an "advanced" view about the shape of Earth, the relationship between Earth and Sun etc.). It reflected the observation that the surface of Earth as sunlight fell on it was flat, not curved—hence a square seemed an appropriate way of representing this fact. The expression "Heaven is round and Earth square" was no more than a felicitous expression of cosmological iconography—it actually stood for the relationship between Time (cyclic reversion) and Space (surface of Earth and directions in terms of compass points) which chapter 10 will explore as the concept of Timespace.

4. East, South, West, North plus the Center added up to 五方/*wufang*, which literally means "five directions/ locations," equivalent, if you like, to the expression 天下 *tianxia* (what is under Heaven) which by Zhou times was used to refer to that part of the universe which fell within their political, cultural, economic, and military orbit.

By Shang times, the Chinese had further developed the above preoccupations. Their Oracle Bone script bears evidence that they had the concept of *wufang*. The script contains expressions such as 中商/Central Shang, 东土/Eastern territory, 南土/Southern territory,西土/Western territory,北土/Northern territory. Their divination records also referred to the winds from the four quarters or directions.[6] One could say, then, that the "five" in *Wuxing* could hark back to times much earlier than the late Warring States Period when Zou Yan 邹衍 (c 305—240 BCE) was commonly said to have first systematized the concept of *Wuxing*.

We have so far mentioned some earlier texts/discourses upon which *Wuxing* might be partially based. Another source is said to come from the term "resources" as in the expression 五材/*wucai* meaning "five resources." This discourse emerged toward the end of the Western Zhou period, and can be found in two texts called the *Guoyu*《国语》and the *Zuozhuan*《左传》. In the former, one *philosopher*, Shi Bo 史伯, said: 以土与 金、木、水、火

杂以 成百物《国语·郑语》, which this author remders as: "(By a judicious) mix (in the use) of these five (resources), namely, earth, metal, wood, water and fire, one would be able to create all things (or forms of artefacts)." In the Spring and Autumn Period, another thinker wrote as reported in the latter text: 天生五材, 民并用之, 废一不可 (《左传》襄公二十七年 which this author renders as: "Nature has engendered these five resources which the people must need use, not missing out on any one."

So how did *wucai*, a term which referred to something quite concrete and physical such as the soil in which one grew things/with which one manufactured bricks, or metal which when melted could be turned into ploughs or axes lead to the concept of *Wuxing*, which appeared to be abstract and theoretical, even downright *metaphysical*? As usual, the ancient Chinese began this process of abstraction and theorization from observations, that is, from an empirical starting point. We can see this process at work in a text called the *Shangshu/Shujing*《书经》, held either to date from the Spring and Autumn or later Period. A relevant passage from the chapter called *Hongfan* (《尚书·洪范》) reads: 五行: 一曰水, 二曰火, 三曰木, 四曰金, 五曰土。水曰润下, 火曰炎上, 木曰曲直, 金曰従革, 土爰稼穡。润下作咸, 炎上作苦, 曲直作酸, 従革作辛, 稼穡作甘, which this author renders as:

> *Wuxing* refers to *Water*, *Fire*, *Wood*, *Metal* and *Earth*. *Water* moistens and seeps downwards; *Fire* burns and leaps upwards; *Wood* can bend and straighten; *Metal* is malleable and can be shaped in anyway one pleases; *Earth* (as soil) is excellent for sustaining cultivation. That which is moist and seeps downwards produces the salty taste; that which burns and moves upwards produces the bitter taste; that which straightens and bends the sour taste; that which is malleable and changes in shape the acrid taste; crops born of soil taste sweet.[7]

The above is evidence for saying that *wucai*, the five physical resources which one may find listed in a discourse about economics or geography had been left behind as the author(s) of the *Shangshu* was/were more interested in detailing the properties of these items and what they were capable of doing—in four out of the five cases, the property named in each is a property pertaining to the study of physics (or what could be said to come under its aegis), such as that water flows downward, fire goes upward, wood straightens or bends, metal when heated or melted is malleable and can take on all shapes and forms. The one exception is *Earth*—the passage was keen to talk about *Earth*'s productivity in terms of cultivation. In any case, when it went on to refer to the respective tastes of *Wuxing*, one knows that here is an abstract schema being put in place, analogous to the construction of the *Yao-gua* Model examined in chapter 6, which aims at introducing systematization, order, economy, and increase in the range of material and information which it could encompass. We shall return to this point later. In the *Yao-gua* Model, although the aim was to assist divination, however, once the model was set up, it could, nevertheless, be used in many other domains as a set of analytical tools—in this case of *Wuxing*, the model appeared to have originated with politics and rulership in mind but once constructed, its remit expanded and could not be confined to political discourse alone but also to other domains of life which involved theory and praxis, such as *medicine*, the military, calligraphy, martial arts, and so on. In a moment, we shall see more clearly why these two models had this tendency to generalise and systematize, no matter that one model developed initially in the context of divination and the other, supposedly, in the context of politics. (For details about the relationship between *Wuxing* and the *Neijing*, see Lee.)

A later text (that is if the *Shangshu* is accepted to be a work of the Spring and Autumn Period), toward the end of the Warring States era, called the *Spring and Autumn Annals of Mr Lü*, in the steps of the *Hongfan*, carried further the process of setting up the schema. This development was incorporated into the *Neijing* and can be found in passages such as the following (*Suwen*, *Neijing*: Chapter 66/《素问·天元纪大论》): 夫五运阴阳者, 天地之道也, 万物之纲纪, 变化之父母, 生杀之本始。This author renders it as: "Nature's Dao is but *Wuxing-Yinyang*, which is the *Law of Nature* followed by *Wanwu*, the *alpha* and *omega* of Change, the *fons et origo* of birth and death (growth and decline)."

Sima Qian in the *Shiji* wrote that during the Warring States Period, two kings of the State of Qi/齐国 (Qi Wei *wang* /齐威王 and Qi Xuan *wang*/齐宣王 , respectively, 358–320 and 319–309 BCE) in the second half of the fourth century BCE initiated a project (which, as a matter of fact, continued for roughly a hundred and forty years, until the State of Qi fell prey to Qinshihuangdi's successful attempt to unify China), convening a group of scholars, of different persuasions, to discuss intellectual matters which included the concept of *Wuxing*. They met by the Ji Gate of the capital city, Linzi 临淄, and hence came to be known as the Jixia Academy 稷下学宫 *Jixia xuegong*, which included Zou Yan 邹衍, Zhuangzi,[8] Menzi 孟子 (c372–289 BCE) and Xunzi (c 310–220 BCE).

Coming later to the Han Dynasty, a clear expression of the concept of *Wuxing* can be found in the *Huainanzi*. A passage from Chapter One, "Originating in the Way," reads: 其德优天地而和阴阳，节四时而调五行。。。《淮南子·原道训》. Translation by Major et al., 2010, reads:

> Their Potency:
> accorded with Heaven and Earth and harmonized yin and yang;
> delimited the four seasons and attuned the Five Phases.

The chapter, from which the passage is taken, as a whole, is an expression of *Daojia philosophy* of the *Laozi*, as it appears to say quite clearly that by adhering to the Dao, which meant following *Ziran*, rulers could become sages, and that not only would this ensure that the natural order continue unperturbed, the political/social order would also be smoothly stable. The passage is itself clear evidence that by early Han times, the concepts of *Yinyang* (of the *Yi*), the Dao of the *Laozi* and the *Zhuangzi* as well as of *Wuxing* had been synthesized and promulgated under the aegis of Liu An, among others.

The synthesis mentioned above makes it much easier to explain the concept of *Wuxing*, as it was not a stand-alone notion but one deeply rooted in *Yinyang*, the *Yijing* and the teachings of the *Laozi* and the *Zhuangzi*. As we have already discussed in some detail for these other concepts, all we need to do here is to remind readers of their salient features, in particular the first two mentioned, as they are foundational for Chinese thought and *philosophy*. It might not be too far from the truth to say that *Wuxing* extracted and thereby extended the implications inherent in *Yinyang* itself, which is nothing more than the mutually interactive relationships between *yin qi* and *yang qi*. Chapter 3 has already established that *Qi* operates in two modes, *Qi*-in-concentrating mode and *Qi*-in-dissipating mode—the former referred to the domain of *xingerxia* (形而下), the latter to that of *xingershang* (形而上). When *Wuxing* elaborated on the concept of *Qi*, it was *apropos* the latter, not the former domain. That was how it distinguished itself ultimately from *wucai* which involved *Qi*-in-concentrating mode, within the domain of *xingerxia*. It appropriately reflected that the five types of *qi* it propounded were really about the processes of their mutual interactions; hence *xing* (行), in the context of *Wuxing*, literally meant, as already observed, movement/motion. To use the language of the *Yi*, they were fundamentally about the processes of change and transformation between the five types of *qi*—*Wood* in the discourse of *Wuxing* was, therefore, not about the physical/economic resource called wood which one could measure in terms of cubic tons and from which one could make artifacts such as boats and bows, but the kind of *qi Wood* stood for, given the time and season of the year in relation to location or space. Similarly, *Water* did not refer to the liquid used for drinking and washing oneself, but the kind of *qi Water* stood for given the time and season of the year in relation to location or space.

In other words, we are here simply re-capping what we have said with regard to the figures shown in the preceding section of this chapter. *Yang qi* would start to emerge toward the end of Winter, slowly to increase, beginning its ascent (represented by the upward arrow on the left) as *yin qi* correspondingly decreased, until it reached its maximum at the height of Summer; then *yang qi* would start to decline on its descent (represented by the downward arrow on the right) while the *yin qi* correspondingly would begin to increase, until the *yin qi* reached its maximum in the depth of Winter, when the cycle of the relationship between the respective ascent and descent of *yang qi* and *yin qi* would start up all over again. In other words, the corresponding increase of the one *qi* varies with the corresponding decrease of the other *qi* and vice versa.

However, to make absolutely clear that *Wuxing* and the trigrams are understood to be intimately related, one could superimpose the one scheme upon the other (as well as on the trigrams and the eight compass points) as shown in figure 7.5.

To complete the above overall account, we set out the relationship between *yin* and *yang* on the one hand and the *guas* on the other in the clearest version possible, in that version constructed by Shao Yong, the Song Dynasty yilogist, in the form of a square/rectangle, with the *gua* system illustrating the alternating succession of *yin gua* and *yang gua* in the trigram and the hexagram series—see figure 7.6.

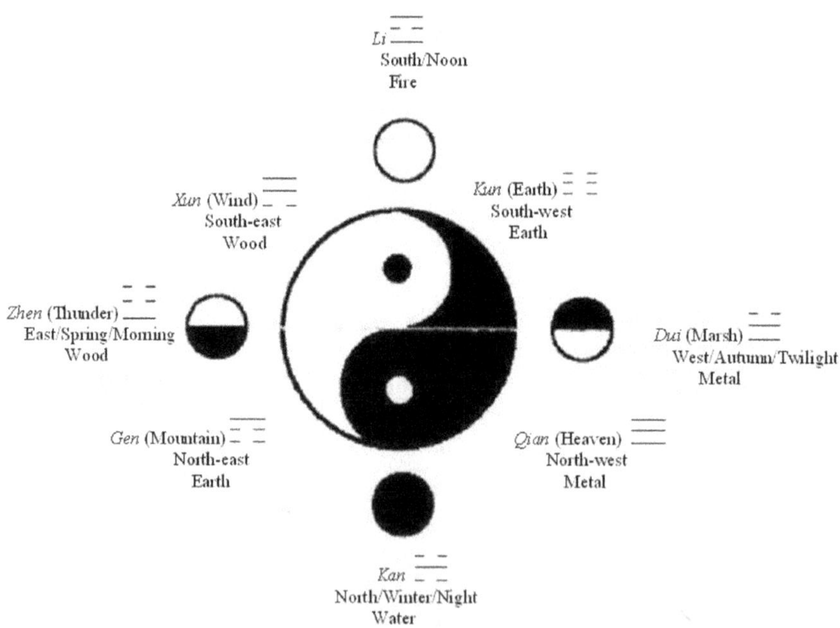

Figure 7.5. Superimposing Wuxing on Yinyang, bagua, and the eight compass points

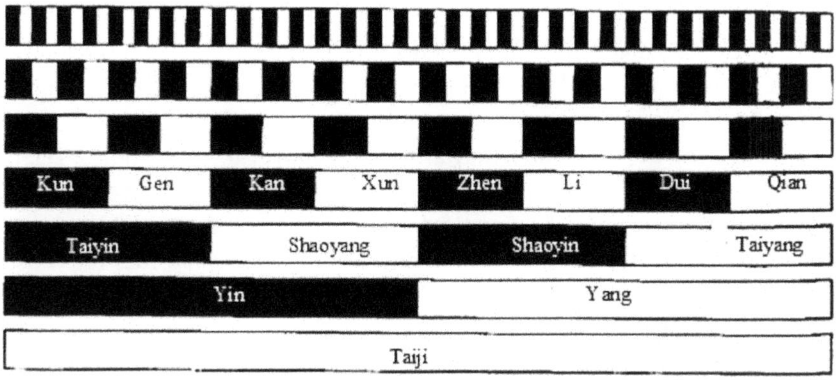

Figure 7.6. The gua system of yin and yang gua

1. *Taiqi* (right at the bottom) has no manifest division between *yin* and *yang*.
2. The second level up shows division into *yin* and *yang* (the level of *liangyi*).
3. The third level shows further division into *taiyin* and *shaoyang* to the left, *shaoyin* and *taiyang* to the right—the level of *sixiang*.
4. The fourth level in turn sub-divides into the eight trigrams, reading as follows from left to right: *Kun* (*yin*) and *Gen* (*yang*); *Kan* (*yin*) and *Xun* (*yang*); *Zhen* (*yin*) and *Li* (*yang*); *Dui* (*yin*) and *Qian* (*yang*)—the level of *bagua*/trigrams.
5. The fifth level is a similar sub-division yielding sixteen possibilities, while the sixth level creates thirty-two possibilities—these are shown as part of the logic of the process of sub-division.
6. Finally, the seventh, that is, the topmost level of the figure shows the level of the sixty-four hexagrams starting from the *Kun gua* (*which* is pure *yin*) on the extreme left to the *Qian gua* (which is pure *yang*), on the extreme right; in between, *yang* and *yin guas* alternate—for instance, the *Kun gua* is followed by a *yang gua*, the *Bo gua*/ 剥卦, while to the left of the *Qian gua* is a *yin gua*, the *Guai gua*/夬卦 .

Another relevant passage from Zhou Dunyi's publication, the *Taijitu shuo*/《太极图说》, following on from the one already cited earlier above regarding *Wuxing* reads: 阳变阴合，而生水火木金土。五气顺布，四时行焉。五行一阴阳也，阴阳一太极也，太极本无极也。五行之生也，各一其性, rendered (by this author) as: "When *yang* changes, so does *yin* correspondingly change—this (mutual interaction) engenders *Water*, *Fire*,

Wood, Metal, Earth. With the five *qi* in place, the four seasons would also be in place. *Wuxing* is but *yin* and *yang* and *Yinyang* is but *Taiji* while *Taiji* itself comes from *Wuji*. *Wuxing* is thus engendered, with each (*qi*) bearing a characterization of its own."

In the light of the clarification attempted above, it would no longer be surprising that both the *Yao-gua* Model and the *Wuxing* Model can each be developed to become a set of generalised analytical tools regardless of the initial context from which each appeared to have sprung. In reality, they are "cousins" from the same stable, so to speak. That stable is *Qi* (its two modes of operation, *Qi*-in-dissipating and *Qi*-in-concentrating modes), as *yin qi* and *yang qi*, as *Yinyang* (the interaction between them). One could perhaps be even more adventurous in seeing the concept of *Wuxing* as no more than an extended elaboration of the cluster of concepts under *Qi*, bringing out with greater clarity (or at least this author would like to argue) the "ecological" or "ecosystem" implications of *Qi* which will be further explored in the next section.

Wuxing and Its Main Modes of Interaction

Given the roots of *Wuxing*, one could perhaps regard the concept as an attempt to organize and systematize knowledge from three different aspects, namely, as physical resources, as functions and as (ecological) information. This systematization yields an account of five different types of *qi* represented by *Wuxing* and the processes involved in their changing from one to the other; to understand the true relationships between them, one must grasp that each stands for a particular stage in the daily and/or yearly cycle (*zhouye jielü* and *sishi jielü*) when *yin qi* and *yang qi* interacts with each other. These stages are:

Water:	*taiyin* reaches its maximum
Wood:	*yin* retreats/decreases while *yang* begins to advance/increase
Fire:	*taiyang* reaches its maximum
Earth:	*yin* and *yang* are at equilibrium
Metal:	*yang* retreats/decreases while *yin* begins to advance/increase

We can, therefore, readily see that *Wuxing* is but an attempt to draw out the implications of *Yinyang*, upon which the trigrams and the hexagrams are themselves founded. We may infer that *Yinyang*, the *guas*, and *Wuxing* form a kind of trinity, leaning upon one another to enrich the meanings and implications for one another. For this reason, it would be appropriate to call them the *Yinyang-Wuxing* Model, for short. Having admitted this much, one must also quickly add that when all is said and done, *Yinyang* remains the foundational concept, as it represents the various processes of change at work between *yin qi* and *yang qi*, resulting in the engendering of *Wanwu*, not only in the more restricted sense of all things found in Nature—biotic and abiotic—but also in the more general sense of all the circumstances and outcomes in the world, including human affairs. Of the various processes of relationship between *yin* and *yang*, two pairs of *guas* stand out, that represented, on the one hand, by the *Li gua* (standing for Fire) and the *Kan gua* (standing for Water), and that represented, on the other, by the *Qian gua* (Heaven) and the *Kun gua* (Earth)—these are the foundational *guas* as the mutually interacting relationships between them ultimately generates *Wanwu* and the circumstances/conditions which would ensure their flourishing.

Wuxing is commonly attributed two major modes of interaction between the five types of *qi*, and this short account will, by and large, concentrate on them, although there are more complicated details than that which cannot be explored for lack of space. The first is the Mutually Engendering or Promoting Mode/Cycle (相生/*xiangsheng* as represented by the thick broken lines of the circle and their arrows) and the second, the Mutually Constraining or Controlling Mode (相克/相胜 *xiangke/xiangsheng* as represented by the thinner unbroken lines and their arrows inside the circle).

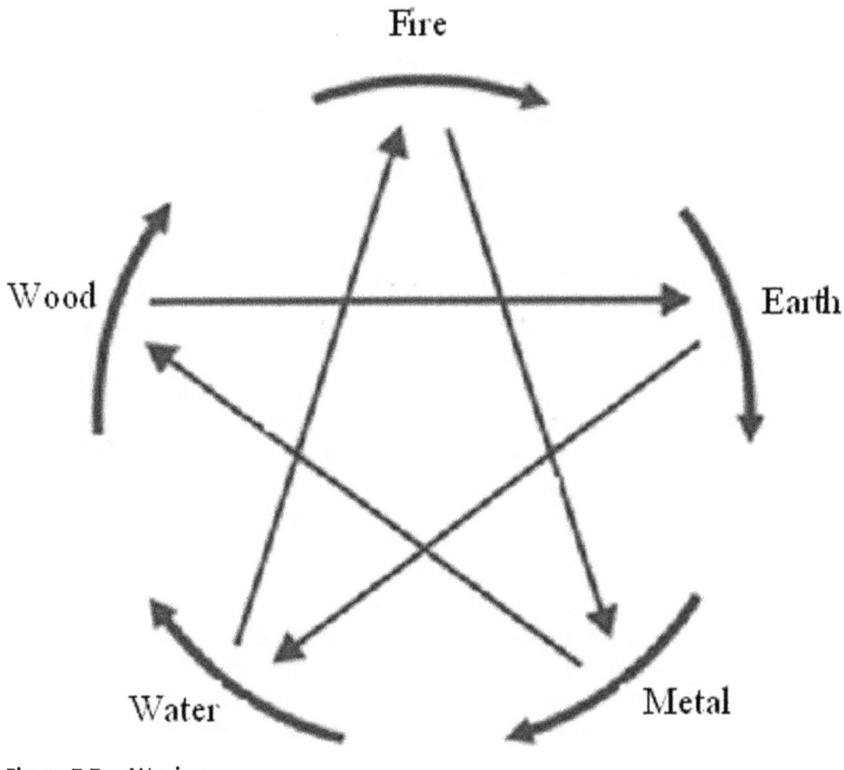

Figure 7.7. Wuxing

The Mutually Engendering/*xiangsheng* cycle runs as shown below:
水生木、木生火、火生土、土生金、金生水 which may be rendered as: *Water* engenders *Wood*, *Wood* engenders *Fire*, *Fire* engenders *Earth*, *Earth* engenders *Metal* (and the cycle begins again).

From the two aspects of *Wuxing* in terms of physical resources and functions, the account for this cycle goes as follows:

The ancient Chinese knew that water was an indispensable requirement for Life and Life's activities. They used *Wood* to stand as a general symbol for all Life and its activities. Hence, it was reasonable to postulate that *Water engendered Wood*. Early humans rubbed two sticks or pieces of wood together to produce friction to generate a spark, to start a fire. It was therefore reasonable to postulate that *Wood engendered Fire*. It was obvious that fire burned-wood down to ashes, literally, adding to the soil. As *Wood* for them was a general symbol for Life and its activities, the extinction of life with death would return all dead forms to the soil, to the earth. Hence, it seemed natural to say that *Wood engendered Earth*. *Earth* supported both the biotic and the abiotic, it could cause things to move/grow in all directions—upward, sideways, downward; it was capable, too, of keeping things which could be found in its bowels. Hence, the ancient Chinese held that *Earth engendered Metal* (with *Metal* standing, not only for the physical objects called metal but for all which the earth could harbor and embody in its bowels). They observed two different kinds of phenomena—drops of water formed on the surface of metal; the Moon seemed to have something to do with the tides. When the Moon was full, the tide was high, and they were particularly impressed by the high tide at the time of the full moon during the eighth lunar month of their calendar. The eighth lunar month was for them the beginning of Autumn, and as the ancient Chinese associated *Metal* with Autumn, hence they thought it reasonable to say that *Metal engendered Water*.

Although this account of *Wuxing* in terms of its reference to physical resources and their functions could explain something, it would be incomplete without reference to the five kinds of *qi* the concept stood for, constituting a *Whole*. This more complete account is already implicit in the incomplete one just given. We can see immediately, for example, why *Water* was said to engender *Wood*, as *Water* stood for the maximum reached by *yin qi* in the Winter. They also knew the *Law of Nature* which said that when *yin* or *yang* reached its limit, *yin* would transform to become *yang* and vice versa. As *yang* gingerly began to re-appear and to increase (as *yin* correspondingly declined), this *yang qi*, giving forth both light and warmth, would herald Spring, which would provide the ideal conditions for plants to begin to grow new shoots, for animals to come out of hibernation, for humans to start to sow their crops. In this way, it was eminently reasonable to say that *Water engendered Wood* in the sense that *Wood* simply stood for that kind of *qi* associated with or necessary for growth.

As *yang qi* continued to increase, with Summer overtaking Spring, it would be reasonable to say that *Wood engendered Fire* (the soaring temperature would ensure that plants would develop rapidly). Such an abundance of *yang qi* would ensure that plants and animals mature, the former forming seeds and fruits, the latter having brought up their young to fend for themsevles—it seemed reasonable to the ancient Chinese to say that *Fire engendered Earth—Fire* simply stood for that kind of *qi* associated with development and maturity, typical of biotic Nature.

When *yang qi* had reached its highest point, it would slowly begin to decline after the Summer solstice, but increasingly so especially after the abundant harvest (not simply in terms of crops but also in Nature at large) yielded by the earth—this process would be represented by saying that *Earth engendered Metal.* However, to understand this point we would now have to refer to geology; the ancient Chinese held that the decline of *yang qi* as Autumn approached could be accounted for not simply by the apparent movement of Sun with regard to the planet Earth but also by *yang qi* being returned to the bowels of the earth where it would remain until the emergence of Spring in the following year. In that sense, one could say that *Earth engendered Metal—Metal* stood for that kind of *qi* associated with the descent/increasing diminution of *yang qi*.

The decrease of *yang qi* and the corresponding increase of *yin qi* would accelerate until the depth of winter was reached, at the Winter solstice, when *yin qi* would have reached its maximum. Water transformed to become ice and snow in the winter, when the temperature dropped drastically; in the language of *Wuxing*, the ancient Chinese would say that *yang qi* had returned to, and become concealed within, the water. (This again is not as unscientific as it might look at first sight, as this account is not at odds with that given by Modern Science.[9]) So it seemed reasonable for them to encapsulate this process of *qi* transformation by saying that *Metal engendered Water—Water* stood for that type of *qi* associated with *yin qi* but within which *yang qi*, nevertheless, lurked in readiness, so to speak, to re-appear in the following Spring with the return of the light and warmth of the sun.

When told from the point of view of (ecological) information, the most important information emerging from *Wuxing* concerns the processes of *qi* transformation behind the five different kinds of *qi* identified by its theoretical framework. The five different kinds of physical resources and their functions were after all, themselves the product of the interactions between *yin qi* and *yang qi*, between *yin* and *yang* and the relationships between them as *Yinyang*.

We briefly note here that *Yinyang-Wuxing* is but the mapping of astronomy upon geography together with an account of the relationship between the two—astronomy yielded knowledge about the predominance of one *qi* over the other *qi* at any particular period either in the annual cycle of the seasons (*sishi jielü*) or the daily cycle of day/night (*zhouye jielü*), while geographical knowledge informed the ancient Chinese about the location upon which the predominant *qi* would fall at a specific moment in the cycle. In the daily cycle of *yin qi* and *yang qi*, the sun rose in the east and set in the west—hence, for them, it was eminently sensible to associate the emergence and increase of *yang qi* with the east, and the decline of *yang qi* (corresponding increase in *yin qi*) with the west. As *yang qi* commenced to increase during Spring while *yin qi* began to do the same during Autumn, the ancient Chinese felt it eminently sensible to associate *Spring* with *East*, *Autumn* with *West*. The same reasoning led them to associate *Summer* with *South* and *Winter* with *North*, given that China was/is a country in the northern hemisphere, such that, as already remarked, the southward face of a house is the aspect which receives the sun while the north side is exposed to the cold winds from the steppes of Mongolia and the frozen wastelands of beyond.

At this point, some readers might feel that this mapping of astronomy upon geography, this superimposing of *Wuxing* on *Yinyang*, raises a problem, as astronomy only showed up four seasons in the annual cycle of *yin qi* and *yang qi*, and geography recognised merely the four main compass points—East, South, West, North, which could be correlated respectively with *Shaoyang*, *Taiyang*, *Shaoyin*, and *Taiyin*. *Wuxing* mentioned five different kinds of *qi* with seasonal mix of *yin qi* and *yang qi* in terms of *Wood*, *Fire*, *Earth*, *Metal* and Water. To prevent a mismatch, when *Wuxing* was teamed up with *Yinyang*, explicitly and systematically by the early Han Dynasty if not before, the ancient Chinese felt obliged, it appeared, to introduce a fifth season to match *Wuxing*. The following super-impositions below were obvious:

Shaoyang/East/Spring/*Wood*
Taiyang/South/Summer/*Fire*
Shaoyin/West/Autumn/*Metal*
Taiyin/North/Winter/*Water*

With what then could one pair *Earth*? One way to solve the problem was to assign *Earth* to the central position; we have already raised the point that even as early as Neolithic times, the people then had talked about *wufang* which included the center as the fifth geographical position/direction (also their political center) in their cosmological map. Hence if one must assign

Earth a similar perspective, then it would be the center, with the other four main compass points as *sifang*/ 四方 (the four directions/regions). That would solve the problem as far as spatial orientation was concerned, but what about temporal orientation? Let us remind ourselves that in *Wuxing* discourse, *Earth* stood for equilibrium between *yin qi* and *yang qi*. It occurred to the ancient thinkers that they could borrow from the *Yi* itself regarding the *Kun gua* which was the *gua* for Earth. The *Zhouyi* attributed to *Kun* the primary characteristic of being hospital and open to *Wanwu*, nurturing and sustaining all. This all-embracing ability to sustain *Wanwu* could be said to imply that it was present in the other four main types of *qi*, set out above. If the year were to be divided into four main seasons, each season would last three months. The last eighteen days of each season could then be said to belong to *Earth*. *Earth* guaranteed the earth's fruitfulness, by holding *yin* and *yang* in equilibrium, and hence being assigned to all four seasons would make sense, as the perennial processes of birth, growth, maturity, and decline/death of *Wanwu* were underpinned ultimately by the equilibrium between *yin* and *yang*. Another way is to split up Summer into two stages with the first stage being the ordinary Summer/夏 and the second, the High Summer/长夏/*changxia*, being accorded the last eighteen days of Summer. Both interpretations are found in the *Neijing*, although, it appears that on the whole, the former is endorsed by CCM.[10]

However, the role played by *Earth* in *Wuxing* was a special one which had something to do with the matter that *Fire* could not directly engender *Metal*, but had to rely on *Earth* to mediate between *Fire* and *Metal*. We have seen that the season associated with *Fire* was *Summer*, when *yang qi* had reached its maximum, and must according to the *Law of Nature* (which stipulated that when *yang qi* or *yin qi* reached its respective peak, then the one *qi* would transform into the other) change to become *yin qi*. However, a critical difference existed between the two contexts of transformation—that of *yang qi* into *yin qi* was considered to be "against the grain" /逆/*ni* whereas that of *yin qi* into *yang qi* was considered to be "with the grain" /顺/*shun*. Hence the latter could proceed without *Earth's* mediation, and *Water* could engender *Wood* directly, whereas in the case of the former, *Earth's* mediation was required. *Fire* was *Taiyang*, the beginning of the process of change to *yin*; however, *Metal* being *Shaoyin* was not the beginning of *yin*—hence *Fire* required the mediation of *Earth* to effect the change to *Metal*. The sequence then went: *Fire engendered Earth*, and in turn *Earth engendered Metal*.

We next turn our attention to the second mode of *Wuxing*, its Mutually Constraining/*xiangke* cycle. Again, we start with an account in terms of the two aspects as physical resources and their functions. The ancient Chinese knew that vegetation was vital to prevent soil erosion and soil loss, especially during heavy rains when exposed soil with no vegetal cover could be washed away; by growing trees on such surfaces, soil erosion would be prevented. So in this sense, they postulated that *Wood constrained Earth*. Heavy rains could cause floods; to prevent flooding, one could use earth to build dykes and dams—they postulated that *Earth constrained Water*. To prevent a fire from spreading, one would need water to damp down the fire—in this sense, it could be said that *Water constrained Fire*. To make implements such as an axe or a sword, one would need fire to melt the metal before one could cast or mould it—they held that *Fire constrained Metal*. An axe (made from metal) would be useful in chopping down trees which in turn would provide wood to fuel fires—in this sense, they postulated that *Metal constrained Wood*.

However, again, for a more adequate account, one must turn to the information the cycle contained in terms of the processes of *qi* transformation and their interactive relationships, which entail a great degree of complexity in the two cycles, the Mutually Engendering and the Mutually Constraining modes. To bring out this degree of complexity, we have, initially, to introduce two more concepts: too much/太过/*taiguo* and not enough/不及/*buji* or不足/*buzu*—to be brief, one can simply say: excess and deficiency. These two concepts in turn entailed a third, that is, normality/平常/*pingchang* in the form of the *qi* which is normal for the season (平气/*ping qi*). In general, to grossly over-simplify a complex matter, let us present the ancient Chinese here to hold that in certain years, the *qi* of any one season could be in excess, that in certain other years, the *qi* of the season would be in deficiency—for instance, years A, C, E, G, I (甲、丙、戊、庚、壬, which are *yang* years) showed excess of *yang qi*, then years B, D, F, H, J (乙、丁、己、辛、癸 which are *yin* years) would show deficiency of *yin qi*. If year A showed excess in *Earth qi*, then in the following year B, *Metal qi* would be in deficiency, and in turn, given this deficiency of *Metal qi* in year B, the following year C would exhibit excess in *Water qi*, and given this excess of *Water qi* in year C, year D would in turn exhibit deficiency in *Wood qi*, and so on in the series of the Ten Heavenly Stems/天干/*tiangan*.

Another context to illustrate what is meant by normality, excess, and deficiency in *qi* at a particular season of the year would be CCM. For instance, if a patient's *mai*/ 脉 (which this author prefers to remain untranslated, although it is often misleadingly, translated as "pulse") were diagnosed in Winter to be more like the *mai* of a normal person in Summer, that is, one could say it showed excess, then the physician would have to prescribe in a certain way in order to correct the imbalance, to restore equilibrium. If a patient were diagnosed as suffering from deficiency in Kidney *qi* (the Kidneys being associated with *Water* in the *Wuxing* system when applied to *medicine*), this deficiency would have to be addressed via therapy in order to restore balance (normality).

We next look more closely at how the concept of excess works in the Mutually Constraining cycle. If *Fire qi* were in excess, this would over-constrain or control *Metal qi*, as *Fire* constrains *Metal*—this specific circumstance is called *xiangcheng*/相乘, which may be called the Over-controlling Sequence—this would provoke the "unexpected" reaction on the part of *Metal*, ironically, to inflict "insult" (反侮, literally meaning "to insult as reaction"/相侮/*xiangwu* which may be called the Insulting Sequence) upon *Water*, the role of which is meant to constrain *Fire* itself.

To grasp this complex chain of inter-relationships, recall that *Wuxing* operates two main cycles, the Mutually Engendering and the Mutually Constraining (Figure 7.7); the reactions and counter-reactions within the two cycles when *Fire qi* is in excess (let us call this Example A):

1. In this cycle, *Fire* constrains *Metal*/我克/*wo ke*); in other words, *Metal* is constrained by *Fire*/克 我/*ke wo*.
2. As the *qi* of *Fire* is in excess, this meant that *Metal* would be over-constrained in the *wo ke*—*ke wo* relationship.
3. This over-constraining by *Fire* would provoke *Metal* to "fight back" not directly against *Fire*, but against *Water* instead, as *Metal* engenders *Water*.
4. In this way, *Metal* would induce the *qi* of *Water* to be in excess, which would in turn undermine *Fire*, as *Water* has the role of constraining *Fire*.
5. One could then say that *Fire* has, ultimately, "met its own come-uppance" or achieved an "own goal."

Using the same instance of *Fire*, let us see what happens when its *qi* is in deficiency/*buzu*—let us call this Example B. This would result in *Water* taking advantage of such a weakness to damage/undermine *Fire* as well as in *Metal* reacting by "insulting" *Fire*, leading ultimately in this chain of reactions to *Earth* being undermined, as *Fire* engenders *Earth*.

1. *Water* constrains *Fire* /*wo ke*; *Fire* is constrained by *Water*/*ke wo*.
2. When *Fire qi* is deficient, *Fire* would be unduly constrained by *Water*/*ke wo*; in that way, *Water* would undermine/damage *Fire*.
3. *Fire* constrains *Metal*/*wo ke*; *Metal* is constrained by *Fire* /*ke wo*.
4. However, as *Fire* itself is undermined and weakened by *Water*, *Metal*, in reaction, would take advantage of *Fire*'s weakness and turn around to undermine *Fire*.

5. In the *Engendering* cycle, we know that *Fire* engenders *Earth/我生/wo sheng*; but here *Fire* itself has been weakened and its weakened state would in turn impact upon its process of engendering *Earth*.
6. *Earth* constrains *Water*, but weakened Earth would let *Water qi* be in excess.
7. *Water qi* in excess, in constraining *Fire*, would weaken *Fire* even more.

These examples touch upon the complex inter-relationships between the two cycles which do not perform in isolation from one another but interactively to produce a multi-factorial, unified theoretical framework for understanding and explaining phenomena. So let us explore a little further this aspect via Example B involving *Fire*, *Water*, and *Earth*. In the Mutually Constraining cycle, *Water* constrains *Fire/wo ke* while *Fire* is constrained by *Water/ke wo*. It follows, therefore, that *Fire* could not impact on *Water* in the *Constraining* cycle. However, in the Mutually Engendering cycle, *Fire* engenders *Earth/我生/wo sheng*; *Earth* is engendered by *Fire/生我/sheng wo*; but in the Mutually Constraining cycle, *Earth* plays the role of constraining *Water/wo ke*. In this chain of reactions involving the two cycles, we can see how *Fire* and *Water* are ultimately inter-related *via Earth*—as *Water* in the Mutually Constraining cycle plays the role of constraining *Fire*.

The sciences of today—cybernetics, systems theory, physiology, ecology and others—are said typically to display feedback mechanisms, both negative and positive. Take this instance from physiology to illustrate negative feedback at work: the human body regulates its temperature via neural feedback mechanisms operating mainly through the hypothalamus to ensure that its core temperature is between 98° and 100° F (36.7°–37.8 °C). One begins to sweat when the temperature of the skin reaches around 37° C; but when the temperature falls below 37° C, sweating stops, shivering begins to increase heat production in the muscles, the flow of heat to the skin is decreased via vasoconstriction, the secretion of norepinephrine, epinephrine and thyroxine to increase heat production, and so on. Such devices then return the body to its normal temperature. We resort to medicine under those circumstances when the body is unable to undertake this function to return to normal on its own. *Wuxing*, when applied in CCM, would offer many examples of negative feedback loops, but for the moment, only one small instance would do to illustrate the same mechanism at work - take the case which we have already cited above of a patient whose *mai* displayed unseasonal characteristics—in Winter, the normal *mai* should be quiet, not vigorous and large/洪 脉/*hong mai*, which would, however, be normal for Summer. But should a patient display a Summer *mai* in Winter, the physician would diagnose trouble during the summer to come. As we have already seen, *yang qi* in Winter retreats into *Water*, with the *yang* hiding within the *yin*, so to speak. *Yin* stands for rest/tranquillity/stillness while *yang* stands for activity/motion. In Summer, *yang qi* in the natural environment would reach its maximum; this *yang qi* would aggravate the person's own condition (when his *mai* even in Winter exhibited not the normal Winter but the unseasonal Summer *mai*), as a result of which his *mai* would get totally out of control, indicating that there be such an excess of *yang qi* that it might overwhelm and kill the patient. Hence medicinals and/or other therapeutic interventions must be prescribed to return the person to normality—the treatment would then be a kind of negative feedback mechanism to restore equilibrium and balance between *yang qi* and *yin qi* where health lies.

Let us now return to Example A above regarding excess of *Fire qi* in *Wuxing*. We can interpret it as negative feedback at work using the language of *Wuxing*.

Fire is not in a normal state as its *qi* is in excess.

The excess *qi* of Fire, as a result, over-controls *Metal*.

Metal reacts by "insulting" *Water*.

Water, upon being insulted, would "work harder" to constrain *Fire*.

In this way, the original excess in *Fire qi* would be reduced, that is, returned to normal.

This would be analogous to the example from modern physiology which talks about the hypothalamus controlling the various nervous feedback mechanisms to ensure that the body's temperature be returned to its normal range.

On the other hand, today's global warming is a perfect illustration of positive feedback loops at work, shown below:

1. Historically, a change in atmospheric temperature occurred (caused by the continuous release of carbon dioxide and other greenhouse gases through burning of fossil fuels), leading to →
2. Melting and shrinking of sea ice cover →
3. Ocean waters absorbing more radiation from the sun (as water has a lesser capacity for reflecting solar radiation than sea ice) →
4. Temperature rising →
5. Further melting and shrinking of sea ice cover →
6. Further increase in atmospheric temperature → . . .

Another example would be from ecology, concerning the relationship among vegetation, earth/soil, and water. One can present it as follows:

1. Cutting down trees excessively causes soil erosion/loss →
2. Less soil brings about less regeneration of tree growth →
3. Fewer trees cause greater loss of water/moisture in the soil →
4. More soil loss/erosion → . . .

One could use the language of *Wuxing*, should we so wish, to encapsulate the same information above:

1. *Metal* constrains *Wood*/*wo ke*. When excessive tree cutting occurs, *Wood* would be adversely affected (with fewer trees left standing—*ke wo*).
2. However, *Wood* constrains *Earth*; with fewer trees around, *Wood*'s ability to constrain *Earth* would be in deficiency (in other words, soil loss/erosion would increase).
3. *Earth* constrains *Water*, but with soil loss/erosion, *Earth* can no longer perform adequately the role of holding back water, owing to deficiency in its *qi*.
4. *Water* engenders *Wood*; but when *Earth* can no longer constrain *Water*, *Water* in turn, in this context, would be in deficiency, and *Water* would be unable to engender *Wood* as normal.
5. When *Water*'s capability of engendering *Wood* is adversely affected, the end result of this chain of *Wuxing* reactions would be an even greater loss/erosion in soil than the initial loss.

This would be like Example B used earlier when we looked at *Fire qi* in deficiency. Extrapolating from the various instances illustrated above, we may tentatively conclude that excess of *qi* in *Wuxing* tends to illustrate negative feedback loops, while deficiency of *qi* to illustrate positive feedback loops at work.

Needham and Wang, 1956: 258 is correct in observing that ecology provides good examples to illustrate *Wuxing* at work. For instance, they cite the case of a predator-prey relationship, say, birds/ladybirds/aphids. Ladybirds are brightly colored, a signal to its enemies to keep away, as they exude a yellow substance (reflex blood), rich in toxic alkaloids. Nevertheless, this does not mean that they are immune to enemies—for instance, swifts and swallows are birds which catch their prey on the wing; these then avoid being poisoned by the toxic chemical of the ladybird. If for some reason, the population of swifts and swallows increase in a particular location (a possible reason being favourable Spring condition for such animals), this would result in more ladybirds being eaten and the ladybird population would decline. This, in turn, would have a beneficial effect on the ladybirds' prey population as ladybirds themselves are predators of aphids—this consequence would constitute bad news for gardeners with aphids eating up their favourite plants.

We can conceivably invoke the *Wuxing* cycles involving *Wood/Earth/Water* to explain the chain of ecological outcome above:

Wood constrains *Earth*; but *Wood qi* in excess (increase of swifts and swallows) would lead to over-constraining in the *wo ke–ke wo* relationship →

Earth qi being in deficiency means decrease of ladybird population →

Earth qi (being deficient) resulting in under-constraining *Water* →

Water engenders *Wood*; *Water qi* in excess leads to increase in population of aphids.

Take another predator-prey relationship. Imagine the population of foxes increasing in a particular habitat. Foxes prey on rabbits; increase of foxes would mean decrease of rabbits; but as rabbits are eaten up by foxes, the predator would suffer from shortage of prey—as a result, the fox population would die back, the rabbit population would no longer decline but increase. As a result, a new equilibrium between predator and prey would be established, equivalent to a negative feedback loop. If one were to cast the above in the language of *Wuxing*, it would run as follows:

Excess of *Wood qi* (increase in fox population) would over-constrain *Earth qi*, via the *wo ke—ke wo* relationship, resulting in decrease in the rabbit population →

Deficiency of *Earth qi* in its state of humiliation would hit back "insulting" the stronger party, resulting in decline in the fox population.

As the *Wuxing* Model necessarily rests on *Yinyang*, we can see even more clearly by now why it is appropriate then to link it with the *Yinyang* Model and consider the two under the *Yinyang-Wuxing* Model.

Table 7.1 below summarizes some of the main points discussed above showing the role *Yinyang- Wuxing* plays in CCM under the concept of *Tianren-xiangying/Tianren-heyi* (Macro-Micro-cosmic *Wholism*, what sinologists call "Correlative Thinking").

Conclusion

The *Yinyang-Wuxing* Model may be said to be an extension of the *Yao-gua* Model explored in chapter 6 as both are ultimately rooted in *Yinyang* and the *guas* themselves. Like its counterpart, it, too shares the following features:

Table 7.1.

The Environment Embedding the Person							*The Human Being/Person*						
Five flavors	*Five colors*	*Five processes of qi transformation*	*Five types of qi*	*Five directions*	*Five seasons*	Wuxing	*Five yin visceral organs*	*Five yang visceral organs*	*Five sense organs & their openings*	*Five tissues*	*Five emotions*	*Five vocalisations*	*Five musical notes*
Sour	Green	Being born, coming to life	Wind	East	Spring	*Wood*	Liver	Gall bladder	Eyes	Tendons/ sinews	Anger	Sighing	Jue/角
Bitter	Red	Growing and developing	Summer Heat	South	Summer	*Fire*	Heart	Small Intestines	Tongue	Blood and its vessels	Joy	Laughing	Zhi/徵
Sweet (not to be confused with sugar-sweet)	Yellow	Transforming	Damp	Center	High Summer	*Earth*	Spleen	Stomach	Mouth	Flesh	Pensiveness	Singing	Gong/宫
Pungent	White	Gathering-in/ harvesting	Dry	West	Autumn	*Metal*	Lungs	Large Intestines	Nose	Skin and hair	Sadness/ grief	Crying	Shang/商
Salty	Black	Storing	Cold	North	Winter	*Water*	Kidneys	Bladder	Ears	Bones	Fear	Moaning	Yu/羽

1. It was rooted in observations and empirical findings, but the ancient Chinese went beyond them to construct a theoretical framework which both encompassed and surpassed them, through processes of extrapolation, abstraction, and generalization.
2. This framework, too, developed into a set of analytical tools for organizing, systematizing information, and knowledge, which satisfies the methodological criteria of unity, economy, and explanatory scope.
3. In terms of the requirement of economy, no suitable alternative can be found (at least by this author) as, for instance, the Greek model in terms of its four elements could not be said to be a comparable alternative. It should be obvious, in the light of the account given above of *Wuxing*, that they are totally different in conception—the Greek account entails substance/thing-ontology, and hence, methodologically relies on Reductionism, whereas the ancient Chinese model entails process-ontology, and rests on *Wholism* as well as a complicated network of inter-relationships between *Yinyang* and *Wuxing*, on multi-factorial causation (to be explored in chapter 11), on negative and positive feedback loops, and so on.
4. However, in terms of the requirement of unity, it is obvious that the model amply satisfies it, as ultimately the Mutually Engendering and the Mutually Constraining modes inter-mesh, as demonstrated above, to create a single internally coherent and structured network of mutual actions and re-actions.
5. In terms of explanatory scope, it would coincide, by and large with that of the *Yao-gua* Model, covering astronomy, rulership, military affairs, martial arts, calligraphy and painting, and so on;[11] however, the most developed domain of its application over time was in Chinese *Medicine*.
6. The account of *Wuxing* in this chapter is partial and therefore incomplete, but other aspects of it will be explored in the sequel to this volume, in the context of CCM itself; also its limitations and resulting criticisms against the framework, starting from its first emergence historically and up to today, would be critically discussed and assessed.
7. A quick re-cap of its key points is called for to emphasise yet again that *Wuxing*, though traceable to the five physical resources (*wucai*, namely, wood, fire, earth, metal, and water), nevertheless transcends that empirical notion, as well as even the attempt to understand it in terms of functional properties, such as *Wood* standing for what can remain upright and bend. Its real reference is to five different kinds of *qi* involving their respective processes of combining *yin qi* with *yang qi*, as well as transforming *yin qi* into *yang qi* (and vice versa) at the appropriate time of the year or day:

Wood: That kind of *qi* associated with coming into existence (birth), not only in the biotic and non-biotic domains in terms of their characteristics and their functions, but for all phenomena, including the domain of human affairs. The key term is "engendering/giving birth"/生/*sheng*, which is a characteristic, predominantly associated with the initial ascent of *yang qi* accompanied by a corresponding diminution of *yin qi*.

Fire: That kind of *qi* associated with warmth/heat, with ascending movement, with going upward, with development. The key term is "growth"/长/*zhang*, associated predominantly with the further ascent of *yang qi* accompanied by corresponding further diminution of *yin qi*.

Earth: That kind of *qi* associated with anything capable of sustaining, engendering, and maintaining, of holding different factors together, of accepting all relevant factors and elements. The key term is "transformation"/化/*hua*; associated predominantly with maintaining equilibrium between *yin qi* and *yang qi*.

Metal: That kind of *qi* associated with anything which is clean (free of impurities). The key term is "to contract and conserve"/收敛/*shoulian*; characteristic of the initial descent or diminution of *yang qi* accompanied by corresponding increase of *yin qi*.

Water: That kind of *qi* associated with cold, moisture/wetness, with seeping downward. The key term is "to store"/藏/*cang*, characteristic of the further descent or diminution of *yang qi*, accompanied by the further increase of *yin qi*.

8. In view of the above, adding *Yinyang* to *Wuxing* as the *Yinyang-Wuxing* Model would no longer make it easy to confuse *Wuxing* with *wucai*, but firmly identify the concept of *Wuxing* with *qi* in terms of *Yinyang*, of *yin qi* and *yang qi* as well as the relations between them.

Notes

1. The author is the Northern Song Dynasty scholar Zhou Dunyi/周敦颐 (1017–1073 CE).
2. For an account in English, see Wang, R., 2012: 32–33.
3. For short accounts in English, see, for instance, Littlejohn, 2012; Henderson, 2003; Kaptchuk, 2000: Appendix F with Dan Bensky; for detailed, theoretical presentations in sinological literature, see Needham & Wang, 1956: 232–268 and Porkert, 1974: Vol. 3, 43–44. For a relatively short account in Chinese, see *Rong, 2013. For detailed exploration in Chinese, see See *Pan, 2013 and *Liu, 1980.
4. See Wang, 2000: 55 also for an image.

5. A famous one is the Li Gui which can be seen at the National Chinese Museum in Beijing; http://chinablog.cc/2009/05/li-gui-a-bronze-vessel-that-recorded-history/ [Accessed September 14, 2016]

6. For further examples, see *Liu, 1980: 83.

7. The word 甘*gan* cannot be equated with "sweet" in meaning, certainly not when it means "sugary sweet." It could be translated as "flavourful," even "delicious"—when something is *gan*, one is not likely to swallow it immediately but to retain it in the mouth to savor its flavor and taste to the full. A deconstruction of this character shows this to be its real meaning—Lee, 2008: 77.

8. There are passages in the "inner" chapters of the *Zhuangzi* which refer to *Wuxing*, such as in chapters 2, 6, and 7—Littlejohn, 2012.

9. For instance, Modern Science recognizes that water can absorb more heat and retain it longer than many other substances.

10. The first interpretation may be found in *Suwen, Neijing*: chapter 29 which raises the issue in the context of the Spleen organ-system.

11. For instance marriage traditionally was arranged by a matchmaker, but the two families involved had to exchange what were/are called the *bazi*/八字 or the specific bio-data (a record of the year, month, day, and hour of their birth in terms of the Ten Heavenly Stems and Twelve Earthly Branches system/天干地支/*tiangan dizhi* of recording time) of the prospective bride and groom to see if they were compatible in terms of the *qi* under which they were born, as determined by the relationships of the five different kinds of *qi* in *Wuxing*. This is because the ancient Chinese believed that the *qi* at the precise time of one's birth would constitute (in great part) the identity of the individual self.

A very famous text on military affairs based on *Wuxing* was the *Six Strategies*《六韬》, also known as the *Tai Gong's Six Strategies*/《太公六韬》, a text whose authorship, today, escaped identification, but whose emergence was probably sometime between the mid Warring States Period and the end of Qin/early Han dynasties (for a relatively more detailed account in Chinese, see *Six strategies, 2013*). Painting was informed by *Wuxing* (for a relatively more detailed account in Chinese, see *Jin, 2013); a very famous novel of the sixteenth century, *Journey to the West*/《西游记》, has characters in it embodying *Wuxing*, each enacting their respective *qi* of *Wuxing*; another very famous novel written in the Qing Dynasty, whose title is normally translated as *Dream of the Red Chambe*/《红楼梦》 is said to have been constructed on the principles of *Wuxing*—for a brief reference on these points, see Littlejohn, 2012.

CHAPTER EIGHT

Process Philosophy/Ontology

In Western Philosophy

Process philosophy (including process-ontology) is but a mere sideshow in the history of Western philosophy from the Pre-Socratics to today. Furthermore, it is even a twentieth-century philosophy, although should one wish to seek out roots in the more distant or recent past, one may find some fragments of thought, here and there. In stark contrast, process *philosophy* has always been the mainstay of Chinese *philosophy* ever since the emergence of foundational texts such as the *Yijing*, the *Laozi*, the *Zhuangzi*, the works of the *Yinyang* School which though lost but, nevertheless, influenced the dominant orientation in the history of Chinese *philosophy* through the millennia.

What then is the dominant model in Western philosophy and therefore of Western science which such a philosophy underpins? That philosophy, emphasising three characteristics—being, permanence, and uniformity—may be summed up as "substance/thing philosophy/ontology." In contrast, its marginalized counterpart and shadow, process philosophy (including ontology) also focuses on three features, namely, becoming, change/motion, and novelty/creativity, standing in direct contrast to those which substance ontology/philosophy focuses on.

We first pause to clarify a matter of terminology. The terms used are "process-ontology/philosophy" and "substance ontology/philosophy." However, this author prefers "thing-ontology/philosophy" to "substance ontology/philosophy" as the term "substance" bears considerable philosophical baggage that may be distracting, whereas the term "thing" is, in the main, both transparent in its meaning as well as free from the usual extraneous load.[1] However, as the term "substance ontology/philosophy" is standardly used, this author cannot entirely ignore this; readers do bear in mind, that in this discussion, "substance" means no more than "thing." (In earlier chapters, the term "thing-ontology" is often used which reflects this author's preference which is explained here.) In chapter 3, we have characterised a thing in terms of its conjoint possession of two sets of properties: Set A refers to its shape and size, Set B to its solidity, impenetrability, and stability. In other words, a thing is something enduring and hard which occupies space.

The philosopher normally credited with having systematically constructed process philosophy in the last century is Alfred North Whitehead (1861–1947). His career is divided into three stages. In his first "incarnation," he collaborated with Bertrand Russell at Cambridge to produce the three-volume magisterial *Principia Mathematica*, 1910, 1912, 1913, in defense of logicism, namely, the thesis that mathematics could be reduced to formal logic.[2] The work remains a towering achievement notwithstanding criticisms against the project.

Next, Whitehead left Cambridge for London, eventually becoming professor of applied mathematics at the Imperial College of Science and Technology in 1914. He tried to improve science education but with no real success; he also busied himself with constructing a philosophical foundation for physics, especially as it became obvious that the work of Einstein had caused revision of the ideas of space, time, and motion.

In 1924, Harvard offered him an appointment as professor of philosophy. Sixty-three years old, he crossed the Atlantic and eventually became a metaphysician, constructing a systematic account of process philosophy first through the publication in 1925 of *Science and the Modern World* and in 1929 of *Process and Reality*, which were based on his Gifford Lectures delivered at Edinburgh University in 1928. In the former book, he gave an account of the rise, triumphal achievements, and impact of what he called "scientific materialism," which is, that the object of study in science is matter in motion. He argued that this materialism was nothing but an abstract system of mathematical physics, which we have mistaken for the concrete reality of nature. For instance, in Euclidean geometry, we take a line to be something which is said to have length but no breadth, that a point has position but no magnitude—such views are erroneous as they are the result of mistaking the abstract for the concrete which he called "The Fallacy of Misplaced Concreteness" (Whitehead, 1925: 64, 72). In reality, a spatial point is more than an abstraction; it involves volume. Indeed, he wrote: "In a certain sense, everything is everywhere at all times. For every location involves an aspect of itself in every other location. Thus every spatio-temporal standpoint mirrors the world" (1925: 114). Any object in real life may be seen as a series of events and processes. By 1929, he went so far as to hold that process, rather than substance, is the basic ontological constituent of the world. If Reality is not enduring substance, then it could be a process of becoming (which he called philosophy of organism). He thought that while substance philosophy/ontology could be adequate for Newtonian physics, Scientific Materialism would not be adequate to cover quantum physics, biology (which appeared to invoke teleology) and certainly not psychology. One would need to work toward a metaphysical framework unifying space, time, matter, events and even teleology.

Rescher, 1997: 20–21 sums up his philosophy thus:

> Whitehead fixed on "process" as a central category of his philosophy because he . . . regarded time, change, and creativity as representing salient metaphysical factors. The building blocks of reality . . . are not substances at all but "actual occasions"—processual units rather than "things" of some sort . . . Whitehead envisions a "philosophy of organism" in that everything that exists not only forms part of the organic organization of nature-as-a- whole but also will itself constitute an organism of sorts—an integrated whole with an organic constitution of its own. But it is the pervasiveness of the growth/decay cycle operative throughout nature that marks this metaphysic of organism as being a metaphysic of process as well.

What impact did Whitehead's process philosophy have on Western philosophy in the last eighty years? It would be no exaggeration to say that it has made very little impression. It has not succeeded in revising the mainstream philosophical framework to support the new post-Newtonian sciences which have emerged in the last hundred years or so. However, he had slightly better luck in theology where his view was taken up in the form of process theology, developed by the philosopher Charles Hartshorne and theologians such as John B. Cobb, as Whitehead held that an essential attribute of God is involvement with temporal processes in contrast with more orthodox forms of Christian theistic claims that God is an entity which is wholly eternal (therefore non-temporal), unchanging (immutable), and not affected by the world (impassible); process theologians while not denying that God possesses such attributes, nevertheless, hold that God in some ways can be said to be temporal, mutable, and passible.[3]

On the whole, process philosophy was better received in the United States than elsewhere; according to Rescher, many American pragmatists could be said to be processists, such as Peirce, James, and Dewey—indeed the friendship between William James and Bergson (of whom more in a moment) bore witness to this. Charles Sanders Peirce (1839–1914), like a lot of thinkers of the period, was impressed by the theory of evolution as expounded by Charles Darwin (and William Wallace), which seemed to exemplify change and spontaneity at work in nature. In other words, the universe (at least in the biotic domain) appeared to be undergoing constant change and development. His countryman, William James (1842–1910) was similarly impressed. To quote Rescher, 1997:15:

> James saw the world as a sea of flux comprising a manifold of changes that are not a clear-cut replacement of one hard-edged state by another but a melting and fusion of boundaryless processes that lead into one another. The blooming buzzing confusion of physical process and the ordinary stream of consciousness that provides for structural awareness provide, as James sees it, the key to philosophical understanding to the world's course of things.

Apart from Whitehead's construction of process philosophy in the United States in the twentieth century and the American pragmatists who appeared to be working towards such a philosophy in a desultory manner in the nineteenth and early twentieth centuries, two or at best three other European philosophers are usually mentioned who could be said to have contributed towards the project in the last four centuries—these are Gottfried Leibniz (1646–1716), possibly G.W.F. Hegel (1770–1831) and Henri Bergson (1859–1941). First, a brief look at Bergson. He rejected the mechanistic view of time in science; in his letter to William James who befriended him, he wrote:[4]

> I had remained up to that time wholly imbued with mechanistic theories. . . . It was the analysis of the notion of time, as that enters into mechanics and physics, which overturned all my ideas. I saw, to my great astonishment, that scientific time does not endure . . . that positive science consists essentially in the elimination of duration. This was the point of departure of a series of reflections which brought me, by gradual steps, to reject almost all of what I had hitherto accepted and to change my point of view completely.

He considered that time, as measured by a clock, which is the conception of time employed by "positive science" to be the spatialized conception of time which allowed for quantification and numbering only, but excluding all other aspects—to him, duration, that is, "real duration"/*durée réelle* or "lived time" should not be identified with extension, succession with simultaneity, and quality with quantity. He distinguished qualitative from quantitative multiplicity—the latter saw homogeneity amongst similar looking objects, whereas the former implied heterogeneity. In his doctoral dissertation, *Time and Free Will* (1910: 76–77), he cited the example of a flock of sheep. The "positive" scientist would see the members of the flock as uniform (or at best as male or female, big or small); he would count them up, note in his record the number "25." He could count them because each animal is spatially separated from its neighbors, each occupying a location whose co-ordinates could be specified. However, if one were studying the flock from another philosophical perspective, one would notice that each member of the flock is somewhat different from its companion, for instance, one male from another male, one female from another female, one lamb from another and so on. (See Lee, 2017a, which argues that while Biomedicine is based on homogeneity, CCM is based on heterogeneity or "qualitative multiplicity" in its account of personalized medicine.)

His thoughts on process philosophy were most clearly expressed in his most popular work, *Creative Evolution* (1907) written under the influence of the theory of evolution. He did not doubt evolution as a fact, but he criticized what he saw to be a mistaken philosophical interpretation of it, as such mechanistic account invariably failed to grasp the importance of duration—instead, he argued that the entire evolutionary process should be understood in terms of a "vital impulse"/*élan vital* which manifests itself continuously through generating new forms. In other words, evolution is not mechanistic but creative, changing and developing all the time. Becoming is, therefore, endemic in the nature of reality but "positive science" distorts and falsifies it by imposing static and discrete concepts upon the study of such a nature. In other words, "positive" or "mechanistic" science grasps reality in terms of material things which are solid, discontinuous, with clear and distinct boundaries among them. As such it leaves out duration and its state of flux. In sum, one could say, he rejected a static universe in favor of one which is in perpetual motion, change and evolution.[5]

Hegel's contribution rests on a triad of terms such as: "being," "nothing" and "becoming." At first sight, "being" appears to be both "immediate" and simple, but upon reflection it may not be so, as it is meaningful only in opposition to another concept, "nothing." "Nothing" in one obvious sense is absolutely distinct from and opposed to "being," yet in another sense, they appear to be the same as no criterion is at hand to differentiate between them. To get out of this difficulty, Hegel proposed a third category, that of "becoming" which contains within itself the two paradoxical concepts, "being" and "nothing"—when something "becomes," it moves from the latter into the former category. In this sense, the third term in the triad contains the first two, overcoming them as two sublated "moments" (stages/phases)—the term in German is *aufhebung* (translated as "sublated"). Hegel's philosophy is often portrayed in dialectical format—thesis leading to antithesis, which leads to synthesis, which in turn itself becomes the thesis, leading to its own antithesis and so on.[6]

Aristotle's logic is about separate, discrete identities related in a deductive structure, whereas Hegelian logic aims, it is held, to replace this static view with a dynamic model involving, not merely parts, but the Whole. The Whole (synthesis) is meant to constitute an overcoming which retains what it has overcome; this then ratchets up the process to the next level of a spiral. This is, therefore, not "mechanical" logic but what may be called an "organic" logic. The dynamic aspect of his logic, he calls the power of "negation" or "contradiction"—it is this "negativity" of thought, which enables one to transcend the static/the habitual to arrive at a another level. Under thesis, a thought is postulated which upon reflection turns out to be incomplete or even contradictory; this leads then to the affirmation or postulation of its negation, the antithesis, which may also turn out to be unsatisfactory and so both thesis and antithesis have to be sublated under synthesis, reaching a higher level of unity.

Again, Rescher, 1997: 13 has summed up the matter succinctly:

> For Hegel, whatever exists in the world of reality or of ideas is never a stable object but a processual item that is in transit and cannot be properly understood through its stable properties or as a successism of stable states, a matter of now this, not that. It is a process, an item constantly reshaped in an ongoing development proceeding through the operation of a dialectic that continually blends conflicting opposites into a unitary but inherently unstable fusion. Historical change is omnipresent. For Hegel, the real in all its dimensions can be understood and accounted for only in processsual terms.

In the history of modern Western philosophy, Leibniz is considered by Rescher, 1997, 2000 to be the pioneer of process philosophy. His basic ontological category is what he called "monads"; the word from Greek means that which is one, has no parts and hence is indivisible. Leibniz was writing at a critical period as a contemporary of Newton; hence his rejection of the atomistic world-view which Newton and others were using to underpin their new science was highly significant. While atoms are defined as the smallest unit of matter, with extension, out of which all other larger material entities in the world are built, Leibniz's monads were meant to be without extension, as he considered that space was an illusion (at least at the metaphysical level).

Leibniz held that a metaphysics, to be adequate, must be capable of giving a complete account of Reality. Only a complete concept could do that;

his monads were meant to fulfil that role. A complete concept must contain within itself not merely all the predicates of the subject of which it is the concept, but must also contain all other predicates to which it is related—this implies a vast unifying network of relationships between monads. As the monad is meant to be a complete concept, it follows that it manifests not only properties contained within it, here and now, but also "potentially" in the future; furthermore, it must also contain within it traces of all the properties it exhibited in the past. As he said, the monad is both "pregnant" with the future and "laden" with the past (see Leibniz, 1714). In other words, his kind of metaphysics encompassed past, present, and future—the historical, temporal dimensions at their fullest. It thereby emphasized time, not space, whereas atomism focused on space, while in the main excluding time. When circumstances are right and ripe, so to speak, these properties, thus "folded up" in the monad, would unfold themselves. But to understand any one manifestation of them at any one moment in time, strictly speaking, one must see it within its full historical context. Hence, Leibniz held that the monad is a substance which is one, simple and indivisible. In this sense, the monad is self-contained—from such a standpoint, the relation between cause and effect are not real, being part of Appearance only—for instance, he held that metaphysically speaking, it did not matter whether we said that the ship pushed the seawater to produce large circles or that the water was caused to produce all these circles, thereby causing the ship to move.[7] If cause and effect do not constitute the basic agency of change, how did Leibniz explain the inter-relatedness of things, which he proclaimed existed? He invoked the theory of pre-established harmony—each monad, being self-contained, could not be said to influence another but it just happened to be the case that every monad is "synchronized" with one another by God in accordance with His conception of the perfect universe.

Leibniz held that Reality must be grasped at different levels, most importantly, at two:

1. At the metaphysical level which is the highest, each monad simply unfolds according to the kind of thing it is—at this level, concepts of causality, even space and time, are not appropriate.
2. The next level down is the descriptive level which is the level at which the finite, imperfect, human mind tries to grasp the world via concepts such as cause, operating in space and time. This is the level at which science operates. At this level, Leibniz appeared to have no quarrel with the mechanistic view of matter; his objection appeared to lie in the claim that at the metaphysical level, Reality is accordingly "mechanistic."

Leibniz distinguished between four different types of monads: matter, plants, animals, and humans. They all have internal properties but also express external relations with one another (in his language, they have "perceptions"). But the last three, unlike matter, have what he called "appetition" (for example, they strive to achieve an outcome—the plant in striving to get sunlight grows taller than the surrounding plants and rocks). The last two have memory (or at least those animals higher up in the animal kingdom do); only the last, namely, humans, have reason (*Monadology* §§ 18–19 and 29).

Just as Reality must be grasped at two different levels, time must be grasped at three levels:

1. Of God who ordained pre-established harmony and is an entity which is eternal, and hence, atemporal or beyond time.
2. Of each monad which is continuously unfolding itself, that is, immanently becoming it-self.
3. Of mere chronology which is the external framework of the "nows."

Our finite human minds can operate only at levels 2 and 3, and hence differ from that of God, which is not a contingent but a necessary being. For humans, level 2 does the "real" work, so to speak, for it is at this level of time that change would be accommodated—each monad embodies the internal principle of change.

The above is but the scantiest of outline that space and remit of this book would permit about Leibniz's philosophy.[8] For the moment, we shall leave Leibniz but return to him a little later and turn our attention now to the contribution toward the articulation of process metaphysics in ancient Greek philosophy to complete this rough history of the subject in the tradition of Western philosophy.

Pre-Socratic Greek philosophy (according to some interpretations) presents us, it is said, with both the static world-view of enduring, unchanging substances as well as its rival, the dynamic world-view of change and flux. The representative of the former is Parmenides (possibly born c. 515 BCE and hence philosophically active from early to mid-fifth century BCE), the latter, Heraclitus (said to have been active around 500 BCE). Parmenides claim to fame rests on a poem of perhaps eight hundred verses (of which only a hundred sixty have survived) entitled "On Nature."[9] Scholars have arrived at the view attributed to him—that there exists only one thing and that thing is undifferentiated and unchanging—by various routes of understanding some key fragments. For instance, the so-called Strict Monist Interpretation argued that Parmenides urged us to rely on our reason, rather than our senses; according to our everyday observations of the world around us, there are indeed many things, changing all the time, but we must trust not our senses but our reason which reveals one unchanging thing. The Logical-Dialectical Interpretation grounded it in logic, that what can be thought and talked about, turns out surprisingly to be something that is absolutely one and unchanging. Another interpretation says that Parmenides focused on understanding necessity (what must be) as opposed to what might be (contingency). Contingent matters are subject to change, but surely genuine conviction cannot rest on things which change; furthermore, if there is also what is (what it is) and cannot not be (what it is), then there must be something which goes beyond what changes, grows, and decays, that is to say, it must embody all the perfections (free from all the imperfections of the world of contingency), of everlasting existence, immutability, completion. However, whatever the interpretation favored by the community of scholars at any one point in history, it remains the case that metaphysically, Parmenides might be said to propose a monism (of immutability, completion, and eternity), whether it be a strict or a generous monism.

Heraclitus is credited with having written one book, which he was said to have donated to the temple of Artemis in his native Ephesus, in today's Turkey. Again, the book did not survive intact but only in fragments, over one hundred; it appeared to have consisted of sayings and epigrams rather than continuous exposition, some about science, others about human affairs as well as theology. He had been seen by different people to hold different, even contradictory views, such as that he was a material monist or a process philosopher, an empiricist, a rationalist, or a mystic.[10] However, this small discussion would focus on that interpretation which sees him as a processist, as propounded by Rescher, 1997, 2000.[11]

He is normally said to have advanced three claims: 1) the flux doctrine; 2) coincidence of opposites; 3) material monism, that fire is the source and nature of all things. The second is held to be an entailment of the first—if everything is changing or flowing, then "every pair of contraries is somewhere coinstantiated; and every object coinstantiates at least one pair of contraries" (Barnes, 1982:70).

Let us take a quick look at the flux doctrine; the most commonly held view seemed to have come from Plato via Cratylus: "Heraclitus, I believe, says that all things pass and nothing stays, and comparing existing things to the flow of a river, he says you could not step twice into the same river." (Plato *Cratylus* 402a = A6).[12] However, the most recent scholarship today holds that Plato and those influenced by him down the ages were not correct, as the most reliable textual evidence from the fragments do not support it;

the reliable fragment reads: "On those stepping into rivers staying the same other and other waters flow."[13] If this is genuine Heraclitus, then it would not support Plato/Cratylus's interpretation, as it seemed to be contrasting the human who stepped into the river as remaining constant with the waters in the river changing, as they obviously would and do, but, nevertheless, with the river remaining constant or the same. Instead, as Graham, 2005 contends, it would mean that Heraclitus was not saying something unacceptable, namely, that all things are changing such that we cannot confront them twice, but something more defensible and more profound. This is that certain things stay the same only by changing. In chapter 7, we cited our own bodies as one such example—the body we were born with, the body which grew from infancy to adulthood, from maturity to decline, is a body that changes all the time, while simultaneously renewing at regular intervals the very cells which constitute our body at any one given moment. On this reading of Heraclitus, flux and constancy are not mutually exclusive, but that paradoxically, change is the basis of constancy. On this last point, compare with the Chinese account given in chapter 3 (about *Qi-in-dissipating* mode and *Qi-in-concentrating* mode) and in chapters 5 and 6 of this book, regarding the three meanings of the term *yi*/ 易.

Ever since Aristotle, Heraclitus had been said to be a material monist—for him, fire is the ultimate reality, that all things are nothing but manifestations of fire. (Other Milesians, such as Thales or Anaximenes respectively held that water or air was the ultimate ontological category.) But if he were, the critics—see Graham, 2011—of such an opinion point out two flaws: first, that as a material monist, his choice of fire would be odd, as fire is the least substantial and the most transient of so-called elemental stuffs; second, if he were really a material monist, then this could not be reconciled with the flux doctrine when that doctrine is understood in a radical way—the change of everything into everything else, that fire can turn into water, water into earth. . . . He must either hold that change is illusory or he must be a material pluralist.

The influence of Heraclitus is measured not so much by the influence which his processist approach had upon his fellow Greek philosophers but more by the reaction which his perspective appeared to have provoked. First, it impelled Parmenides to retort with universal stasis against his universal flux; Plato, via Cratylus, thought his account was fit only for characterizing the sensory world where change was obvious and endemic, but opted to embrace Parmenides for his world of the Forms, of Reality. In an ironic sense, Heraclitus could be said to have performed an immense service to Western *philosophy* when Plato rejected him, thereby bestowing on Western philosophy his *imprimatur* of substance-/thing-ontology. (Whitehead was held to have said words to the effect that all philosophy after Plato is but a footnote to Plato.) Aristotle tried his best to "naturalise" Plato's substance-/thing-ontology of unchanging forms, and in that very limited sense, to accommodate the Heraclitean view of flux, but his compromise did not bear too much fruit either. Rescher, 1997: 11 says that Aristotle's half-way house ontology "was less one of substances pure and simple than one of substances-in-process."

Thing-ontology and Process-ontology: A Contrast

It bears reminding the reader that the discussion here is not about how philosophers through the ages have understood the notion of substance; nor is it within its remit to explore the issues in detail whether the fundamental entities in the world are substances or events (or properties) or whether a thing can ultimately be reduced to events or properties. Its aim is, in the main, to present a quick contrast between two contrasting metaphysics which may conveniently be labeled respectively as thing-ontology and process-ontology as well as a brief account of the problems which confront the former but which the latter claims to be able to overcome in a more satisfactory manner.

To complete this Cook's tour of ancient Greek philosophy, one must next turn to the atomistic materialism as well as the mechanistic philosophy of Leucippus (during the fifth century BCE)[14] and his pupil, Democritus (c. 460–c. 370 BCE), which were developed to overcome an objection mounted against Parmenides.[15] However, this contribution laid more or less dormant for nearly two thousand years (as Aristotle/Aristotelianism reigned supreme) until Modern Western philosophy/science were forged in Western Europe from the seventeenth century onward.[16]

The physical and cosmological doctrines of Democritus invoked two notions: Space/the Void on the one hand and Being, on the other. The Void was like a vacuum, amounting to an infinite space within which an infinite number of atoms moved. These atoms constituted Being, that is, the physical world; they were the smallest bit or unit to which matter could be reduced no further (in Greek *atomon* means "indivisible"). Hence atoms are very small, so small as to be invisible to the naked eye (it was not until the invention of the electron microscope in the 1930s that they became visible to humans), absolutely full (no pores or any holes inside them), and incompressible (cannot be squeezed any further), and as such fill the space they occupy. Hence they are qualitatively homogenous but quantitatively they differ in shape, position, in size, and arrangements. Macroscopic objects, such as rocks, trees, and humans are all made of atoms, except that their combination and arrangement are different. However, they do appear to our senses to differ qualitatively but this is not Reality—it is simply the case that different combinations and configurations of atoms cause our sense organs to have certain impressions, such as being something is hard or soft, bitter or sweet, cold or hot. Reality is such that there are only homogeneous atoms, whether these are the atoms of water (soft) or of granite (hard)—the difference between water and granite, say, lies in their difference in shape, one is smooth and round (the water atoms roll past one another), the other jagged and uneven (the granite atoms hook on, clump together to form a solid body). Atoms are eternal but the macroscopic objects embodying them are not. Although the actual piece of granite may over a geologically long period of time decay and perish, the atoms of which it is made do not perish—these live on to form ultimately other compounds, to constitute other things/objects. "Death" and "birth" in that sense are also only apparent.

According to Democritus, the atoms are not only eternal but also uncaused; there is no need for a god/God, an external intelligent cause to account for them. So too is their motion. Originally, the atoms moved in all directions, involving collisions and hence producing "vibrations," during which the atoms (of a certain shape, say) came into contact with similar atoms in this rushing about of atoms—in this way, larger bodies and worlds were formed. There was no design or purpose of any kind involved, whether human or divine—all these movements and motion happened in a purely mechanical manner. Furthermore, there was change, but all change was merely change of place. Hence, the emphasis is on space but does not appear to make room for time.

The above, by and large, provided the ontological underpinning for Modern Science, beginning in the seventeenth century, with Newton's achievements rapidly being elevated to the iconic pedestal of such a science and such a philosophy behind it.[17] The operative phrase is "by and large," as the remark is not intended to deny other philosophical inputs to embellish and add further dimensions to it, such as that of Descartes, in particular his dualist philosophy.[18]

Rescher, 1997: 2 has provided a succinct contrast between substance-ontology and process-ontology, which justifies quoting his account:

> Process metaphysics as a general line of approach holds that physical existence is at bottom processual; that processes rather than things best represent the phenomena that we encounter in the natural world about us. The doctrine takes a position within the spectrum of competing following contentions:
>
> 1. Process has *primacy* over things. Substance is subordinate to process: Things are simply constellations of processes.

2. Process has *priority* over substance. Things are always subordinate to processes because processes inwardly engender, determine, and characterize the things there are. But processes as such transcend the realm of things since there are also substance-detached processes.
3. Substance has *priority* over process. The only sort of processes there are those involved in the doings and comportment of things.
4. Substance has primacy over process. Indeed, substance is all there is; all processes and changes are simply a matter of how things appear to certain (mind-equipped) substances.

The first two of these competing contentions represent process philosophy respectively in its stronger (Heraclitean) and weaker (Empedoclean) versions. By contrast, the substance approach which process philosophy rejects is represented by the last two contentions. This approach also has a weaker (Democratean) and a stronger (Parmenidean) version.

As the Newtonian sciences over the last four centuries have scored so many triumphs, there is no need to rehearse them here. Thing philosophy, as a result, basks in similar lights of glory. So if process philosophy is intended to be a serious rival, the key questions to pose are the following:

1. Can it do what substance philosophy can now do, and as well, if not better?
2. Can it accommodate some of the more spectacular sciences which have appeared since the beginning of the last century, but which its rival cannot?
3. Can it solve certain outstanding problems which substance/thing philosophy has so far been unable to solve in a satisfactory manner?

Processists answer "yes" to all the questions—see Rescher, 1997, 2000. To questions 1 and 2, they would argue that it could give a more adequate account of time and change than its rival as substance-/thing- ontology focuses on space in the Newtonian sciences. Einstein's special theory of relativity (1905) challenged the classical notion of invariant time interval for two events with the notion of invariant space-time interval, introducing the notion of space-time or space-time continuum. This model which combines space and time into a single continuum sees space as existing in three dimensions (up/down, left/right, forward/backward) with time as the fourth which is considered to be a different sort from the three spatial dimensions—this four-dimensional space is the space-time continuum. Another example: certain areas of scientific investigation involve the notion of field, such as a magnetic, electromagnetic, or gravitational field which cannot readily be fitted into the restrictive framework of substance-/thing-ontology. A field is not a thing that does something or performs certain actions—they do not answer to the paradigm of one billiard ball hitting another billiard ball, imparting motion to it. Yet "a physics of fields and forces that operate on their own, without an embedding in things, is the quintessence of a process phenomenon of nature" (Rescher, 2000: 11). Processes, unlike things, are necessarily historically linked together to constitute a coherent "bundle" (the present leads back to the past and feeds into the future)—in this way, they give rise to laws/regularities/patterns. In the words of Rescher, 2000: 11: "the idea of law is inherent in the very concept of a process."

We have already cited one example how Einstein's theory of relativity has broken through the boundaries laid down by the space-dominating framework of Newtonian science and the atomistic/mechanistic philosophy supporting it. Another obvious example to cite is quantum physics, where at the sub-atomic level, thing-ontology becomes irrelevant, as there are no enduring things/objects, that is to say, no particulars to which one could ascribe a continuing descriptive identity in the way one can with macroscopic things/objects such as Mount Everest or Queen Victoria. At such a level, we can measure many "events" which exist in reciprocal interaction with one another, "with no stable characteristics in and of themselves but only come to exhibit spatiotemporally stable aspects at the level of statistical aggregates" (Rescher, 2000:12). Far from it being the case that atoms combine and arrange themselves in a particular manner to produce processes such as windstorms, lightning, and so on, quantum physics appears to show that very small processes (at the quantum level) adhere/combine to produce standard, that is, macro objects, which we call things. We shall be returning to this example when we look at the thoughts of Bohr on this matter.

As to question 3, we can argue that the examples already cited above are illustrations of how they raise problems which cannot be solved within thing-ontology but could readily be accommodated within process-ontology. Another supporting example is self-identity, a long-standing problem within the framework of thing-ontology. The human person obviously has a body which lends itself readily to the thing paradigm. But yet talk about the body cannot exhaust talk about the human being as such a being is also the subject of many mental activities and experiences. The unity of the self appears to be more than the unity of the body. Here is not the place to discuss the long philosophical history about the mind-body relationship. Suffice it to say, that if the self were held to be a "thing," then Hume was right to say that whenever one looked for "it," "it" cannot be found. However, if we shift the perspective, from thing to process, then the unity of the self/mind becomes more readily graspable. (Rescher, 1997: 107) puts it thus: " . . . the unity of a person resides neither in the physical body as such nor in the psychic unity of custom and memory but in a synoptic unity of process"; and in (2000:16), he writes:

> The unity of self comes to be seen as a unity of process—of one large mega-process that encompasses many smaller ones in its makeup. Such an approach wholly rejects the thing-ontologists' view of a person as an entity existing separately from its actions, activities, and experiences . . . the unity of mind (is) a unity of functioning—of operation rather than operator. A "self" is viewed not as a thing but as an integrated process.

Process-ontology appears to run against a fatal criticism, mounted by Strawson, 1964 which claimed that things are ontologically prior to processes, as things satisfy what may be called the "identifiability-dependence" criterion, whereas process cannot. Rescher, 2000 attempts to show that Strawson opened himself to objection by singling out identifiability-dependence as the sole legitimate criterion to use for determining ontological priority, while dismissing other possible candidates for identification which rest instead on non-conceptual, dependence relationships. This then amounts to begging the question.

It is fitting to conclude this section about process philosophy/ontology via the following theses:

1. The historical dimension; it privileges time over space.
2. The present looks back into the past, the present leads into the future.
3. Events, unfolding, are interrelated, not merely temporally but also functionally/causally.
4. Such interactions/inter-relations form a coherent network of events.
5. The world is not static but dynamic.
6. Such a dynamic network constitutes a Whole. (Wholism will be explored at greater depth in chapter 10.)
7. It is the antithesis of the atomism/mechanism/stasis of Democritus and others who followed centuries after him.

Process *Philosophy* in the Chinese Tradition As Understood by Leibniz and Bohr

Rescher is careful to point out that process philosophy should not be understood to stand for homogeneity; instead, it would be fitting to use the Wittgensteinian concept of "family resemblances" to refer to different versions or attempts to articulate it. For instance, process theology is one such version. In contrast, the ancient Chinese had long secularized their thinking, and if process philosophy were to be applicable, then it would be addressed to the natural, rather than the supernatural domain.

It is plausible to make the claim that the *Daojia* tradition, as explored in the key texts such as the *Yi*, the *Laozi*, the *Zhuangzi*, the *Huainanzi*, and the *Neijing*, is an articulation of a version of process philosophy. It was systematically applied in numerous domains—at the level of one particular type of organism, namely, the human being in CCM, in *ecology*, in the relationship between astronomy (Time) and geography (Space), among Heaven-Earth-Human (in the triad of *sancai*), in the relationship between ruler and ruled, between exponent and opponent (in military affairs, in martial arts) and so on via the crucial concepts and models of the Dao, *Yao-gua*, *Yinyang-Wuxing*.

However, perhaps the best initial way to approach this claim is via two eminent Western thinkers who have recognized and acknowledged the contribution of the ancient Chinese to what we, today, call *process philosophy*. These are Leibniz and Bohr (1885–1962). However, this is not to say that the ancient Chinese on the one hand, and Leibniz and Bohr on the other, used the language of process philosophy as set out in the section above, as they (with the exception of Bohr) lived long before the term "process philosophy" was coined in the West. All the same, their thoughts could be said to amount to an implicit endorsement, in general, if not in detail, of the various theses of process philosophy as enumerated above.

Rescher, 1997, 2000 has explicitly proclaimed Leibniz to be a processist in early modern Western philosophy. Indeed, Whitehead, the acknowledged prime architect of process philosophy in the twentieth century, has said his own thoughts on the organic view of nature owed much to Leibniz.[19] However, Whitehead had not, and neither has Rescher for that matter, drawn attention to the fact that Leibniz himself perceived a remarkable resemblance between his own monadology and the ancient Chinese tradition of *philosophy* in which *Yinyang* played a crucial role. This is not the place to set out in detail Leibniz's monadology, but simply to say that Leibniz, himself, more than any commentator of his philosophy was well aware that his own pre-occupations as well as the cultural context[20] did not coincide with those of the ancient Chinese when each side respectively constructed their own version of what today we call process philosophy. The thing to grasp is that Leibniz had insightfully realised that Chinese *philosophy* (at least in what this author has called the *Daojia* tradition and insofar as it had influenced the Confucian tradition) was, as Lach, 1945 puts it, "simply an alien counterpart of his own monadology." As such, it is beside the point to "prove" that Leibniz came to his views without the benefit of the Chinese texts[21] and had articulated his system even before he got to learn about them.[22] Leibniz's insight amounted to this: he questioned the adequacy of the Cartesian and

Newtonian world-views based on the mechanical conception of nature. Wiener, 1951 writes: "One might, as John Herman Randall, Jr. has suggested, derive the whole of Leibniz's metaphysics from his life-long polemic against the Cartesians. Their view of the conservation of motion was attacked by Leibniz because it failed to take into account the internal, dynamic interplay of natural forces." In trying to do justice to the organic, dynamic, purposive features as well as their inter-relatedness of life and thought, his grand ambition was to provide a unifying framework to account for all phenomena, at the physical, biological, as well as psychological levels. Leibniz was fond of two analogies—the optical one in which the monads were like mirrors reflecting one another with each embodying its own degree of energetic scintillation, while the other was to see the world as a pond full of living organisms. The two analogies illustrated the following abstract principles: "the interrelatedness and reciprocal causal action of bodies and life processes as well as the evolutionary continuity of species of graded complexity and internal organization" (Wiener, 1951). Given Leibniz's intellectual impulse and motivation, it is therefore not a mystery that he saw in the tradition of ancient Chinese thought a striking resemblance to his own efforts in perceiving the universe, not as a static entity but as a dynamic Whole, displaying a network of inter-relatedness in functional and causal terms.

Leibniz, following the early Jesuit missionaries in China, had adopted the principle of charity in understanding foreign cultures. Its default axiom is not that what these cultures have to say is necessarily gibberish but that they could embody something rational and sensible provided the European interrogator was prepared to keep an open mind. For instance, Father Bouvet with whom Leibniz had long corresponded and from whom he learnt about Chinese culture in a serious fashion had written to Leibniz that he saw the trigrams and hexagrams "as universal symbols invented by some extraordinary genius of antiquity . . . in order to present the most abstract principles in all the sciences" (Lach, 1945).

Bohr is acknowledged to have significantly contributed to the emergence of quantum physics. Rutherford's model of the atom with a cloud of more or less weightless electrons floating around a dense nucleus had run into a problem—the electrons in orbiting the nucleus would be losing energy until eventually they would simply spiral down into the center, collapsing the atom. In 1901, Max Planck had put forward the notion quanta; Bohr borrowed it from Planck, modifying the Rutherford account such that electrons operated at fixed distances from the nucleus, at set levels of energy. When the atom absorbed energy, the electron would jump to a level farther from the nucleus; when the atom radiated energy, the electron would fall to a level closer to the nucleus. This revamped model, bar some minor inaccuracies, turned out to be correct and could do justice to the experimental evidence coming in from other physicists. (The role played by Bohr is only relevant to this early history of quantum physics, not in its later developments to which Bohr did not contribute.) For this, he was bestowed the Nobel Prize in physics in 1922 at the age of thirty-seven.

What is significant is not so much his Nobel winning work on quantum physics *per se*, but his realization that quantum phenomena cannot be accounted for within the standard philosophical framework of atomism and mechanism which underpins Newtonian science so well. The world of sub-atomic phenomena appears not to conform to Newtonian boundaries, as such phenomena are not simply one moment, particle (a thing) and the next, wave, but that they are at once both wave and particle. If this, indeed, is quantum Reality, then that Reality appears to be incompatible with the whole tradition of Western philosophy constructed on thing-ontology, from Parmenides, Aristotle, Leucippus, Democritus, Descartes, and Newton to the emergence of quantum physics. Not only is quantum Reality incompatible with thing-ontology, it appears to be incompatible also with the logic which thing-ontology entails, as it violates the principle of excluded middle, which forbids one to claim that a state of affairs can be both p and not-p at one and the same time. What this book calls the *Yinyang/Yao-gua* Model permits just that—this set of topics will be further explored in chapter 9, which assesses the relationship between classical two-valued logic, fuzzy logic and the implicit *logic* embedded in the *Yinyang/Yao-gua* Model via an assessment of Aristotle's three laws/principles of thought.

However, his work did not stop there. In 1947 the monarch of Denmark awarded Bohr, a commoner, for his outstanding life-long contributions to science and scientific eduation, the highest order of the realm, one bestowed on members of the royal family or rarely on famous military personnel. The merit was called the Order of the Elephant. As a result, Bohr needed to design a coat of arms. None of those available at the College of Arms appealed to him; a friend suggested the *Liangyitaijitu* which he, with alacrity, accepted, agreeing that it captured exactly what he had been trying to say in prose, via his notion of complementarity. He incorporated it into his coat of arms and added in Latin: *Contraria sunt complementa* (opposites are complementary) to make explicit the *philosophy*/ontology embodied in the *Liangyitaijitu*. He died in 1962; on his tombstone is carved his coat of arms.[23]

The Dutch-American physicist/historian of science, Abraham Pais, wrote about Bohr and his physics. When Pais was rescued from the Nazi pogrom, he became Bohr's assistant. He could be said to be someone who knew Bohr personally as well as professionally, yet in his book on Bohr (1990: 24), he gave the following account of how Bohr came to light upon his coat of arms:

> I should note that Bohr never cared much for, nor knew much of, what professional philosophers had to say. . . . Occasional attempts to trace the origins of Bohr's complementarity to their writings are without basis in fact. . . . In particular the occasionally expressed belief that Bohr's views on physics were influenced by oriental philosophy is unfounded. These speculations have an amusing origin. In 1947 Denmark's highest distinction, knighthood in the Order of the Elephant, was conferred on Bohr . . . tradition demanded that he now acquire a coat of arms. So he consulted others about a choice of emblem. One friend reported that he had browsed without success in the Royal Library. Then Hanna Koblinski, an expert on Chinese history, the wife of Bohr's close co-worker Stefan Rozental, had an idea: use the Yin-Yang symbol. Formally known as Tai-Ji-Tu. This is the diagram of the supreme poles: Yang, the active, male, and Yin the receptive, female, principle. Bohr thought that this was a great idea.* And that is how Yin-Yang was chosen, with the added motto: *Contraria sunt complementa* (opposites are complementary).
>
> (* This refers to Endnote 32 in which Pais claims that this account comes from S. Rozental's *Erindringer om Niels Bohr*, 1985: 31 (Gyldendal, Copenhagen). Unfortunately, no English translation of this book exists which this author could track down.)

Obviously, Pais regarded the matter as a bit of a joke. As a historian of science and colleague of Bohr, he had performed a disservice to the subject of his biographical study, for the truth of the matter lies elsewhere. Pais was not as conscientious a biographer as he should have been in tracking down documentary evidence which puts beyond reasonable doubt that Bohr had read the *Laozi* in his youth, when his philosophy tutor presented him with a Danish translation of the text. One such document, as pointed out by Allinson, 1998 is a reply to a letter of inquiry from someone called Svend Hugo Jügensen who had sent to Bohr a manuscript entitled *Daodejing/Tao Te Ching and the Idea of Complementarity*. Bohr's reply was dated March 26, 1958:

> I thank you for your letter and the enclosed little note about *Tao Te Ching*, which I have read with great interest. I believe what you say about the old Chinese philosophy is in many ways quite to the point. In my youth I received a beautiful impression of it through Ernst Møller's book 'Oldmester,' and at a visit to China twenty years ago I learned how highly the memory of Lao-Tzu is still valued.[24]

Møller's *Laozi* was first published in 1909 when Bohr was twenty-four. Such early exposure to Chinese *philosophy* appeared to have made a deep impression on the young Bohr, so that his later identification of the notion of complementarity within the *Laozi/Yinyang* tradition was no mere whim or happenstance.[25]

Stefan Rosental (quantum physicist) and his wife (Hanna) escaped from Poland and the Nazis, upon which Bohr made Rosental his personal assistant, a post Rosental retained for nearly fifteen years. Hanna was a philosopher (pupil of Husserl) and sinologist. They were therefore well placed to appreciate what Bohr was doing when he invoked the notion of complementarity. Furthermore, according to Allinson (1998), Bohr's grandson, Christian, had said that his grandfather would have liked to use the Dragon on his coat of arms, but his wish was turned down because the Dragon was not a heraldic animal recognized by the Danish College of Arms; in any case, his award was the Order of the Elephant. However, the Dragon is a key symbol in Chinese culture. Allinson also pointed out that Bohr's favorite line of poetry was from Schiller's *Sayings of Confucius*: "Only wholeness leads to clarity." The preceding chapters of this book have established that the *philosophy* of the *Yi*, the *Laozi* and other such texts is but a celebration of *Wholism* (for further discussion see chapters 9 and 10), of harmony and unity between polar contrasts.

Blaedel, 1988: 193 says that a colleague reported Bohr as having said to him one morning:

> I have made a great discovery, a very great discovery: anything which any philosopher has ever written is sheer nonsense. . . . No one who calls himself a philosopher understands the significance of the complementary mode of description. . . . Those who thought that Copernicus' system was elegant were killed, Bruno was burnt and Galileo was compelled to retract his words. But in the next generation the school children did not find anything crazy in it, and thus a situation was created where the new ideas had to be taken for granted. I believe the same thing will happen with the complementary mode of description.

Bohr, 1961: 19–20 in his 1937 "Biology and Atomic Physics," wrote:

> For a parallel to the lesson of atomic theory regarding the limited applicability of such customary idealisation, we must in fact turn to quite other branches of science, such as psychology, or even to that kind of epistemological problems with which already thinkers like Buddha and Lao Tse[26] have been confronted, when trying to harmonize our position as spectators and actors in the great drama of existence. Still, the recognition of an analogy in the purely logical character of the problems which present themselves in so widely separated fields of human interest does in no way imply acceptance in atomic physics

> of any mysticism foreign to the true spirit of science, but on the contrary it gives us an incitation to examine whether the straightforward solution of the unexpected paradoxes met with in the application of our simplest concepts to atomic phenomena might not help us to clarify conceptual difficulties in other domains of experience.

It is very important to note that in his entire corpus of writing, Bohr never called complementarity the principle or the theory of complementarity, as he thought that would produce misunderstanding "regarding the sort of thing he intended complementarity to be. "Complementarity" never labels any principle or theory, and searching for such merely obscures the fact that it is a conceptual framework from which to view physical principles or theories." (Flose, 1986: 19). Flose is, by and large, correct, but this author would like to enter a modification, namely, that Bohr was not so much invoking a new conceptual framework as a new ontological one. He did not invoke the notion (and its process-ontological framework) simply because of his co-operation with Heisenberg leading to the latter's formulation of the Uncertainty Principle. He had envisaged this new ontological framework to accommodate not only quantum physics but also other domains of scientific enquiry such as biology, psychology—in this, one could say that perhaps Bohr died disappointed for no such initiatives had obviously come to fruition by 1960 (see Saunders, 2005).

Bohr and Einstein did not see eye to eye about the new physics; Einstein had hoped that quantum physics would one day be replaced by something which would not require an overhauling of the classical framework and its criteria for an acceptable description. Given the choice between rejecting quantum theory or abandoning classical descriptive ideals, Einstein had opted for the former; Bohr believed that quantum theory and phenomena do constitute the world out there at the sub-atomic level, hence rejecting it would not be scientific. Einstein endorsed the idea that one should cling to the framework by rejecting the experimental evidence which challenged it (saying that it is incomplete); confronted by Heisenberg's Uncertainty Principle, many physicists including Einstein, constructed thought experiments to show that the results were absurd, or that the results were to be explained in terms of perturbations caused by observation itself—in such ways, they hope to preserve classical realism. In contrast, Bohr considered such a move dogmatic. Quantum physics is here to stay, and has stayed for about eight decades, and could not be wished away. It is not the quantum measurement process *per se* that disturbs the results, but that science can only ascribe numerical values to the quantum phenomenon as a whole including the measurement interaction itself. This means that scientists have a choice in the questions they would like to ask of the system and in the kind of measurement they would want to perform. This is totally unlike classical physics where the complete description of the system as it "objectively" is can be given independent of the choice of how it is to be observed.—on these points, see Prigogine and Stengers, 1985: 224–25. What is required, according to Bohr, is a different framework altogether for grasping quantum phenomena; furthermore, Bohr could proffer an alternative through the notion of complementarity which would remove the paradoxical character of quantum theory. For his part, Einstein was reported to have said: "Despite the expenditure of much effort, I have been unable to obtain a clear understanding of Bohr's principle of complementarity" (Saunders, 2005).

Part of Einstein's failure to do so might lie in his calling it the "principle of complementarity." "Complementary" refers to the view that polar terms are not mutually exclusive but complementary to each other, just as *yin*, through the polar contrast of *yang*, nevertheless harmoniously combine to form *Yinyang*, as well as that in *yin*, is found *yang*, in *yang*, is found yin—in other words, *yin* and *yang* are not mutually exclusive. A profound ontological gulf (and from this gulf also followed other gulfs such as logical and methodological ones) existed between Einstein and Bohr—unlike Bohr, Einstein had never been exposed to the "complementarity *philosophy*" of the *Laozi*.

To grossly oversimplify matters, Bohr was attempting to grapple with the wave-particle duality of light, electron, and other phenomena at the quantum level. It seemed impossible to distinguish properly between the actual behavior of "objects" at this level and their interaction with the instruments which measured that interaction and which served to define the conditions under which the phenomena appeared. Take light—measure it with one instrument, and it appears like a wave; measure it with another and it appears to scatter like a particle. Bohr concluded that such evidence obtained under different experimental conditions could not be understood within a single picture; instead they could be regarded as complementary and together they could be said to exhaust the information obtainable about the quantum state. In lay language, one would say that light is both wave and particle, paradoxical though that might sound. At the macroscopic level, large-scale particles or waves such as billiard balls and water waves are incompatible rather than complementary, but at the sub-atomic levels, one's knowledge of phenomena is necessarily incomplete until both aspects are taken into account.

Bohr's notion or philosophy of complementarity first made its appearance, albeit in a fragmentary form, in 1927 when he delivered his lecture at the international physics congress at Como, Italy; his fellow physicists were not impressed, complaining that Bohr's argumentation had been far too "philosophical," with nothing new to offer in physics itself—Folse, 1985: 37–38. Later he revised it, spending a great deal of time and energy in the 1930s to develop it. He remained faithful to it for the rest of his life; nor could he be accused of inconsistency or incoherence—see Saunders, 2005.

The above account, though limited in scope, shows, all the same, that Pais is just wrong in holding or implying the following:

1. Bohr was not interested in, had little or no time for, little or no knowledge of philosophy of any kind, at any stage of his life.
2. He was never exposed to, did not know anything about ancient Chinese *philosophy* until Hanna Rosental (Koblinski) suggested the *Liangyitaijitu* to him.
3. His exploration of the notion of complementarity with which he was pre-occupied since 1927 for the rest of his life did not amount to "doing philosophy" in its own right.

Exploring Some Differences Between the Western and Chinese Traditions

This discussion will only single out three articulations from the Western tradition for comparison with the Chinese version, namely, Heraclitus, Leibniz, and Bohr.

Rescher, by making the important point that process philosophy is not homogeneous, alerts one to the fact that there are commonalities as well as differences between the various versions on offer. Limited space here will only permit a brief exploration, in the main, of their differences.

Heraclitus's doctrine of universal flux is capable of two interpretations—the extreme view of Plato (that one cannot step into the same river/water twice) and the more subtle one argued by Graham, 2011, making Heraclitus closer to the Chinese version, that behind change also stands constancy. For both Heraclitus and the Chinese, there appears to be something even more fundamental than change itself, namely, what drives change. However, in this matter, the two versions part company—Heraclitus (see *The Fragments of Heraclitus*) saw polar contrasts in terms of conflict, and that it was conflict between them which propelled change in the world. He said: "Thunderbolt steers all things" lightening, as part of thunder, symbolized that power; fire and the changes it wrought governed the world. He said that war is the father of all and king of all; and some he manifested as gods, some as men; some he made slaves, some free. Opposites—such as king/ruler and ruled, slaves and free men, war and peace, satiety and hunger, winter and summer, and day and night—exhibited conflicting powers. This conflict was the basis of change and variety in the world. On the other hand, the Chinese saw polar contrasting states of affairs, not in terms of conflict, but of harmony and *Wholeness*, for instance, that *yin* and *yang* are both ontologically as well as functionally/causally entwined, propelling each other forward to achieve the next level of dynamic equilibrium. The Chinese also held that in the case of human beings, neither the male is exclusively male/*yang* nor the female exclusively female/*yin*—as the *Liangyitaijitu* displays so clearly, the eye of the so-called white fish (*yang*) is black (*yin*) while that of the black fish (*yin*) is white (*yang*). *Yin* separated from *yang* would not endure, nor would *yang* separated from *yin*. The endurance of *Wanwu* in the universe depends on the entanglement, the mutual support of the two polar contrasts in *Yinyang*. We shall be returning to these points in a further exploration in chapters 9 (setting out what this author considers to be modes of thinking unique to Chinese culture/civilisation) and 10 (how *Wholism* is understood in Chinese *philosophy*).

Leibnizian monadology was conducted within a framework in which God played a clear role, not merely in theological terms, but also in terms of the requirement of its own system, in which God was invoked, *deus ex machina*, which enabled Leibniz to account for how his monads could form a harmonious Whole. Ancient Chinese *philosophy* was conducted, as observed numerous times before, within a secularized context; as a result, there was neither room nor necessity for a transcendent being to play the role of producing harmony in the world. In the natural domain, if harmony and *Wholeness* were to be found, they must come from within the naturalistic framework itself. This, the ancient Chinese *philosophers* endeavored to achieve. Their *metaphysics* is a naturalistic, not a theological one. In contrast, Leibniz for all his efforts, in the end, found theology indispensable; the Chinese had no theology to fall back upon. The history of Western philosophy shows a deep involvement with theology which even Enlightenment philosophy did not entirely free itself; the Chinese were free of this intellectual burden and encumbrance.

Leibniz differed from the Chinese in an even more profound respect. His monads involved a "closed" system, while the Chinese account was essentially an "open" system. By this, one means the following: each monad appears to be self-contained, its components intricately internally related, but to have nothing to do with one another, and that is why pre-established harmony between them was invoked via his *deus ex machina*. Wiener, 1951, rightly observes: "His monads are "without windows" reflecting each other's inner nature but opaque to external influences." This could not be further from the Chinese version which permitted exchanges not only between the so-called internal components of any system identified and labeled as such, but also between such a system with other systems, either at the same level of analysis and operation or at a higher level of analysis and operation. For such and other related reasons, this author prefers to characterize the Chinese version as "ecosystemic;" chapter 10 explores this characterization.

However, to make the point intelligible and a little clearer for now, a quick example would be used. The model of harmony and *Wholeness* between polar contrasts, such as the *Yinyang* pairing can be invoked at any level of analysis which the scientist/thinker would care to use. In studying the human person, at the physiological level, one could, if one so wishes, begin at the level of the cell, where one cell would interact with another neighbouring cell, which in turn would interact with yet another neighboring cell. A network of such cells would constitute a certain kind of tissue; this tissue would interact with neighboring tissue until a network of tissue relations is established which could be said to constitute an organ, another identifiable system at another level of operation. One organ mutually interacts with another organ, thereby establishing a network of relations and operations at the level of the entire human individual. The human individual is not a closed system either—s/he needs inputs of various kinds for sustenance, maintenance, development. These inputs range from food, water (other non-damaging liquids), solids (vegetables, meat, fruit, bread/rice), oxygen in the atmosphere, an ambient range of temperature within which the human person would find comfortable, clothes and shelter for protection and comfort, to emotional bonds with fellow humans (in early years with those bringing up the young human, and when mature, with others in the community), to psychological, economic, political, and other social ties with the wider society at large. On the level of health, the human person at all the levels mentioned thus far would have to cope on occasions with external pathogens, such as the flu virus, the TB bacillus, the malaria parasite, and so on.

According to the Chinese version, any system selected for understanding is not like a Leibnizian monad which is "without windows," shutting out what is external to it. On the contrary, that system necessarily has mutual relationships with yet other systems. Such systems are not "opaque to external influences."

We next look at Bohr. As he was exposed to and influenced by the *philosophy* of the *Laozi*, it is, therefore, not surprising to note that his notion of complementarity is closest to the Chinese version. Bohr, too, like the ancient Chinese, confined himself to the phenomena of this world, and was not distracted by the supernatural world of a transcendent being which Leibniz was. Unlike Heraclitus, he did not understand conflict to be the "engine" which drives change; rather, he held (just like Chinese process *philosophy*) that polar contrasts or opposites are complementary, mutually helping each side of the contrasting pair to achieve harmony and *Wholeness*. He had grasped that the shift in ontological paradigm opened up a whole new vista on scientific research, just as the ancient Chinese had done. The difference between Bohr and the ancient Chinese is that by the time of Bohr's death in 1962, the world of Modern Science had not listened to his clarion call, whereas in the long history of Chinese *philosophy* and Chinese *science*, such an ontological perspective had yielded rich harvests in numerous domains such as in agriculture, architecture, astronomy, calligraphy, defense (military affairs), ecology, engineering (especially hydraulics), ethics, geography, martial arts, *medicine*, mining, novel writing, opera, painting, politics (rulership)[27] and today even in management, systems theory, and other cutting-edge domains of knowledge (both "knowing how" and "knowing that").

Prigogine and Stengers, 1985 argue that while some natural phenomena are amenable to being treated as a closed system, Nature displays many other phenomena which are not, but occur within an open system. They imply that Modern Science, since Newton, has so far achieved such brilliant results by plucking the low-hanging fruit which display behavior susceptible to being understood within the domain of the closed system; but increasingly, science is reaching and has to reach out to the more difficult "higher-hanging fruit" which display behavior in the domain of the open system. Their book provides examples of argumentation which show this to be the case, beginning with the science of thermodynamics, chemistry, even molecular biology and DNA genetics, where the causal/functional relationships between components of a system cannot be captured by the straightjacket of linear, Humean, mechanistic causation, but which are non-linear, reciprocal, leading to outcomes which cannot be accounted for in terms of the former model—these are subject to fluctuations, and hence to instability. Prigogine and Stengers call these dissipative structures; furthermore, they identify irreversibility in such processes, thereby introducing the notion of time, as key in its own right, and not simply as an adjunct to space, since Einstein's theory of special relativity. (This matter will be further pursued in the case of Chinese process *philosophy* when we look at the concept of Timespace, rather than Spacetime in chapters 9 and 10.)

In this sense, we can say that the work of Prigogine and Stengers continues the program which Bohr had enunciated, but which within his own lifetime, alas, did not bear sufficient fruit to console him about his vision for science. On the other hand, Prigogine was awarded the Nobel Prize in 1977 for "his contributions to non-equilibrium thermodynamics, particularly the theories of dissipative structures;" in other words, the scientific community even by the late 1970s had recognised that the more exciting horizons in scientific investigations lie in studying dynamic processes involving understanding the role of time in complex systems. And what system could be more complex than biological systems? Yet on one level, the double helix discovered by Crick and Watson in 1957 (for which they were awarded the Nobel Prize in 1963) was simply perceived as a triumph for thing-ontology as that DNA- double helix molecule transmits genetic information from one generation to another, via the four bases, adenine, thymine, guanine, and cytosine (usually abbreviated A, T, G and C).[28] However, on another level, Prigogine & Stengers, 1985: 153–167 show that beneath the identification of things so to speak, of the proteins and how they are structured by way of the double-helix, lies something even more complex, namely, the functional relationships and the dynamic processes which they involve, phenomena which do not appear to conform to thing- but to process-ontology instead. (Note that in their book, Prigogine and Stengers do not use the language of thing- or process-ontology.) In this respect, Bohr could derive "posthumous" comfort from both physics (quantum, thermodynamics, not to mention chemistry) as well as biology as they are all instances of complex systems at work displaying "non-linearity, instability and fluctuations" (in the language used by Prigogine and Stengers).

One more point regarding Chinese process *philosophy*: it does not entail choosing process-ontology over thing-ontology—it can accommodate both, as it does not subscribe to the principle of excluded middle at any level of analysis and discourse. Both process- and thing-ontology may be regarded as complementary to each other. Chapter 3 sets out how Chinese *philosophy* understood that *Qi* operates as *Qi*-in-dissipating mode and *Qi*-in-concentrating mode—the latter manifests itself as thing, within a certain given duration, after which it reverts back to *Qi*-in-dissipating mode which in turn under certain sets of conditions would again manifest itself as *Qi*-in-concentrating mode. The cyclic reversion from one to the other repeats itself, and the processes endure, and so do *Wanwu*, as a result. It would be a mistake therefore simplistically to regard *Qi* either as a form of materialism (taking the cue from *Qi*-in-concentrating mode), or as energism (taking the cue from *Qi*-in-dissipating mode)—it is neither the one nor the other, but as Bohr's philosophy of complementarity says, it is both at once. Chapter 3 offers the barbarism "Em-ism" to capture this dyadic characteristic of

Qi. At one level, it may be correct to say that surely *Qi*-in-dissipating mode is more basic than *Qi*-in-concentrating mode—existentially speaking, the former would have preceded the latter. However, the fundamental characteristic of Chinese process *philosophy* could only be captured by saying that ontologically, the two polar contrasting modes are complementary, they harmonise to form a *Whole*. *Yin* cannot be grasped or endure in the absence of *yang*, and *yang* cannot be grasped or exist in the absence of *yin*; in a similar way, one could also argue, as chapter 6 has done, that empirically speaking, *yang qi* provides the driving force for the flourishing of biotic *Wanwu*, yet ontologically *yin* and *yang* form a harmonious *Whole* as *Yinyang*. Just as at the quantum level, Reality is wave-particle duality, similarly in the case of *yin* and *yang*, of process-ontology and thing-ontology, the concept of *Yinyang* and that of thing/process are expressions of their respective duality (to be understood as dyadism, not dualism—see chapter 9). In the case of the latter two concepts, one could recognise the existential priority of *yang* over *yin* and of process over thing by, perhaps, saying that *yang* is *primus inter pares* in the *Yinyang* pairing, while process is *primus inter pares* in the thing/process pairing. (Chapter 10 will explore these and other pairings, such as Timespace, in this spirit, in greater detail.)

Conclusion

In this chapter, we have taken a Cook's tour of the history of the two ontological paradigms which have so far emerged, thing-ontology and process-ontology, and discussed briefly the role played by each in the respective traditions of Western philosophy and ancient Chinese *philosophy*. While process-ontology is but, so far, a marginalized perspective in the Western tradition, it has always been the dominant perspective in the Chinese tradition until the recent arrival of Western philosophy/science and its embedded thing-ontology which serves on the whole to undermine it. However, all may not be doom and gloom for process-ontology both in the West and in China—if Bohr were alive today, he might take heart from the new directions which so many cutting-edge sciences are taking, going down the route signposted "process philosophy" itself. The twenty-first century could well be ripe for the ship of process-ontology to come safely to port—see chapter 5 for some shoots of enthusiasm in some of the newer or new scientific disciplines. Biomedicine, too, in some aspects finds that it is (in spite of itself) more hospital to the model of causation which is multi-factorial and non-linear, embedded in process-ontology rather than adhering rigorously to the linear, billiard ball, Humean model entailed by thing-ontology—a theme which will be examined in chapter 11.

This conclusion would, therefore, end on a mildly optimistic note. We have looked at the thoughts of Bohr as a case study of the relationship between quantum physics and ancient Chinese process *philosophy*. That brief investigation establishes that such a link exists. The evidence proffered is sufficient to explain convincingly that Bohr invoked the notion of complementarity to account for quantum phenomena; there is less evidence that Bohr used the *Laozi* consciously, at least, to guide his scientific investigations in the quantum world. However, it remains true that Bohr and Heisenberg worked together, leading in 1927 to the formulation of the Uncertainty Principle (but commonly attributed to Heisenberg, as it is referred to as Heisenberg's Uncertainty Principle). This principle states that the pair of variables, position (x) and momentum (mv) of a particle cannot be determined simultaneously with certainty. This limit is fundamentally inherent in the properties of all wave-like systems; it arises because of the wave-particle nature of all quantum objects. Hence the two variables x and mv are called complementary variables. As already observed, it was also in 1927 that Bohr introduced to fellow physicists the notion of complementarity. However, unless more evidence is forthcoming in the future, Bohr's input via the process mode of the *Laozi* remains under-determined in this respect. All that one is entitled to infer given present evidence is that Bohr could have sub-consciously been inspired/guided by the impressions which the *Laozi* had made on him in his younger days.

Chapter 4 distinguishes between the context of hypothesis-generation which may be metaphysically/ontologically inspired and the context of finding empirical support for such hypotheses and ascertaining the implications of such generation. The Bohr case-study seems to address the second context more than the first, based on presently available evidence. Is there a case in recent scientific research activity which could point to the relevance of the first context as far as process ontological thinking is concerned? This author cannot immediately think of a clear-cut case. However, as process philosophy comes increasingly to be seen as the correct as well as the fruitful ontology in which to understand and conceive non-linear sciences dealing with complex systems, more scientists in the near future may find themselves consciously being guided by process-ontology in the context of hypothesis-generation than up to the present. In this respect, the writings of Prigogine and Stengers could play a crucial role, as their work is informed not simply by philosophy/philosophy of science (as Rescher's are) but also as practitioner of science in the case of Prigogine himself.

This author would like to end the chapter on yet another encouraging note—encouraging on the grounds that another physicist who was keenly interested in such philosophical issues had written:

> In this movement, there is NO Thing. Rather, things are abstracted out of the movement in our perception and thought, and any such abstraction fits the real movement only up to a point, and without limits. Some 'things' may last for a very long time and (are) fairly stable, while others are ephemeral as the shapes abstracted in perceptions of clouds (Bohm, 1976:40).

Bohm further pointed out that thing-ontology, which he (1980: 15) called "a fragmentary self-world view," is strongly entrenched in language, at least in many languages such as European ones, which portray reality in terms of things—nouns are primitive in such linguistic systems, verbs are derivative. He proposes the "rheomode" as an experiment in language and thought, which he holds would give us access to the idea of Wholeness which is masked by the noun/substantive mode, and which is carried to such an extent that a noun is used even when there is nothing (no-thing) to which it can possibly be pointing or referring to, such as "It is raining." The pronoun "it" is a "dud" noun, yet in English, we feel its use to be natural, whereas a more accurate representation of reality would be "rain is going on" or even better "raining is going on" as the latter would show that a process is underway, which yields a thing we call "rain." Furthermore, Bohm, 1980: 54 points out that even the word "reality" refers to thing-hood, as it comes from the Latin "res" which means "thing:" "To be real is to be a 'thing.' 'Reality' in its earlier meaning would then signify 'thinghood in general' or 'the quality of being a thing.'" Such is the dominance of thing-ontology in Western philosophy, language and thought.

Bohm's world-view chimes excellently with that of the *Yijing* whose basic meaning of *yi* is change (see chapter 5), pointing out that while things of a macroscopic kind with which we are familiar are perceived to be stable and permanent, yet behind them, processes of change occur. "I regard the essence of the notion of process as given by the statement: not only is everything changing, but all is flux. That is to say, what is the process of becoming itself, while all objects, events, entities, conditions, structures, etc., are forms that can be abstracted from this process." Furthermore, he cites the flowing stream as the best image of process: ". . . one may see an ever-changing pattern of vortices, ripples, waves, splashes, etc., which evidently have no independent existence as such. Rather, they are abstracted from the flowing movement, arising and vanishing in the total process of the flow."

Notes

1. For one account of the philosophical baggage, see Robinson, 2014.
2. For a brief account, see Irvine, 2010.
3. See Stengers, 2011.
4. See *Bergson's letter to William James*, 2014.
5. See *Bergson on process philosophy*, 2014 (for a brief account); see also Lawlor and Leonard, 2013.
6. See Rescher,1997: 13; Redding, 2012. See *Controversy regarding Hegel's dialectics*, 2013; *Phenomenology of Spirit*, 1807; *The Science of Logic*,1812-1816; *Philosophy of History*,1830-1831.
7. "Draft letter to Arnauld," December 8, 1686—see Burnham, 2005.
8. For a succinct, detailed though relatively brief but accessible account, see Burnham, 2005.
9. For a brief but clear account of some of the scholarship surrounding Parmenides' poem, see Palmer, 2012.
10. For an accessible account, see Graham, 2011; see also Robinson, 1987.
11. See also Popper, 1945: 179-182 (Notes 1-12 in chapter 2).
12. As cited by Graham, 2011.
13. This author knows no Greek, classical or modern, and so relies entirely on those scholars and commentators who do.
14. Berryman, 2010; Graham, 2008.
15. Berryman, 2010.
16. See Lee, 2012b; on the history of the atom in the history of Modern Science, see Walker, 2013; Mokeur, 2013.
17. For an account of Newtonian science and conception of space, see Rynasiewicz, 2011.
18. See Lee, 2012b, for one account.
19. See Wiener, 1951.
20. For brief accounts of what some of these differences amounted to, see Lach, 1945 and Wiener, 1951.
21. For instance, Leibniz never read the *Yi*, as a translation of the text into Latin did not happen till the eighteenth century. However, he did learn about the trigrams and the hexagrams from Father Bouvet who sent him an account drawn up by a fellow Jesuit, which Leibniz/Bouvet claimed had anticipated binary logic—see chapter 9.
22. For instance, see Cook and Rosemont, 1981.
23. For an image, access via "Bohr's coat of arms."
24. Allinson says that this letter can be found in the Niels Bohr General Correspondence, and that Finn Aaserud, Director of the Niels Bohr Archives had drawn it to his attention as well as provided him with the translation. On his visit to China in the summer of 1937 which Bohr referred to, this author has managed to track down some details of that visit. He met one of China's leading theoretical physicists of the time, 束星北 Shu Xingbei (known in English as Hsin. P. Soh). Shu's son has

written an account of the discussion between his father and Bohr on the subject of the liquid drop model (which laid the basis for nuclear fission) which Bohr had put forward. Bohr and Shu apparently got on very well indeed and in the 1950s, Bohr made attempts to get in touch again with Shu but unfortunately without success as political conditions of that time had caused Shu to drop physics to turn his attention to another area of research in which he excelled (radar) and he was no longer at his pre-war university in Jiangnan—see *Shu Xingbei*, 2013.

25. There is a view that Bohr might have got inspiration for the notion of complementarity from Kierkergaard, but there is no documentary evidence of any kind so far unearthed to support this claim—see Blaedel, 1988: 47.

26. He kept referring to them after 1937—see Honner, 1987: 94.

27. For one discussion of such fruitfulness, see *Liu, 2008.

28. For one quick account about the details of the discovery from the perspective of the history of science as well as that of the philosophical implications of such a discovery both for science and technology, see Lee, 2005.

CHAPTER NINE

Modes of Thinking

Chinese *philosophy* did/does not appear to have a branch designated "Logic" in the way that such a subject exists in Western philosophy as formal logic.[1] However, although it is undoubtedly true that Chinese *philosophy* did not engage with formal logic, it may be precipitous to dismiss the notion of logic (short of formal logic) as irrelevant to the various Chinese modes of thinking. This chapter will explore the cluster of related themes listed below:

1. Why did the Chinese not engage with formal logic? The Contextual mode of thinking is key to understanding how their *philosophy* and world-view were shaped.
2. The distinction between dyadism and dualism: the Chinese mode of thinking is dyadic, not dualistic as modern Western philosophy is.
3. The ancient Chinese operated with an implicit *logic*, which may be called *Yinyang/Yao-gua logic*.
4. Two-valued and many-valued logic; classical logic in the West is two-valued, while it could be argued that embedded in *Yinyang/Yao-gua* metaphysics and its model of thinking is an implicit *logic* which is many-valued.

However, one must enter a caveat regarding the title of this chapter. It must not be interpreted to mean that the assessment here of ancient Chinese implicit *logic* was exclusive to the *Yijing-Daojia* tradition—on the contrary it held true for all forms of Chinese *philosophy*, including the dominant

Confucian *philosophy*. The reason for singling out the *Yijing-Daojia* tradition for analysis is that their foundational texts could be said to have explicitly commented (either in terms of their texts or in terms of their actual models of thinking) upon the subject called in this context implicit *logic*, whereas the Confucian tradition, by and large, simply accepted and presupposed such an account. This chapter attempts to make explicit this implicit *logic* in its various modes and aspects.

Contextual Thinking

It is not an exaggeration to say that contextual thinking[2] was/is truly foundational to Chinese thought, laying down the framework in which *Yinyang/Yao-gua* thinking and what this author calls *Yinyang/Yao-gua* implicit *logic* were to be understood. So what is contextual thinking in the ancient Chinese context? The clearest relevant passages can be found in *The Zhuangzi* :

> a) Chapter 17, "Autumn Flood" 秋水 is all relevant; selected passage is just an illustration. (Admittedly this is one of the Outer Chapters and hence is considered to be not as reliable as the seven Inner Chapters.)
>
> 河伯曰: 「然則吾大天地而小毫末可乎? 」北海若曰: 「否。夫物，量無窮, 時無止, 分無常, 終始無故。是故大知觀於遠近, 故小而不寡, 大而不多, 知量無窮; 證曏今故, 故遙而不悶, 掇而不跂, 知時無止; 察乎盈虛, 故得而不喜, 失而不憂, 知分之無常也；明乎坦塗, 故生而不說, 死而不禍, 知終始之不可故也。計人之所知, 不若其所不知；其生之時, 不若未生之時。以其至小, 求窮其至大之域, 是故迷亂而不能自得也。由此觀之, 又何以知毫末之足以定至細之倪! 又何以知天地之足以窮至大之域!
>
> The earl of He said, "Well then, may I consider heaven and earth as (the ideal) of what is great, and the end of point of a hair as that of what is small?" Ruo of the Northern Sea replied, "No. The (different) capacities of things are illimitable; time never stops, (but is always moving on); man's lot is ever changing; the end and the beginning of things never occur (twice) in the same way. Therefore men of great wisdom, looking at things far off or near at hand, do not think them insignificant for being small, nor much of them for being great: knowing how capacities differ illimitably. They appeal with intelligence to things of ancient and recent occurrence, without being troubled by the remoteness of the former, or standing on tiptoe to lay hold of the latter: knowing that time never stops in its course. They examine with discrimination (cases) of fullness and of want, not overjoyed by success, nor disheartened by failure: knowing the inconstancy of man's lot. They know the plain and quiet path (in which things proceed), therefore they are not overjoyed to live, nor count it a calamity to die: the end and the beginning of things never occurring (twice) in the same way. We must reckon that what men know is not so much

as what they do not know, and that the time since they were born is not so long as that which elapsed before they were born. When they take that which is most small and try to fill with it the dimensions of what is most great, this leads to error and confusion, and they cannot attain their end. Looking at the subject in this way, how can you know that the point of a hair is sufficient to determine the minuteness of what is most small, or that heaven and earth are sufficient to complete the dimensions of what is most large?" (Translation by James Legge as reproduced by The Chinese Text Project)

This author understands the above (and the two other passages to follow) to imply a discussion of the Contextual Mode of Thinking; however, this should not be interpreted to mean that other interpretations are unsound or mistaken. For instance, Schwarz, 1985 looks at *The Zhuangzi* from a somewhat different perspective.[3] An alternative translation of the last sentence provided by Watson as cited by Schwarz, 1985: 219 may make this author's reading clearer; it reads: "From the point of view of their difference, if we regard a thing as big because there is a certain bigness to it, then among all the ten thousand things, there are none that are not big. . . . If we know that heaven and earth are grains and that the tip of a hair is a range of mountains, then we have perceived the law of difference."

b) Chapter 2, 齐物论 "The Adjustment of Controversies" (an Inner Chapter):
毛嫱、丽姬, 人之所美也, 鱼见之深入, 鸟见之高飞, 麋鹿见之决骤。

Legge's translation: "Mao Jiang and Li Ji were accounted by men to be most beautiful, but when fishes saw them, they dived deep in the water from them, when birds saw them, they flew from them aloft, when deer saw them, they separated and fled."

c) Another passage from Chapter 2:
物無非彼, 物無非是。自彼則不見，自知則知之。故曰: 彼出於是，是亦因彼。彼是，方生之說也。雖然, 方生方死, 方死方生; 方可方不可, 方不可方可; 因是因非, 因非因是。是以聖人不由, 而照之于天, 亦因是也。是亦彼也, 彼亦是也。彼亦一是非, 此亦一是非。果且有彼是乎哉？果且無彼是乎哉？彼是莫得其偶, 謂之道樞。樞始得其環中, 以應無窮。是亦一無窮, 非亦一無窮也。故曰「莫若以明。

Legge's translation: "All subjects may be looked at from (two points of view), from that and from this. If I look at a thing from another's point of view, I do not see it; only as I know it myself, do I know it. Hence it is said, "That view comes from this; and this view is a consequence of that:"—which is the theory that that view and this (the opposite views) produce each the other. Although it be so, there is affirmed now life and now death; now death and now life; now the admissibility of a thing and now its inadmissibility; now its inadmissibility

> and now its admissibility. (The disputants) now affirm and now deny; now deny and now affirm. Therefore the sagely man does not pursue this method, but views things in the light of (his) Heaven (-ly nature), and hence forms his judgment of what is right. This view is the same as that, and that view is the same as this. But that view involves both a right and a wrong; and this view involves also a right and a wrong - are there indeed, or are there not the two views, that and this? They have not found their point of correspondency which is called the pivot of the Dao. As soon as one finds this pivot, he stands in the centre of the ring (of thought), where he can respond without end to the changing views; without end to those affirming, and without end to those denying. Therefore I said, "There is nothing like the proper light (of the mind)."

The Contextual Mode in general amounts to this: the two values, truth and falsity, have no proper application in the abstract or in a vacuum—they only have application and meaning relative to a particular context. They are context-bound. The two instances of female beauty cited above make clear this point—they embodied beauty in the human context. If the beholder were not a human, but a fish, a bird, or a deer, they would even be repelled by such a sight which would inspire in them fear and flight. It makes no sense to discuss beauty or ugliness (truth or falsity) in a vacuum, free of a particular context. These values, even in a human context, would not necessarily yield fruitful discussion unless the disputants are fully aware of the context in which the claim of beauty, say, is made, and when the contexts are made clear, the dispute would lose purchase as each side would have realized that it would be futile to continue to maintain that only one's own candidate for beauty/truth/falsity constitutes the winner, while rival claims are the losers. For instance, the paradigm of female beauty in the Tang was very different from that of the Song Dynasty just as the paradigm of female beauty today in the modern world (as displayed by models along the catwalk) is very different from that of the Renaissance period in European history.

Focusing on context renders the respective criteria or standards used by the disputants in contesting their case visible and obvious. These criteria may be incommensurable—if the most significant criterion for determining female beauty is to be thin as a rake for Party A but to be as amply endowed as a Tang or Renaissance lady for Party B, then it becomes obvious that argument is fruitless. Of course, this is not to say that all disputes entail incommensurable criteria or standards.[4] Whether a dispute does or not itself involve incommensurability depends on the context of the dispute—this is indeed the key thing to grasp about the Contextual Mode of Thinking.

In turn what is the key implication of the Contextual Mode? It is this: its incompatibility with formal logic, whether as traditional syllogistic logic or as modern propositional logic since the twentieth century, as the latter implies the intelligibility of studying relations between assertions looked at solely through their formal relations as extreme abstractions, with no reference either to content or to context.[5] In contrast, in evaluating an argument, the ancient Chinese were interested not merely in the concept of validity but also in the truth of what was said. For them, as the passages from the *Zhuangzi* make clear, they held that truth depended on context, that truth could not be understood in abstraction or extrapolation from the context in which the assertion is embedded. Hence from the standpoint of the Contextual Mode, a project such as formal logic would be absurd, impossible, fruitless, and pointless. Hence the ancient Chinese had steered clear of it. This is the most important conclusion to draw from the brief discussion here of the Contextual Mode of Thinking as the over-arching mode in ancient Chinese thinking. The next section deals with an embellishment of this fundamental mode of thinking, marrying it to dyadic as opposed to dualistic thinking. The section, which follows it, will then explore more fully the implications of what this author calls the Contextual-dyadic Mode for *logic* in Chinese *philosophy*.

Dualistic Thinking

To put things baldly, ancient/traditional Chinese thinking is dyadic whereas European/Western/modern thinking is dualistic. Unfortunately, the distinction cannot be spelled out in a sentence or two right at the beginning of this exploration, but suffice it to say here that both forms of thinking deal with terms which constitute polar contrasts but which each respectively understands in very different ways.

We start first exploring dualistic thinking. It generally means that in any particular domain, there are two fundamentally different kinds of things, categories or principles. For instance, in many forms of theology, such as Christianity, there are two basic entities, God and the Devil or God and human beings. In philosophy, ever since Descartes, a human being is said to be constituted of two entities or substances, mind/soul and body. In biology/sociology/psychology/anthropology, human beings are divided into male and female. In geo-politics, humans are divided into White (European) and non-White (non-European). In environmental philosophy which deals with the relationship between Man and Nature, there is the culture (human) and nature (non-human) divide.

Table 9.1.

	God (Optional for Secularism) *Nature (c)*			
Level 1	Nature (h)		Nature (nh)	
Level 2	Human		Non-human	
Level 3	Mind	Body	Conscious Higher animals	Non-conscious Lower animals & plants
Level 4	Man	Woman	Subject-of-a-life/ capable of suffering	Non-subject-of-a-life/ not capable of suffering

A slightly more elaborate schema is shown below about dualistic thinking: In the table above:

Nature (c):	Nature in the cosmological sense—the universe which came into existence after the Big Bang and what has evolved since the Big Bang
Nature (h):	That part of Nature which refers to humans and their unique type of consciousness; it is also referred to as Culture (that is, human culture and civilization)
Nature (nh):	That part of Nature which is excluded by Nature (h) or Culture
Subject-of-a-life:	Higher animals, in particular mammals, such as chimpanzees, lions, elephants. Such animals, though they do not possess the kind of sophisticated language humans possess which makes possible abstract thinking, are held, nevertheless, to have memories, capable of forward planning (in a non-linguistic manner), in some cases are said even to possess a sense of the self
Capable of suffering:	Animals which though not capable of what chimpanzees and elephants can do, nevertheless, are like them (and like humans) sentient and hence are capable of feeling pain. The lower animals and plants, however, are not capable of suffering pain as they lack the kind of nervous system possessed by humans and the higher animals, and hence are Non-subject-of-a-life.

Theses which can be inferred from the above representation of dualistic thinking are:

1. What is to the right is inferior and subordinate to what is on the left at each level; what is to the right is inferior and subordinate to what is on the left within each subdivision at each level.

2. Each level is subordinate to the level above it, such that ultimately all levels are subordinate to God in the religious/Christian version, although in the secular version, God drops out of the scheme.
3. What is on the right at each level (and each subdivision at each level) either has less or no value in themselves (no intrinsic value).
4. The religious as well as the secular versions are both compatible with extreme anthropocentricism (the view that only humans have intrinsic value and non-humans only have instrumental value for humans (see Lee, 1999, for details).
5. In other words, 1 through 4 above imply that dualistic thinking is hierarchical thinking. As such, it is ideological thinking writ large, either designed intentionally or co-opted wittingly/unwittingly to entrench a political (in the wider sense of the term) order, celebrating unequal power relationships. In such pairings, the higher/superior class denigrates the "Other;" the two categories are not purely factual or empirical in character, but are heavily impregnated with moral/social meaning and significance. For instance, the human male is not simply a human being born with a certain kind of reproductive organ system, just as the female is not simply a human being born with a different kind of reproductive organ system.
6. It is Reductionist thinking—the inferior member of the pair is but an appendage, a mere shadow of the superior member. In the case of humans, the latter enjoys the status of being the epistemological/methodological authority, laying down criteria for what constitutes a "proper"/"good" specimen of the former. Feminism complains bitterly on these two fronts.[6] Historically, in the Mind/Soul and Body pairing, the former was privileged over the latter; this held true in Christian theology; in Descartes's view, this remained true, thereby releasing the Body as inert matter, fit for scientific investigation while retaining the Soul/Mind for higher things beyond, thereby escaping empirical/scientific probing. However, after Descartes, Materialism as the new metaphysics began to undermine this version of the Cartesian accommodation, turning the relationship upside down, with Body as Matter becoming the superior category while Mind was/is to be reduced to Matter. In Modern Medicine/Biomedicine, the human being is even conceived as machine, as artefact, no longer a naturally-occurring organism.[7] Dualism in this sense is the rival of Monism which may take the form of either Materialism (when Mind is reduced to Body) or Idealism (Body/Matter is reduced to Mind).
7. It is embedded within the framework of entity or thing-ontology. In chapter 8, the term "thing-ontology" is used as the context there makes

it appropriate to do so. However, in this section, it may be more appropriate to use the term "entity ontology," as God/Devil, Mind/Soul are not physical things but non-physical entities. (In other words, the class of entities is larger than that of things, as things—physical objects—are a special sub-set of entities.)

Contextual-dyadic Thinking: The Fuxi-Nüwa Myth

The term, "dyadism"/"dyadic thinking," is only used in the sense which can be found in Lee, 1999 and used in opposition to those of dualistic thinking summarised in the section above, and should not be confused with other usages of the term by other writers. Lee, 1999 has introduced it specifically to oppose it to dualism, especially in the context of environmental philosophy and the philosophy of technology in the pairings of Human and Non-human as well as in the pairing of Culture (human) and Nature (non-human). Lee, 1999, 2006, 2012b in common with other critics of dualism, reject theses 1 and 2 set out above, while holding the denial of them to be constitutive of dyadism/dyadic thinking. It is time to spell out what it amounts to in the context of Chinese modes of thinking:

1. Dyadism, here, should be understood and discussed within the overarching framework called Contextual Thinking. As Contextual Thinking is much more fundamental than even complementarity (of polar terms) in Chinese culture and civilization, let us call it Contextual-dyadic Thinking.[8]
2. In dyadic thinking, strictly speaking, a term presupposes its opposite. For instance, "cat" implies the class of "non-cat." An oppositional pair may then be drawn out, namely, cat and non-cat.
3. However, in the real world beyond that of strict logic, the class of non-cat is a very large class indeed, as it includes dogs, buttercups, humans, indeed, virtually everything else in the universe other than cats.
4. In the real world, therefore, depending on the context, that negative category is delimited to say dogs, such as when we are talking about a cat show as opposed to a dog show, or when we discuss the merits of keeping cats as opposed to dogs as pets. How we pick out "the other category" depends on the context; contextualism, in turn, means that the oppositional pair created is not a dualism but a dyadism.
5. Dualism implies permanence, as it is context-independent—hence, men are (in all contexts) superior to women, mind/soul is superior to body (or body to mind in Biomedicine), humans are superior to non-humans, and so on. Under dyadism, as it is context-dependent, men are superior to women in certain contexts such as, in general, possessing

greater physical strength, while women, in general, are superior to men, for example, in grasping nuances in emotional relationships; women can bear children but men cannot, and in this sense, men may be said to be "inferior" to women. Inherent inferiority or inherent superiority is not part and parcel of dyadic but only of dualistic thinking.

6. In dyadic thinking, the two terms in opposition in any one pair—"men"/"women" or "mind"/"body"—simply refer to different clusters of characteristics or functions in any one given context. The difference(s) focused on would not necessarily be carried over to other contexts. For example, a cat can catch mice, a dog cannot; so in the context of exterminating vermin, cats are opposed to dogs and are superior to dogs in this respect. But in the context of animals as pets, dogs and cats are both pets and so are different from and, therefore, opposed to cattle or chickens which are kept and then slaughtered for the market.
7. All oppositional terms, according to dyadism, involve contextualism, and can also be said to involve perspectivism, in the case of particular terms such as "big"/"small," "above/below," "tall"/"short." When judged from a great distance, an object appears small, but nearer, it appears to be much larger. Relative to *y*, a is tall or above, but relative to *z*, *a* is short or below. Relative to a chicken, a human is large but relative to an elephant, a human is small. What is above or below, big or small depends on the position of the viewer and the kind of viewer it is, on the distance between the viewer and the viewed, on the value standpoint of the viewer. Other pairings are sweet/bitter or hot/cold: if the person first eats a very sweet piece of milk chocolate, then a piece of dark chocolate, then the latter would taste even more bitter than if it were taken on its own without first having eaten the former and vice versa; if you first plunge your hand in cold water followed by plunging it into hot water, the hot water would feel less hot than it would otherwise be. Take weeping/laughing: we associate weeping with something sad or tragic and laughing with something happy or funny—yet sometimes the most tragic of circumstances would elicit not weeping but laughing, and the laughing is to be understood as weeping but in another mode. This simply confirms the claim that perspectivism is context-dependent; hence, the significance of Contextual Thinking as the over-arching framework in the Chinese Mode of Thinking.

The examples earlier cited from the *Zhuangzi* are instances of perspectivism at work; *the Laozi* is also full of similar pairings such as big and small, up and down, inside and outside, beginning and ending, level and sloping, light and dark, sweet and bitter, advancing and retreating, gain and loss, weeping and laughing, and many others. Smith, 2008: 24

observes that "the line texts are peppered with dozens of rhythmic two-character juxtapositions . . . " In chapter 2, we find the following:

天下皆知美之為美, 斯惡已。皆知善之為善, 斯不善已。故有無相生, 難易相成, 長短相較, 高下相傾, 音聲相和, 前後隨。是以聖人處無為之事, 行不言之教; 萬物作焉而不辭, 生而不有。為而不恃, 功成而弗居。夫唯弗居, 是以不去。

Legge's translation:

> All in the world know the beauty of the beautiful, and in doing this they have (the idea of) what ugliness is; they all know the skill of the skilful, and in doing this they have (the idea of) what the want of skill is. So it is that existence and non-existence give birth the one to (the idea of) the other; that difficulty and ease produce the one (the idea of) the other; that length and shortness fashion out the one the figure of the other; that (the ideas of) height and lowness arise from the contrast of the one with the other; that the musical notes and tones become harmonious through the relation of one with another; and that being before and behind give the idea of one following another. Therefore the sage manages affairs without doing anything, and conveys his instructions without the use of speech. All things spring up, and there is not one which declines to show itself; they grow, and there is no claim made for their ownership; they go through their processes, and there is no expectation (of a reward for the results). The work is accomplished, and there is no resting in it (as an achievement).The work is done, but how no one can see; 'Tis this that makes the power not cease to be.

8. Perspectivism emphazises that there is a conceptual link between the contrasting terms in the pair—that the concept inside (x) implies that of outside (y), far implies that of near, tall implies that of short, beautiful that of ugly. The concept *x* could only be properly grasped/understood by relating it to its conceptual contrast *y* as well as the situation and attitude of the individual in deploying the contrasting terms in the pair.
9. It means one cannot depart form context. Hence, the Contextual-dyadic Mode of Thinking is basic and fundamental. In particular, the *Yinyang* pairing which does not involve perspectivism but is pervasive in Chinese *philosophy*, *science*, and culture, through the ages, has come to be taken as paradigmatic of this kind of thinking. However, it could be that more humble pairings such as above/below, tall/short, or large/small involving perspectivism could have laid the foundation for its appearance; at least they all fall under the same (implicit) logical heading. Smith, 2008:24 observes: "(t)hese contrasts suggest a major source of inspiration for, if not the actual origins of the pervasive notions of yin and yang."

10. The *Yinyang* pairing serves to bring out, more strongly than some of the other pairings, that the relationship between *yin* and *yang* goes beyond a mere conceptual relationship; chapters 6 and 7 have demonstrated the complicated relationships between them, namely, that empirically, causally, and ontologically, they are inextricably entwined with each other, acting as a harmonious *Whole*. The pairing and the harmonious *Whole* are empirically based because processes in Nature exhibit them—day is followed by night, night by day, Winter by Summer, Summer by Winter, heat by cold, cold by heat, life by death, death by life. *Yuzhou* (universe) and *Wanwu* (especially organisms) repeat this cycle in an enduring manner. The pairing is ontologically grounded because the fundamental category in *Yuzhou* is *Qi* and *Qi* exists and operates in two modes, *Qi*-in-dissipating and *Qi*-in-concentrating modes—together they form a harmonious *Whole* as Em-ism, neither only energy nor only matter (to use modern language). The pairing, under *Wuxing*, functions causally in terms of the Mutually Engendering and Mutually Constraining Modes (in the language of science today, the pair could be said to demonstrate feedback mechanisms at work). *Yinyang* does not refer to concrete things set in stone but on relationships in any given context—in the *zhouye* (daily) sequence, relative to night, day is *yang* and night is *yin*, but relative to day itself, the first half is *yang-in-yang*/阳中之阳, and the latter part of the day when sun gets weaker, it is *yin-in-yang*/阳中之阴. Relative to night itself, the first half is *yin-in-yin*/阴中之阴, and the second half is *yang-in-yin*/阴中之阳. (See *Liu, 1980: 48.) In *Neijing/Suwen*, Chapter 4/《素问· 金匮言论》, this passage occurs: 阴中有阴，阳中有阳。平旦至日中, 天之阳, 阳中之阳也; 日中至黄昏, 天之阳, 阳中之阴也; 合夜至鸡鸣, 天之阴，阴中之阴也; 鸡鸣至平旦, 天之阴, 阴中之阳也。As rendered by this author: "In *yin* there is *yin*, in *yang* there is *yang*. From sunrise to noon, the *yang* of the sky is *yang*-in-*yang*; from noon to sunset, the *yang* of the sky is *yin*-in-*yang*; from midnight to dawn (when the cocks crow), the *yin* of the sky is *yin*-in-*yin*; from dawn to sunrise, the *yin* of the sky is *yang-in-yin*."

Another example comes from the *Yao-gua* Model of the *Yijing*. Here is a version of the sequence of the *Xiantian* gua (according to the Shao Yong) which reads *Qian*(1), *Dui* (2), *Li* (3), *Zhen* (4), *Xun* (5), *Kan* (6), *Gen* (7), and *Kun* (8) as shown below.

This arrangement shows the trigrams as polar contrasts: the *Qian gua* occupying South and the *Kun gua* occupying North; the *Li gua* East and the *Kan gua* West; the *Zhen gua* Northeast and the *Xun gua* Southwest; the *Dui gua* Southeast and the *Gen gua* Northwest. The *Houtian* (After-Heaven) ar-

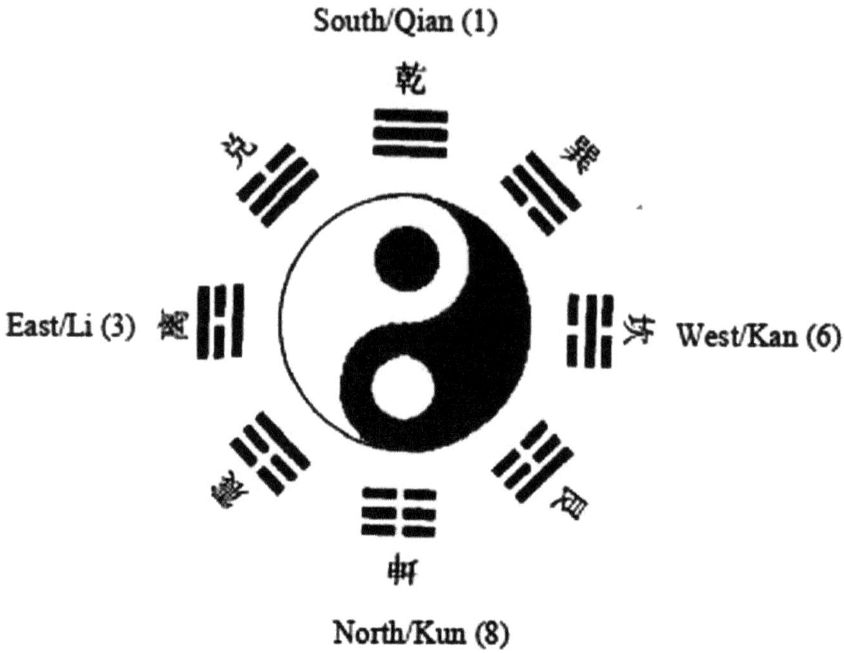

Figure 9.1. Sequence of the Xiantian gua (according to the Shao Yong)

rangement (see chapter 5) illustrates the relationship between the trigrams and *Wuxing*. Here, the *Li gua* now occupies due South and its polar contrast the *Kan gua* due North; the *Zhen gua* due East and its contrast the *Dui gua* due West; the *Gen gua* occupies Northeast and its contrast the *Kun gua* Southwest; the *Xun gua* Southeast and its contrast the *Qian gua* Northwest. The trigrams could be arranged differently depending on the context of their application; they could occupy different positions in terms of Timespace—for instance, a different *gua* than the *Qian gua*, the *Li gua* could be used to stand for East/Summer/Heat/*Yang* depending on context. This accords with the over-arching Contextual Mode of Thinking; its account of polar-contrast pairings is dyadic, not dualistic as according to the latter, the respective status of the superior/privileged/the dominating and that of the inferior/non-privileged/dominated half of the pairing remained hierarchically unchanged, set in stone. Under the Contextual-dyadic Mode, the pairings form a harmonious *Whole* and so could, therefore, be argued to be a distinctive form of thinking, indeed, unique to Chinese civilisation and its culture.

11. Let us now reinforce the analysis above by looking at an image of the pro-creation myth in Chinese folklore. The first image which appeared in Chinese history could be dated to the Han Dynasty;[9] the one reproduced below is a

much later version. The myth itself in its various forms has been found in texts between the Warring States Period and the Han Dynasty.[10] Furthermore, the concepts it represents are in accordance with the foundational texts such as the *Yijing* as well as the *Ten Wings*, the *Laozi*, and the *Zhuangzi*. This is the myth about Fuxi 伏羲 and Nüwa 女娲, the Chinese creation myth. See image below:

In keeping with the Contextual-dyadic Mode, note the following:

(a) Fuxi is not consistently *yang* and Nüwa is not consistently *yin*.

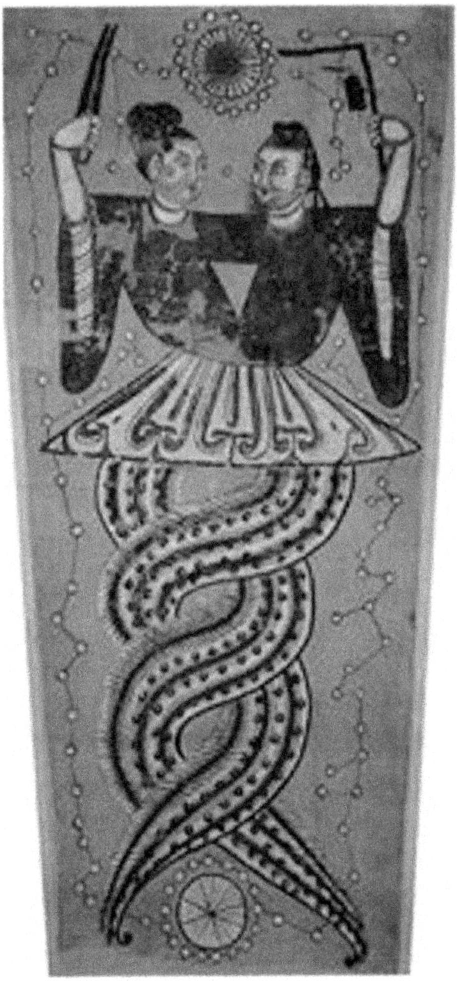

Figure 9.2. The Fuxi and Nüwa pro-creation myth

(b) Processes in *Ziran* are simply never purely *yang* or purely *yin*—these are constantly changing in the configuration of *yin* and *yang*.
(c) Both *yin* and *yang* are necessarily present in generating order and life in the world.
(d) Fuxi and Nüwa form a *Whole*; they are pictured with the top half of their bodies separate while their bottom halves intertwine to form a spiral.
(e) Polarities are inter-dependent, mutually supportive, and inter-acting in producing an outcome which is spiral in nature. The spiral form may be said to be significant in an additional way, to indicate that processes in *Ziran*, in *Wanwu* repeat and replicate themselves but not in an exactly identical manner each time—Summer which had just gone would come round again the next year, but the summer of the past years would not be identical with the summer of this year, or with the summers of years to come. Cyclical reversions occur but each cycle achieves a slightly different equilibrium.
(f) The above exemplifies process-ontology, not thing-ontology.
(g) We can also analyze the image in terms of different levels:

Level 1: Fuxi, being male, is *yang*, while Nüwa, being female, is *yin*—the *jing* 精 (sperm) of the male and the egg/uterus of the female are required for procreation.[11]

Level 2: Fuxi is pictured holding a set-square; the set-square, an instrument used by carpenters, is the symbol of Earth/*Di*—in this sense, Fuxi is no longer simply *yang* but also *yin* and, therefore, embodies *Yinyang*. (Chapter 7 shows how the Chinese developed the concept of *wufang*, namely, the four points of the compass together with the centre to form five key positions/orientations which can be distinguished on Earth). Nüwa is shown holding a pair of compasses; that instrument is used to draw a perfect circle which is the symbol of Heaven/*Tian*/*yang* (as astronomical phenomena such as day/night, the four seasons are cyclical in nature). Hence, Nüwa, too, is not simply *yin* but is also *yang*, embodying *Yinyang*.

Level 3: Fuxi's set-square is no longer associated with something *yin*, such as the carpenter's tool but now stands for something *yang*, as in this context, the instrument stands for kingship which is *yang*. Nüwa's pair of compasses, in this context, is associated with *yin*, with bringing about ordered space following the chaos caused by the flood of mythology—see Lewis, 2006:125–27; Wang, 2012:101.

(i) In generating cosmic order, *yin* and *yang* must co-exist and interact as *Yinyang*; as such the set-square and the pair of compasses stand for *Tiandi*/Heaven and Earth, that is, the universe. Furthermore, *Tian* is about time and *Di* is about space; hence *Tiandi* is about Timespace, a notion to be further explored in chapter 10.

(ii) In generating political order, Fuxi holds the set square, the symbol of kingship—the character for this instrument is *ju* 矩. Nüwa holds the set of compasses, standing for natural order on Earth[12]—the character for this instrument is 规. The two instruments themselves, since the

Warring States Period, stand for rules and standards "that impose order on unruly matter"—Wang, 2012: 101. The two respective characters for the set-square and the compasses are combined to form the word *guiju*/规矩 which refers to any rule or convention for setting up and maintaining order in society/community/organisation. The Eastern Han Dynasty historian and scholar, Ban Gu 班固 (32–92 CE) in *Hanshu*/《汉书》 explicitly identified these two implements with *Yinyang*; he wrote: "The compass is used to standardize circles so they attain their *lei*; the square is used to standardize squares so that they do not lose their form. The compass and square are mutually dependent. When *yinyang* are in order and position, the circle and square will be completed." (Ban Gu, *Hanshu* (*The Book of Han*), Beijing: Chinese Press, 1955) as translated and cited by Wang, 2012:102.

12. However, the analysis above can be challenged by those who care to cite Confucian Thought. The latter, as is well-known, seems to support dualism rather than dyadism (as here defined). Chapter 5 has shown *en passant* that a new set of social relationships of a specific kind or a new interpretation of an extant pairing had been mapped on to the original series of pairings. There we noted that the humanistic tendency as represented by Confucian thinking was super-imposed on the naturalistic tendency of *Daojia* thinking, turning polar contrasts from being understood in dyadic terms only to being understood in dualistic terms in the social/moral domains, in particular. In table 9.2, what is in bold font stands for the humanistic/Confucian/dualistic tendency):

In the naturalistic tendency, Earth being compliant, is taken to mean the following:

(a) Earth can take a lot "seemingly" without protesting and complaining (when we treat it with respect and not abuse its generosity). As elucidation, we can take our present predicament, being confronted with crises regarding our Environment on a scale not seen earlier in human history, of which global warming is one. Since the second Industrial Revolution based on fossil fuels, humankind has been throwing a lot at Earth, which seemed to have coped so marvellously well. This lulled people into complacency. However, we now know that Earth has its

Table 9.2.

Unbroken yang yao	*Broken* yin yao - -
Yang 阳—Sun/brightness/warmth/Summer	*Yin* 阴—the Moon/moonlight/darkness/cold/Winter
Qian 乾—*Tian* 天 Heaven/**Male/Ruler/Superior Man**	*Kun* 坤—*Di* 地 Earth/**Female/the Ruled/the Common Man**
Gang 刚 hard (such as rock/**Ruler/Husband**)	*Rou* 柔 soft, such as water/**Official/Wife**)
Jian 健 strong (**Ruler/Husband**)	*Shun* 顺 compliant* (**Ruled/Wife**)

limits, that its capability for forbearance is not infinite when we abuse it (or at least not, given the time-scale we humans operate with).
(b) In the *Ten Wings*, one finds: 至哉坤元, 万物资生, 乃顺乘天。坤厚载物。德合无疆。含弘光大, 物品咸亨。《周易·象》, for which this author offers as interpretation: The essence of the virtue of *Kun*/Earth lies in its boundless and generous capacity to sustain *Wanwu* (including what today we call biodiversity).

For centuries in Chinese history, Confucius's teaching was not well received by the rulers of the land; its moment of ascendency only came with the establishment of the Han Dynasty which succeeded the short-lived Qin empire (221–206 BCE). The first Qin emperor, like the rulers of the many states (which appeared following the fragmentation of Zhou dynastic rule since the Spring and Autumn Period) relied in the main on Legalist *philosophy*[13] to inform its statecraft. However, the quick demise of the Qin empire prompted reconsideration on the part of the early Han rulers, the most important of which was Han Wudi 汉武帝 (156–87 BCE) who, on the one hand tried to overcome the Xiongnu (a normadic tribe from the north persistently raiding Chinese territory, disturbing the peace of 中原/*Zhongyuan*) through military campaigns, and on the other to consolidate the Han empire so that it would not suffer the fate of the preceding short-lived Qin empire as well as his own power against rivals who invoked *Daojia* teaching. At long last Confucian thought/values came in from the cold and were co-opted to construct a new ideology to underpin Han imperial rule. In earlier chapters we have already seen the Confucian tendency appropriating the *Yijing* by adding the *Ten Wings*, thereby creating the text which the Chinese called/call the *Zhouyi*—*Tian* was no longer simply Heaven, and *Di* was no longer simply Earth but became that supremely important pair of polar contrasts called *Qian* and *Kun* as *Qiankun*, which then bore the heavy weight of supporting what came later to be the ideology of feudal values, derived from

Table 9.3.

Emperor	Officials
Officials	The Common People
Husband	Wife
Father	Son
Older Brother	Younger Brother

Confucian teaching. For instance, from *Qiankun* one could derive the five relationships to illustrate the dualistic spirit at work as shown in table 9.3.

In today's critique of feminism, we would say that this schema would embody patriarchy in its paradigmatic expression as all those with power were consistently Male; hence its polar contrast Female would consistently be the underprivileged and the oppressed. According to feudalistic values through the centuries of Chinese history, since Han times, a woman must first obey her father, then her husband upon marriage, then her eldest son when widowed. Emperor/Official/Male (Husband/Father/Son/Brother) were categorized as *Qian*; Officials (*vis-à-vis* Emperor), the Common People (*vis-à-vis* Emperor/Officials), Offspring (*vis-à-vis* Father), Younger Brother (*vis-à-vis* Older Brother) were all *yin* or *Kun*. The Female alone was consistently *Kun* in all contexts. In this way, *Qiankun* in the Confucianist context took on dualistic significance, with *Qian* standing for "all things bright and powerful" and male, *Kun* for "the powerless," the female. Male and Female were no longer about the mere division of labor, about the different roles each played in human existence but forming a complementary harmonious *Whole* based on equal though different contributions to the *Whole*. Instead, it came, by and large, to stand for an unequal power relationship between men and women, and should unity result it would be based on the female acceptance of the unequal relationship imposed on it through acculturation, education that strenuously instilled in women and men of their respective different roles and statuses within a clearly defined hierarchical structure of their existence. In dyadic thought, men and women were equal but different; in dualistic thought, men and women were different and therefore unequal.

The logic of patriarchy based on the dualistic mode of thought carried to an extreme as noted above is clearly spelled out by Plumwood, 1993: 49–52 who calls this strategy "hyperseparation" or "radical exclusion:"

> For distinctness, for non-identity or otherness, there need be only a single characteristic which is different, possessed by the one but not the other, in order to guarantee distinctions according to the usual treatment of identity (e.g. in Leibniz's Law). Where items are constructed or construed according to dualistic relationships, however, the master tries to magnify, to emphasise and to maximise the number and importance of differences and to eliminate or treat as inessential shared qualities, and hence to achieve a maximum separation. . . . denial or minimisation of continuity is important in eliminating identification and sympathy between members of the dominating class and the dominated, and in eliminating possible confusion between powerful and powerless. . . . A major aim of dualistic construction is polarisation, to maximise distance or separation between the dualised spheres and to prevent their being seen as continuous or contiguous. . . . A further important feature of dualisti-

cally construed opposition is that the underside of a dualistically conceived pair is defined in relation to the upperside as a lack, a negativity.

When the dualistic replaced the dyadic mode in the context of social/political/moral relationships in the history of Chinese *philosophy*, it was significant that the term for harmony (*he*$_1$ 和) was replaced by another character with the same sound but different meaning, namely, (*he*$_2$合), which as a verb could mean "to put things together" and as a noun "unity," but a unity which is deliberately obtained among different (disparate) things through human intervention/manipulation. The meaning of *he*$_2$ is ontologically of a different kind from that of *he*$_1$ which is based on polar contrasts being complementary to each other, thereby forming a harmonious *Whole*. However, this dyadic tendency had to be given a different ontological interpretation when polar contrasts were co-opted by certain thinkers in the human social sphere.

To be fair, the schema constructed above was not exactly the officially sanctioned famous five relationships under Confucian values (from Han times onward). These are shown in table 9.4.

It is immediately obvious that only four of the five (that is with the exception of the last) were intended to involve unequal power relationships and hence embodied dualistic rather than dyadic thinking. The last between Friend and Friend escaped the Han Confucianist revisionist reach which permitted, say, an older/richer/more talented friend to complement harmoniously on an equal footing with another friend who is younger/poorer/less talented.

The introduction of *Qiankun* in the *Ten Wings*, in a sense, laid the groundwork for the more explicit *volte-face* from dyadic to dualistic thinking which entered the scene, especially in the writings of Dong Zhongshu 董仲舒(179–104 BCE), the leading Confucianist of Han Jingdi (汉景帝, 157–41 BCE) and Han Wudi's time who began (explicitly) to change the dyadic mode into the dualistic mode; indeed, he could be said to be the main architect of Confucianism as an official ruling ideology.[14] First, politically, as minister to

Table 9.4.

Emperor/King/Ruler	The Ruled/the Common People
Husband	Wife
Father	Son
Older Brother	Younger Brother
Friend	Friend

the Emperor, he persuaded the emperor to get rid of all non-Confucian scholars from government—this policy was 独尊儒术，罢黜百家 / "only honor the Confucian arts, eliminate all other schools of thought;" to establish an imperial college of learning (太学/*taixue*) trained in Confucian thought (as understood by him) from which appointments to government posts would be selected (later this became the famous civil service examination system).

From the standpoint of this book, Dong Zhongshu's most striking philosophical contribution was his attempt to turn the dyadic mode into the dualistic mode of thinking, thereby abandoning Contextual-dyadic Thinking. Instead, he used the dualistic mode to construct an ideology which was intended to underpin the new Han imperial rule. According to Dong, society was divided into two major categories, the category of superior persons and that of inferior persons, each containing three sets as members. The first included Ruler/Father/Man which constituted the superior people; the second included Ruled/Son/Woman which constituted the inferior persons *vis-à-vis* the first category. They could be sorted out in terms of three pairings: Ruler/Minister (Officials), Father/Son, Husband/Wife. As they were intended to be dualistic pairings, the first mentioned member in each pair was the privileged/dominating member, and the second the non-privileged/dominated member. The respective inferior member simply owed loyalty, filial piety, obedience/subservience to the respective superior member of the pairing. These three unequal power relationships were what Dong called *sangang*/三纲/the three bonds of norms and relationships between the categories of superior and inferior persons. A later work, *Comprehensive Discussions in the White Tiger Hall*/《白虎通议·三纲六纪》by the Han historian, Ban Gu 班固 made clear the reference of the term *sangang* (three bonds): 三纲者，何谓也？君臣、父子、夫妇也, rendered by this author as: "What does *sangang* refer to or mean? It refers to three contrasting pairs, Ruler/official, Father/son, Husband/wife." The passage continues: 君臣、父子、夫妇。六人也。所以称三纲何。一阴一阳谓之道。阳得阴而成。 阴得阳而序。刚柔相配。 故六人为三纲, rendered by this author as: "Ruler/Minister, Father/Son, Husband/Wife involving six people. Why call them the three bonds? That is because in each contrasting pair one is *yin* and the other *yang*, thereby instantiating the Dao. When *yang* partners *yin*, completion occurs; when *yin* partners *yang*, order ensues. These happen because the hard (*yang*) and the soft (*yin*) match (and complement) each other."

Dong Zhongshu had appropriated the concepts of *yin*, and *yang* as well as that of *Yinyang* for his project of constructing a new ideology for the Han emperors—the concept of *yang* was simply to be equated with the superior member and that of *yin* with the inferior member of his three dualistic pairings (*sangang*). In this sense, he could be said to have systematically replaced the Contextual-dyadic mode with the Contextual-dualistic Mode of thinking.

Furthermore, he seemed to have at the same time embraced an extreme form of essentialism where the status of *yang* was bestowed on the superior member irrespective of whether the person exhibited behaviour in accordance with the meaning of *yang* as "bright," "warm," "noble," "external/manifest" and the status of *yin* was bestowed on the inferior member irrespective of whether the person exhibited behavior in accordance with the meaning of *yin* as "dark," "cold," "internal/hidden or latent," "ignoble." Indeed, this was what he said at least with regard to the Husband (Man) / Wife (Woman) pairing: 丈夫虽贱皆为阳, 妇人虽贵皆为阴。《春秋繁露·阳尊阴卑 第四十三章》 which this author renders as: "Even if the husband behaves in a base manner, he is still *yang*, even if the wife behaves nobly, she is still *yin*." (*Chunqiu fanlu*, chapter 43 conspicuously entitled "Venerating *Yang* and Disdaining *Yin*.") This standpoint is precisely that which one finds in racism: a person's superior or inferior status in society is determined by something the person is born with, such as a lighter or a darker skin pigmentation. Moral/political categories of superiority/inferiority under the hierarchical dualistic mode are simply imposed on phenomena which are part of the natural processes of life on Earth.

In the same text, he continued in the same vein in another chapter, chapter 49: 天地之常, 一阴一阳, 阳者, 天制之德 也阴者, 天之 刑也。。。《春秋繁露·阴阳义· 第四十九章 》 which Wang, 2005 translates as: "Heaven and earth are constant and there is one *yin* and one *yang*. *Yang* is *tian*'s virtue (*tiande* 天德) and *yin* is *tian*'s punishment (*tianxing*天刑). Here *tian/yang* was said to involve virtue (that is, what is good) while *yin* to involve punishment—*tian* that which was virtuous/good/*yang*/bright had the task of meting out what was bad (punishment), identifying it with *yin*."[15]

Here in this chapter, he actually repeated what he said in the earlier chapter 43 as can be seen especially in the first part of the quotation: 在善恶，恶之属尽为阴，善之属尽为阳，阳为德，阴为刑。。。阳，天之德，阴，天之刑也，阳气暖而阴气寒，阳气予而阴气夺，阳气仁而阴气戾，阳气宽而阴气急，阳气爱而阴气恶，阳气生而阴气杀。。。。贵阳而贱阴也。《春秋繁露·阴阳义 第四十三章》which this author renders as: "In the benevolent/malevolent contrasting pair, malevolence is *yin* and benevolence is *yang*; *yang* aims at virtue while *yin* at punishment. . . . *Yang* is *Tian*'s virtue and *yin* is *Tian*'s punishment. *Yang qi* is warm while *yin qi* is cold; the former gives, the latter grabs. *Yang qi* embodies *benevolence* while *yin qi malevolence*; the former is generous and relaxed, the latter harassing.

Yang qi radiates love while *yin qi* emanates hate; the former is life-giving and life-enhancing, the latter life-denying, death-foreboding. . . . (Hence) *yang* is valued and *yin* disvalued."

This brief discussion leaves one in no doubt that Dong Zhongshu had systematically transformed the Contextual-dyadic Mode into dualistic thinking. The true impact of his philosophy as far as patriarchy was concerned was profound, reaching new heights by the time of the Song Dynasty when physical restrictions increasingly were ordained to confine female existence (at least upper class females) to the domestic sphere alone.

His turn to the dualistic hierarchical mode in turn raises a question which, though not germane to the pre-occupation of this book, must be briefly addressed. Was he a follower of Confucian thinking, strictly speaking? What he had written as examined above appeared not to be in accordance with texts such as the *Analects* and the *Mengzi*. For instance, if we were to follow the logic as laid down by the dualistic Husband (Man)/Wife (Woman), then it would imply that the Ruler in the Ruler/Official pairing would always be *yang* in virtue of the privileged role assigned to the Ruler irrespective of how vile, vicious, and ignoble his conduct would be toward the Common People. It would imply that the Official would simply be the inferior other; as such, they would have only unswerving obligations to obey the Ruler's will, regardless of the nature of his behavior in discharging his duties embodied as part of his rule. However, this implication would be incompatible with either the *Analects* or the *Mengzi*; hence from this perspective, there should be at least one very big question mark against the claim that Dong Zhongshu was a proper Confucian scholar.[16] Furthermore, as already mentioned, Confucius himself and those who followed the Master's teachings up to the time of Dong did not quite step over the boundary from the Contextual-dyadic Mode to the dualistic mode.

One may conclude this section thus: Confucian thought following the Han ideological project as initiated by Dong Zhongshu was based on turning Contextual-dyadic Thinking into the dualistic-unequal-inflexible-hierarchical mode, which came to dominate social/moral/political *philosophy* in China through the centuries since the Han Dynasty.[17] However, this is not to say that the transformation had also affected all other domains of intellectual/practical activities—for instance, CCM remained faithful to Contextual-dyadic Thinking, which is embedded in process, not thing-ontology.

Leibniz, *l'arithmétique binaire* and *Yinyang/Yao-gua* Implicit *Logic*

We need now to look at Leibniz's claim that his binary arithmetic was but a version of what this book calls *Yinyang/Yao-gua* implicit *logic*. We must first address a matter of terminology which seems to vitiate the claim. Commentators, on the whole (even the most sensitive) use the term "duality" or "binary system" to evaluate it—see Ryan, 1996; Schönfeld, 2006. These terms, unfortunately, obscure the fundamental distinction between the dualistic as opposed to the dyadic mode of thinking. Once grasped, this distinction would enable us to throw light on the relationship between Leibniz's binary arithmetic and *Yinyang/Yao-gua* implicit *logic* of the *Yijing*.

Today's information technology and computing software are based on two-valued logic, the values of Truth and Falsity being represented by the logic gates of 1 and 0. Leibniz is often credited with being a founding father of this new technology (the other, is Charles Babbage). Leibniz saw himself as initiating a new way of processing information which he had described in his April 1679 letter to Johann Friedrich, Duke of Hanover, setting out his entire philosophical program:

> My invention contains the application of all reason, a judgment in each controversy, an analysis of all notions, a valuation of probability, a compass for navigating over the ocean of our experiences, an inventory of all things, a table of all thoughts, a microscope with which to prove the phenomena of the present and a telescope with which to preview those of the future, a general possibility to calculate everything. My invention is an innocent magic, a non-chimerical Cabbala, a writing, which everyone can read and which everyone can very easily learn. . . .

Leibniz also held that the ancient Chinese had already tumbled to it well before he did when the *Yijing* emerged with its *Yao-gua* Model of thinking. Well, Leibniz's generosity of spirit toward the ancient Chinese notwithstanding, was he correct in attributing the discovery of two-valued logic to them? This is the set of issues we need to disentangle to get to the bottom of the truth.

Leibniz at the age of twenty (c 1666), published his *habilitation* dissertation called *De Arte Combinatoria/On the Art of Combinations* in which he admitted where he got the combinatorial method from, namely, two people, one Ramon Llull (Catalan, 1232–1315), and the other Athanasius Kircher (German, 1602–1680, who in 1669 published his book *Ars Magna Sciendi, Sive Combinatoria*).[18] However, having promptly acknowledged them, he started to criticize them. Furthermore, at the beginning of *De Arte Combinatoria*, he had incorporated a figure.[19] Where could this figure have come from? A claim has been made that this was but an attempt on the part of Leibniz to reproduce the *Xiantiantu* (Former Heaven configuration) of the *Yijing*, but using Latin instead of the original Chinese.[20] Is this correct? First let us translate his Latin (roughly) into English. According to Leibniz:

Contraries are: Fire and Water; Earth and Air
Possible combinations are:
Dryness and Heat
Dryness and Cold
Cold and Humidity
Humidity and Heat
Impossible combinations are:
Dryness and Humidity
Cold and Heat

The way that Leibniz had set out the relationships reminds one of Aristotle's Square of Oppositions.[21] It also reminds one of the Greek Four Elements Theory. Leibniz also seemed to have been influenced by the eight trigrams of the *Yijing*, although it appears that he might have been inspired more by the *Houtiantu* (Later Heaven)—figure 5.3—rather than the *Xiantiantu* (figure 5.2) as in the Leibniz figure, Fire and Water occupy the same position as Fire and Water in the *Houtiantu*.

According to Needham, 1956: 497, at the age of twenty (1666), Leibniz had already begun reading Chinese *philosophy*, and through formal and informal channels would have come to hear about the *Yao-gua* system of the *Yijing*.[22] He certainly pursued the subject further with Father Bouvet, a correspondence which lasted from 1697 to 1707 (Ryan, 1996: 83, note 4). Bouvet was chosen by his Jesuit superiors as special missionary and envoy to the Qing court because of his mathematical skills and knowledge, in order to impress the Chinese ruling house of European scientific and technological advances with the aim of converting it to the one true faith—he was the *mathematicien du Roi*. Bouvet at the court in Peking/Beijing (acting, for some time, also as tutor to the children of the emperor Kangxi) received a letter in 1701 from Leibniz which told him that he, Leibniz, had discovered some years ago (in 1666) "binary" or "dyadic" arithmetic.

In response, Bouvet supplied Leibniz with a copy of Shao Yong 邵 雍 (1011–1077 CE)'s *Xiantian cixu* (Former/Earlier Heaven sequence) with the xiantian trigrams arramged as a circle enclosed within the much larger hexagram circle.[23]

Upon digesting Leibniz's letter, he said he immediately recognized that both circles could be read as examples of the latter's binary system which admitted only 0 and 1.[24] Bouvet then worked things out as follows:

1. He rendered the unbroken lines/the *yang yao* of each trigram or hexagram as 1s and the broken lines/the *yin yao* as 0s.

2. The first *gua* with a *yang yao* counted as 1, and each successive 1 doubled the value of its predecessor, thereby giving 2, 4, 8, 16, etc.
3. He began at the bottom of the circle, with the *Kun gua* and then went up its right side to the top, to the *Qian gua*, before descending diagonally down to the bottom, and then continuing up the left side to the top (that is from the *Kun gua* to the *Qian gua*).
4. He also read the successive lines of each trigram or hexagram from the outside in.
5. Thus, he found that the numbers represented by the *yaos* of the trigram in the trigram circle ran consecutively from 0 to 7 (the sequence then reads 000 as 0 in the decimal system, 001 as 1, 010 as 2, 011 as 3, 100 as 4, 101 as 5, 110 as 6, and 111 as 7), while those represented by the *yaos* of the hexagrams in the hexagram circle ran from 0 to 63 (the sequence reads from 0 to 111111).

Below shows a slight adaptation of Leibniz's own rendering of the trigrams (with the names of the trigrams shown on the left hand side starting with the *Kun gua* as 0 and the *Qian gua* as 7) in binary terms (taken from his *Explication de l'arithmétique binaire*)—table 9.5:

The above manner of reading the trigram and hexagram circles convinced Bouvet that Leibniz's binary arithmetic was nothing less than the *Yinyang/Yao-gua* Model of the *Zhouyi*. Hence, on November 4, 1701, he wrote that the mathematician/thinker/inventor of Chinese remote antiquity called Fuxi (traditionally believed by the Chinese to be the author of the trigrams and hexagrams) had already discovered binary arithmetic more than two millenia before him. Bouvet confessed that he had himself overlooked the possibility

Table 9.5.

Kun	000	0	0
Gen	001	1	1
Kan	010	10	2
Xun	011	11	3
Zhen	100	100	4
Li	101	101	5
Dui	110	110	6
Qian	111	111	7

of recognizing the Fuxi-*gua* Model as a binary system until he read Leibniz letter. (According to Bouvet, Fuxi was not originally a Chinese cultural hero anyway, but was in reality Hermes Trismegistos—the Greek name for the Egyptian god Thoth—who, somehow, wandered into Chinese history in the dim and distant past—see Cammann, 1991). At the same time, Bouvet also sent a version of Shao Yong's diagram. On receiving these, Leibniz became convinced that Bouvet was correct in demonstrating that his binary arithmetic and the *Yinyang/Yao-gua* Model were identical. This made Leibniz feel that he had been anticipated by Fuxi by several millenia and by Shao Yong[25] by some six and a half centuries. In 1679, Leibniz published "*De progressione dyadica*," and then later in 1703, *Explication de l'arithmétique binaire*.[26] In that publication and elsewhere in his letters to other savants, he conscientiously acknowledged that Fuxi, not to mention Shao Yong, had long anticipated his own discovery, that Bouvet had recognized and drew his attention to its identical nature with the *Yinyang/Yao-gua* Model, so to speak, and that, therefore, his own account was but a re-discovery of an ancient discovery.

In spite of Leibniz's generosity of spirit, was he correct in agreeing with Bouvet's view? The answer to this question, upon analysis, turns out to be neither a straight-forward "yes" nor "no." Those who answer negatively, A, put forward certain reasons which B counterclaim as follows:

(a) A hold that Bouvet had misread the way in which a *gua* and its three or six *yaos* are read. As already pointed out in earlier chapters, the bottom *yao* is the first *yao*; in other words, a *gua* is always read from the bottom up, not top down. When *guas* are arranged in a circular fashion, the *yao* nearest the center of the circle is the first *yao*, and the one farthest away is the topmost *yao*. Bouvet got to his "discovery" through reading the *yaos* upside down, so to speak.
(b) Bouvet had also misread the way in which the trigrams in the *Xiantiantu* are sequenced, as already mentioned. The Shao Yong's sequence is different: it begins with *Qian*/South, moves down the left side of the circle to *Dui*, then *Li*/East, *Zhen* before crossing diagonally upward to *Xun*, *Kan*/West, *Gen* (on the right side) and finally down to *Kun*/North.

Some sinologists (B) such as Mungello, 1985: 319[27] argue that this reversal of reading does "not invalidate the correspondence in principle;" they think that it is the formal isomorphism which is crucial.
(c) It is also the case that the digit 0 did not appear and was not used in any of the Chinese texts down the millennia regarding the *Yinyang/Yao-gua* Model. The digit 0 is Indian in origin and was imported into Europe via Islamic Arabic[28] scholarship. However, B could retort that although the digit 0 itself was absent in ancient Chinese texts, the concept of zero was available, and therefore, there was no harm on the part of Bouvet/Leibnitz to invoke it in elucidating the *Yinyang/Yao-gua* Model.

(d) The move above would only be innocuous if numbers were understood in exactly the same way both in modern European and ancient Chinese cultures. It is obvious that they are not. The former considers numbers to be important as part of quantification and precise calculation only, while the latter endowed numbers with cosmological significance (in their foundational texts) although it also used numbers in technical contexts much as modern Europeans did and do. For instance, nine (9) in the digital sequence of 1–9[29] represents the highest—hence, *Tian* is nine/*jiu*/九. In Yiology, it is said that "*yang* commands odd numbers and *yin* even numbers 阳奇阴偶/*yang ji yin ou*." *Tian* is one, three, five, seven, nine while *Di* is two, four, six, eight, and ten; in particular nine and six stand for *Yinyang*, and any *yang yao* can be said to be nine, and any *yin yao* can be said to be six (天一地二，天三地四，天五地六，天七地八，天九地十。并且特以九、六为阴阳的代表，凡阳爻皆称为九，凡阴爻皆称为六). Hence nine/*jiu* is used to talk about the *Qian gua* and six/*liu* the *Kun gua*—for example, the first *yao* of the former is referred to as *chu jiu*/初九/first nine while that of the latter is referred to as *chu liu*/初六/ first six. This critique, B counter-claim, overlooks the fact that in the history of European thought, from the ancient Greeks (Pythagoras) to the Renaissance humanists (Nicholas of Cusa), to the modern mathematician, George Cantor (1845–1918), numbers, too, were held to possess mystical/cosmological/ theological significance.

(e) As the earlier chapters have shown, according to A, the *Yijing* and the *Yaogua* Model which emerged are all to do with *yin qi* and *yang qi*, with the constantly changing relationships between them, with the renewable and renewed cycles of such relationships, with the concept of *Yinyang* as expressed so clearly in the eventual emergence of the *Liangyitaijitu*, and so on. All these constitute not only a cosmological but also a *philosophical*/metaphysical/ontological framework and the methodology it entails for doing *science*, for understanding and explaining natural phenomena, and the place of humankind in the natural processes of change.[30] A crucial *xiang*—figure 7.3—is that with the *yang qi* ascending to its maximum on left and descending with its diminution (but with corresponding increase of *yin qi*) on the right.

The *Yinyang* concept is not a dualistic but a dyadic one, where the two components cannot be detached or separated one from the other, where they co-exist, complementing each other. The term "binary" *simpliciter* should not therefore be used, as it masks the critical distinction between polar contrasts as dualism and polar contrasts as co-existing/co-operating dyadism to form a harmonious *Whole* under the over-arching mode of Contextual Thinking.

(f) When all is said and done, Leibniz, in spite of his open-minded, generous, ecumenical spirit towards Chinese culture, nevertheless, operated within a European framework with his own agenda. On the one hand, his system was not concerned to challenge Abrahamic theology, but rather to reinforce it—for Leibniz, 1 stood for God, 0 for nothing (*nihilo*), as

God, the omnipotent created the world from nothing. As such, it implied dualism—God is the master while the created world including humankind would be his slaves, should one care to invoke the Hegelian master/slave image to characterize such a relationship. On the other hand, Leibniz was also a giant in the creation of modern (European) science—one should not forget that mathematical scholarship in the West now recognises that both Newton and Leibniz invented differential and integral calculus, the difference between them being that the former was what one would, today, call an applied mathematician while the latter a pure mathematician.[31] His other great contribution from the standpoint of today was his binary arithmetic which provided the basis for information digital technology. He also invented a computing machine called the Step Reckoner (designed in 1671 but first built in 1673), which did multiplication by repeated addition and shifting; he developed ideas put forward by Blaise Pascal (1623 -1662), French mathematician/physicist/inventor/thinker. Although his Step Reckoner used the decimal, not the binary system, nevertheless, he strenuously advocated the binary system—one could say he was prescient in recognizing its suitability and appropriateness for calculating machines.[32]

(g) The two logic gates, 1/0, or T/F are paradigmatic of classical two-valued logic in European logic and science. On the other hand, one could perhaps make a plausible case for saying that the *Yinyang/Yao-gua* Model appears to be many-valued, that it shares greater affinity with today's fuzzy logic, although, obviously, it is not identical with it as section below will argue.

(h) Given (e, f, g) above, it seems reasonable for A to conclude that Leibniz contributed to establishing the basis for digital technology and not the ancient Chinese.

(i) Against A, B could counter-claim as follows: The ancient Chinese might not have articulated "binary"/two-valued logic explicitly as a clear and distinct mode of thinking in its own right which they could endorse; it remains the case that they were not totally unaware of such a possibility which was, after all, embedded within the *Yinyang/Yao-gua* Model itself. In this sense, Leibniz was correct—they did anticipate him in inventing the binary number system. The *Yinyang* pairing (*yin* of the *Kun gua* and *yang* of the *Qian gua*) itself as well as the other pairings in the trigrams (*Li/Kan*, *Zhen/Xun*, *Dui/Gen*) and in the hexagrams, the *Tai gua* and the *Pi gua* (see chapter 5) are exemplars of binary pairings. So, too, is the fundamental pairing of *you/wu* in the *Laozi*—see chapter 4. The formal isomorphism between that Model and Leibniz's is not a fatal criticism. Furthermore, the fact that the *Yinyang/Yao-gua* Model is embedded in the Contextual-dyadic framework, while Leibniz's is embedded in an abstract/content-free theoretical framework which simultaneously operated within theological dualism, does not undermine the claim of formal isomorphism. Polar pairings/contrasts are neutral with regard to dyadism or dualism.

(j) It follows that B's counter-claim cannot be dismissed so readily, and that Leibniz and Bouvet were not altogether wrong in giving credit to the ancient Chinese for having pioneered the binary system, even though it remains true that they did not embrace it themselves in the way that modern Western philosophy/science had/have done.

Modern non-classical Logic and *Yinyang/Yao-gua* Implicit *Logic*[33]

The reader may be surprised to see *Yinyang/Yao-gua logic* in this section, as so far this book has argued that the ancient Chinese did not engage in formal logic. This apparent inconsistency will be explained below.

The preceding sections have argued that the basic mode of thinking in Chinese *philosophy* is what may be called the Contextual-dyadic Mode. As already pointed out, an obvious implication of the Contextual Mode would be the futility or irrelevance of formal logic (as understood in Western philosophy); hence Chinese *philosophy* (except possibly for the Mohists—whose *Mohist Canons* were a Warring States Period text[34]) seemed to have not been thus pre-occupied.[35] Contextual Thinking means that form and content cannot be separated; formal logic in Western philosophy *ex hypothesi* is about form extrapolated from content (and context).[36] Form is the polar opposite of content—to Western formal logic as such (though perhaps not in philosophy, in general) they are mutually exclusive—either you have form or content, but not both. Formal logic therefore has nothing to do with content. In contrast, Chinese *philosophy*, true to its fundamental spirit, does not consider polar contrasts to be mutually exclusive; instead they are perceived to be compatible and complementary to form a harmonious *Whole* (chapter 10 explores the notion of harmonious *Whole* in various forms in Chinese *philosophy*). Nisbett, 2003/2005: 166 has cited the Chinese *philosopher*, Shu-Hsien Liu thus: " . . . it is precisely because the Chinese mind is so rational that it refuses to become rationalistic and . . . to separate form from content." (However, we beg to distance ourselves from the assessment proffered not because it is primarily wrong but because Liu and Nisbett have failed to realize that it is not so much that the ancient Chinese were "so rational;" it is the case rather that they and the modern Europeans each had their own respective paradigms of rationality.)

As for the Western paradigm, to recap, two points must quickly be made. First, logic in Western philosophy, as already observed, is exclusively about form, systematically divorced in principle from content; second, such classical logic is two-valued; it recognizes only two values, T(rue) and F(alse). Today in the age of digital information technology, the analogue of these two values are represented by the logic gates of 1 (T) and 0 (F).[37] The principle of bi-valence says that every proposition is either true or false. In other words, a proposition under examination has exactly one truth value, either true or false. The history of formal logic is a long one, starting with ancient Greek philosophy to the present, but naturally, too, with periods when the subject fell into decline. Fortunately, this vast subject is outside the remit of this work.[38] Having observed that classical logic is two-valued, let us jump to the twentieth century when logic started to depart in many ways from its classical standards. This section briefly considers the main directions of such departure, which will show that modern non-classical logic is much more compatible, in comparison with its classical predecessor, with the Chinese way of thinking.

Aristotle is generally held to have articulated three well-known principles or laws of thought in Western philosophy. He is said to have regarded them as regulative principles of thought[39] (whereas, later, classical formal two-valued logic recasts them as tautological elements of a formal system[40]). These are:

> Principle of identity: A is A. Or, in a more refined formulation, if $A=B$ then for any referential expression F, $F(A) = F(B)$, and for any proposition p, $p(A) \equiv p(B)$ where '≡' is the operator of logical equivalence
> Principle of non-contradiction (also referred to as the principle of contradiction): two propositions p and $-p$ cannot both be true (at most one is true); in classical propositional logic, it appears as $\neg \_(p \wedge \neg p)$
> Principle of excluded middle: among two propositions p and $\neg p$ at least one is true; in propositional logic, it appears as $p \vee \neg p$

The first direction of departure of logic from its classical standards in the twentieth century has to do with the rejection of the principle of exluded middle leading to what today is called many-valued logic. Doubts as regards the validity of the principle of excluded middle go back as long ago as Aristotle himself; however, the first axiomatized many-valued logical calculus was proposed by the Polish logician and philosopher, Jan Łukasiewicz; his calculus was also the first axiomatized system of non-classical logic. The third value, "possible" was invented in order to deal with Aristotle's paradox of the sea battle which is a classic example of what is called the problem of *futura contingentia* (future contingent events). In 1921, the American mathematician, Emil Leon Post, introduced a logic with n truth values, where $n \geq 2$. These results were later developed by Łukasiewicz, Alfred Tarski, Hans Reichenbach, and Kurt Godël in the 1920s and 1930s. An important new step was taken in 1965 when a branch of many-valued logic called fuzzy logic appeared, with the now classic paper "Fuzzy Sets" by Lotfi Zadeh.[41] The term "fuzzy logic" comes from that paper's development of fuzzy sets. Fuzzy logic seems to bear the closest resemblance to what this work calls *Yinyang/Yao-gua implicit logic*. This is not the place to pursue the technical details about fuzzy logic;[42] let us here simply make a few points:

> (a) Fuzzy set is such collection of elements that each element belongs to it to a certain fixed extent. More precisely, a fuzzy set is a pair (U, m) where U is a set and m is a membership function that assigns to each element a number from 0 to 1 which characterizes the degree of its belonging to the set.
> (b) This allows one to treat any predicates such as "wealthy," "young," "old" or "beautiful" as fuzzy predicates. Thus a person can be estimated as 10 percent, or 70 percent wealthy. The extreme cases are 0 percent wealthy (that is, totally poor) and 100 percent wealthy (maximally wealthy).
> (c) Accordingly, propositions may be assigned a degree of truth, such as being "very true," "very false," or some intermediate degree between these two extremes. It follows that one proposition may be "more true"/"less false" than another. If 100 percent represents Truth and 0 percent Falsity, then there could be 75 percent, or 50 percent of truth or whatever in between the two extremes.
> (d) Fuzzy logic can be applied in technology, such as robot control, soft-computering, in engineering and so on, where one wants to achieve simple, quick and what may be considered to be "sufficiently good" solution to a problem. Technically, it is a form of formal/symbolic logic, that is, a branch of many-valued logic which deals with inference under vagueness.

Given the very brief and simplistic clarification above of classical two-valued logic and of fuzzy logic as a form of non-classical logic, can one be so bold as to venture to say that the *Yinyang/Yao-gua* Model may be considered to be an ancient implicit version of many-valued *logic* (implicit, precisely because obviously it was not set out in a manner which could satisfy the rigours of symbolic logic today when fuzzy logic is understood in the narrow sense)? The *Yao-gua* Model has sixty-four hexagrams; for the purpose of making the point above, it is best to confine ourselves to the eight trigrams and interpret them as an analogue of degrees of truth, with the *Qian gua* to stand for "true," the *Kun gua* for "false," and the other six trigrams each respectively for some intermediate degree between being true and being false. Let us look afresh at the *Yinyang-Xiantian gua* arrangement reproduced again below but with amendments, merely as an exercise in making explicit the *logic* embedded in it. Here we wish to emphasize that *Yinyang philosophy*—see earlier chapters—is much more complex than that. However, if one were to bear in mind the very important point that *Yinyang logic* is never content free, then there is no harm in undertaking the exercise in order to demonstrate the plausibility of the implicit Chinese version of multi-valence, so to speak.

The exercise of identifying degrees of truth with trigrams is conditioned by the basic definitions of the semantics of fuzzy logic, according to which (1), we have to include 0 (falsity) and 1 (truth) in the list of ascribed numbers, (2) all other numbers should appear as the result of the division of the segment [0,1] into equal parts. In order to get eight numbers for the eight trigrams, we have to divide the distance between 0 and 1 into seven equal parts; so we shall have truth-degrees 0, 1/7, 2/7, 4/7, 5/7, 6/7, and 1.[43] On the other hand, the exercise is conditioned by the idea of representing the binary nature of things in terms of the polar contrasts of the trigrams. That means (3), the trigrams should form four pairs of polar contrasts. Our proposal is that the polarity should be reflected in such a way that, and (4), in each pair, both numbers should have the same distance to 1/2 which is the point of balance between *yin* and *yang* or between truth and falsity. Below illustrates how the *Yinyang-Xiantian gua* (trigrams) can be adapted to show multi-valence—figure 9.3a.

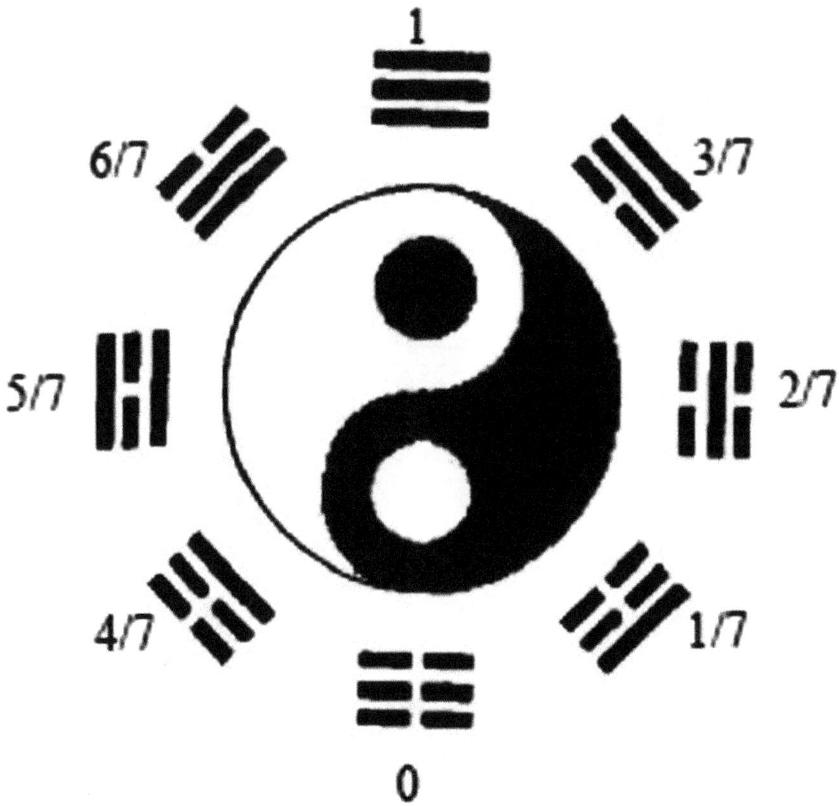

Figure 9.3a. Yinyang-Xiantian gua (trigrams) adapted to show multi-valence

Bearing the conditions (1) through (4) in mind, let us make the *Qian gua* stand for "true" or 1, the *Kun gua* for "false" or 0. All other degrees of truth are represented in the figure by simple fractions with the denominator 7 (where 7 is the total quantity of different positive numbers which can be represented by trigrams). On the left hand side of the diagram, remember *yang qi* is ascending, the first *gua* after the *Kun gua* is the *Zhen gua*, where you can see the inner (bottom) *yao* as a *yang yao*—so let us say this stands for the value of one step toward 1 where 1/2 is the point of balance between *yang qi* and *yin qi*, or between truth and falsity; hence numerically it should be marked as 4/7. The next *gua* (*Li*) up has to be marked as 5/7; the third *gua* up (*Dui*) as 6/7. On the right side of the figure, the *yang qi* begins to descend toward the *Kun gua* and so the first *gua* on the descending arm, the *Xun gua* has an inner (bottom) *yin yao* and should be marked as one step toward 0 from the point of balance, that is, 3/7. This continues with the second and third *guas* to follow marked as 2/7 and 1/7 respectively until one reaches the *Kun gua* marked as 0.

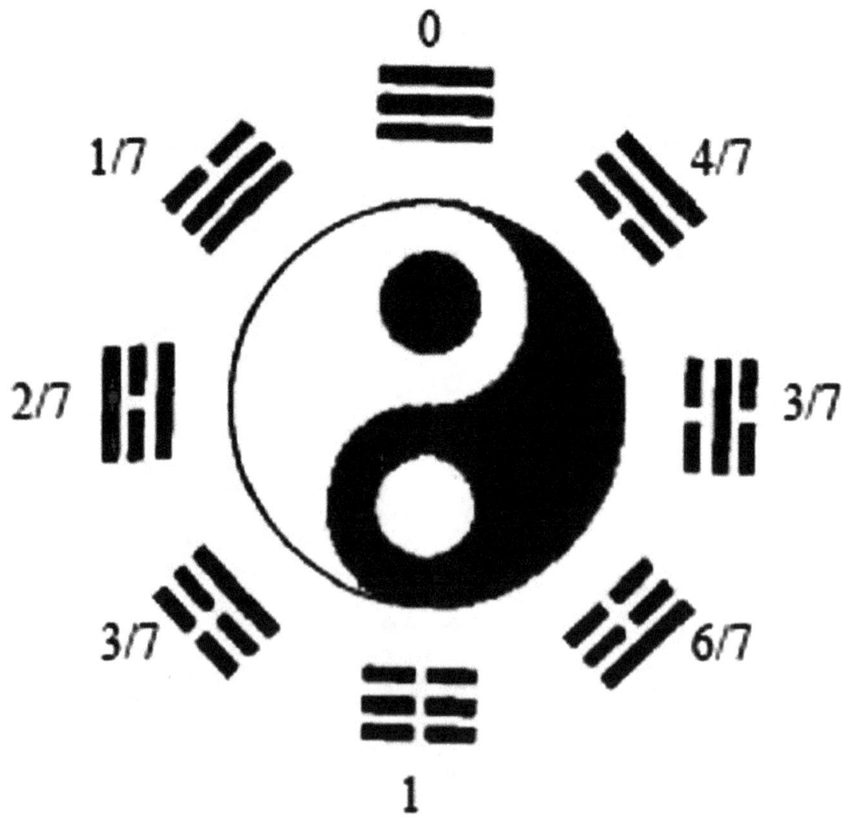

Figure 9.3b. Complementary way to show multi-valuence using Yinyang-Xiantian gua

Remarkably, the numerators of truth values constructed in this way exactly correspond to Leibniz's binary codes of the corresponding trigrams (see table 9.1). Another remarkable feature of figure 9.3a is its symmetry regarding the center of the picture. To fully appreciate this symmetry, let us change our strategy and make the *Qian gua* stand for "false" and the *Kun gua* for "true." Then we can adjust the remaining six trigrams accordingly as shown in figure 9.3b.

Now we can claim that for any given proposition p, figure 9.3a represents the degrees of its truth while figure 9.3b represents the degrees of truth of its negation, ¬p, if we apply the standard definition of negation in fuzzy logic as additive complement, according to which for an arbitrary proposition t(¬p) = 1—t(p) where t is a (many-valued) truth function. Taking these considerations into account, one can state that this exercise in extracting fuzzy logic from the *Yinyang-Xiantian gua* model has been successful; it is easy to see that the same method of extraction can be successfully applied to the hexagrams circularly arranged as mentioned in Shao Yong Former/Earlier Heaven sequence mentioned earlier.

The above analysis of the *Yinyang-Xiantian* model in terms of fuzzy logic is not complete unless one shows that the logic of the model rejects the principle of excluded middle. The standard semantic definition of disjunction in fuzzy logic treats its truth value as the maximum of the truth values of the disjuncts: t(q ˇ r) = max(t(q), t(r)). Then it is evident from figures 9.3a and 9.3b that for any p, the truth value of p ˇ ¬p is equal to 1 only in the extreme points of the *Qian gua* and *Kun gua*. For all other trigrams, t(p ˇ ¬p) is less than 1; for example, the *Li gua* gives t(p ˇ ¬p) = 5/7 and the *Xun gua* 4/7. So generally speaking, the principle of excluded middle does not hold. The standard semantic definition of conjunction in fuzzy logic states that its truth value is equal to the minimum of the truth values of the conjuncts: t(q ˆ r) = min(t(q), t(r)). Then again, t(¬(p ˆ ¬p)) is equal to 1 only in the *Qian gua* and *Kun gua*, but more, generally, it is less than 1; for example, in the *Li gua*, it is 2/7 and in the *Xun gua*, it is 3/7.

Once again, it is important to note that our analsysis of the *Yinyang/Yao-gua* Model does not affirm the identity of the *Yinyang/Yao-gua* implicit *logic* with its fuzzy interpretation. It does not claim in any way that the ancient Chinese *philosophers* themselves had formalized a system of logic called *Yinyang/Yao-gua logic*, analogous to the formal system of binary logic, established by Russell, Whitehead, and Frege, or that of Zadeh's fuzzy logic. It is simply to say that they implicitly used and invoked such a *logic* in their thinking and conceptualization of the world, and that, today, should one wish to make it more explicit, then it could begin to look like a many-valued logic, of which "fuzzy" logic is a type.[44] While our analysis grasps some aspects of the implicit *Yinyang/Yao-gua logic*, its other aspects remain beyond the reach of this fuzzy interpretation. Crucially, the interpretation fails to represent the very fact that each *gua* is itself a combination of *yin* and *yang yaos* which are polar opposites.

This brings us to the second direction of non-classical development in twentieth-century logic, related to the questioning of the Law of Non-contradiction. There are various ways of going beyond the principle; most of them are more far-going and more technically refined than the way in which fuzzy logic does it. Thus as we have seen, in fuzzy logics $\neg (p \wedge \neg p)$ is no longer a universal truth; however p and ¬p still cannot both be (fully) true at the same model. Logics in which this is possible are called paraconsistent logics (see Priest, Tanaka and Weber, 2015). A leading author today in this field is Graham Priest who has coined the term "dialetheism" (Priest, 1986) for a kind of philosophy which claims that contradictions can be true. Motivation for dialetheism initially comes from logical paradoxes, but also from cases of apparent inconsistency in transition states, local motion (such as considered in Zeno's paradoxes), borderline cases of value predicates, multi-criterial predicates, and so on (see Berto and Priest, 2013).

Does paraconsistent logic—in the strong sense of paraconsistency, that is, logic allowing true contradictions—play any significant role in Chinese thinking? To answer this question, we have to remember that, in Chinese thinking, polar opposites presuppose each other and are considered as co-present. Thus, from our analysis of the Fuxi-Nüwa myth, we can see that on some general level *yang* and *yin*, the most *philosophically* significant polar opposites, are co-present in Fuxi; that is, on some level, Fuxi is both *yang* and *yin*. It is natural to interpret *yang* and *yin* for that case as complex or multi-criterial predicates, one of which is symbolically represented as the negation of the other. However, on another level where the issue of balance between the opposites is critical and therefore the degree of presence of each opposite matters, many-valued or fuzzy logic can be the more appropriate instrument of analysis. For instance, a Chinese physician may diagnose a *zheng*/证 as *han bao re*/寒包热/"cold enveloping heat," invoked to account for, say, a case of gum inflammation; *han* and *re* are polar opposites, yet they are co-present in the condition of the patient. According to classical Chinese *philosophy*, everything in the world appears as a particular combination and a fragile balance of polar opposite elements.

One of the stimuli for the development of paraconsistent logics in the twentieth century was the awareness of the fact that scientific theories happen to involve contradictions. It is well known generally that relativity theory and quantum mechanics are mutually inconsistent. Or, to consider the case of a more particular inconsistency: according to the Copenhagen interpretation of quantum superposition, a radioactive atom exists in a combination of mutually exclusive states until its state is observed. A popular version of this paradox is Schrödinger's cat whose life is dependent on the state of an atom—the cat turns out to be both alive and dead until it is observed.

Perhaps the most salient example of a paraconsistent theory in Modern Science is Niels Bohr's account of complementarity observed earlier in the chapter 8. We have noticed an influence of *Yinyang* philosophy on Bohr's interpretation of quantum phenomena—as he was influenced or inspired consciously or sub-consciously by what he knew about the *Laozi* and the *Daojia* tradition as a young student, he invoked the notion of complementarity to make sense of light being at once a wave as well as a particle. Bohr had grasped that according to *Yinyang philosophy*, duality is a built-in feature in understanding natural phenomena. There are reasons to think that not only was Bohr aware of what we call today 'paraconsistency' of his theory but also what we call paraconsistency was an important part of his philosophical world-view. His son, Hans Henrik Bohr, has testified: "One of the favorite maxims of my father was the distinction between the two sorts of truths, profound truths recognized by the fact that the opposite is also a profound *truth*, in contrast to trivialities where opposites are obviously *absurd*" (Bohr, 1967: 328). Or, to use the slightly different Frank Wilczek's formulation: "Niels Bohr distinguished two kinds of truths. An ordinary truth is a statement whose opposite is a falsehood. A profound truth is a statement whose opposite is also a profound truth" (Wilczek, 2008: chapter 2).

It may be pertinent here to cite an episode reported in Blaedel's biography of Bohr in which he recounted the comment of a Japanese theoretical physicist who had, at one time, visited Bohr and his institute. This physicist was Hideki Yukawa who was awarded the Nobel Prize in 1949 for his prediction of the existence of mesons. When asked in 1961 in Kyoto by Léon Rosenfeld (a former colleague of Bohr) whether Japanese physicists had encountered the same difficulty as Western ones in comprehending and coming to terms with Bohr's notion of complementarity, Yukawa said: "Bohr's argumentation has always appeared obvious to us. . . . You understand, in Japan we were never led astray by Aristotle" (Blaedel, 1988: 196–197).

One may conclude that the *Yinyang/Yao-gua* Model of reasoning appears to challenge both the principles of non-contradiction and excluded middle. Perhaps another way of putting the matter which is more in keeping with the spirit of Chinese *philosophy* based on the premises that form and content cannot be separated as well as that the Contextual-dyadic Mode is foundational is as follows: it is not so much that the *Yinyang/Yao-gua* implicit *logic* denies the principles of non-contradiction or of excluded middle *simpliciter*, but that it implies that these principles do not obtain in all contexts. They obtain only in certain limited contexts, namely, at the polar extremes of the *Yinyang* spectrum (as represented by the *Qian gua* at one pole and the *Kun gua* at the other and which stands for 100 percent and 0 percent of *yang*/0 percent of *yin* and 100 percent of *yin* respectively), but not in other contexts indicated in the rest of the basic set of eight trigrams. This would then be consistent with the claim that *Yinyang/Yao-gua* implicit *logic* may be said to be a many-valued *logic* and that, therefore, it is a more comprehensive *logic*, as binary logic is but a subset within that wider many-valued framework. Furthermore, according to *Yinyang philosophy*, the *Qian gua* at one end of the spectrum and the *Kun gua* at the other are at best abstractions only, as in reality even they do not totally exclude their polar counterparts, even when they are represented in terms of three unbroken *yang yaos*, three broken *yin yaos* respectively. Perhaps it is best to regard these two "pure" *guas* to be no more than ideal (logical) types, as in reality, they do not and cannot exist and endure—in that sense they are purely formal and exist only in formal logic textbooks (except that the ancient Chinese did not believe in writing any).

The third direction of non-classical development in modern logic concerns the abandoning of the principle of identity. A point of departure here is given by a famous puzzle of Frege which draws our attention to the fact that, although Hesperus and Phosphorus are the same thing (the planet Venus), the statements "Alex sees Phosphorus" and "Alex sees Hesperus" are not logically equivalent: their truth values can differ. Quine used to call such co-referential terms that cannot be substituted *salva veritate* "referentially opaque" terms. One natural way to deal with Frege's puzzle (proposed by Frege himself in *Sinn und Bedeutung*) is to distinguish between the meaning or reference of a given expression, on the one hand, and its sense, on the other. These considerations gave strong impetus to the development of intentional and modal logics in which the principle of identity was not valid. The central achievement of this line of development is perhaps the invention of possible world semantics. The notion of possible world is a formal analogue of what we call "context" or "situation." Thus the principle of identity, while being violated globally in modal logic, remains valid locally in each possible world. Modal logics with their possible world semantics can be regarded as the paradigmatic tools for exploring intensionality and contextual thinking. The main ideas of possible world semantics, anticipated by medieval philosophers and summarised in modern times by Leibniz, in the mid-twentieth century obtained their formalization in the works of Rudolf Carnap, Saul Kripke, Jaakko Hintikka, and others philosophers.

Technically, possible world is an additional argument or parameter of truth-value function. That is, a proposition can be true in one possible world and false in another. Semantically a proposition can be associated with the set of possible worlds that make this proposition true. Possible world semantics allows us to consider a proposition as necessary in a possible world w if and only if it is true in all possible worlds accessible from w, and consider it as possible if and only if it is true in some possible worlds accessible from w, where accessibility is a binary relation defined on the set of all possible worlds. Further, we can define necessity and possibility on a model (a set of possible worlds with a relation of accessibility defined on it) as, correspondingly, truth in all possible worlds and truth in some possible worlds of this model—see, for example, Priest, 2008a for technical details.

Possible world semantics reflects some of our deepest intuitions about the diversity of the ways the actual world is, was, will or could be. This is why modal logic equipped with this semantics turns out to be a perfect tool for the explication and analysis of metaphysical theories.[45] The metaphysical significance of possible world semantics can be appreciated fully if we take into account the following principle of modal plenitude usually assumed in its metaphysical applications: the truth values of any involved propositions vary arbitrarily over possible worlds, subject only to the constraints imposed by the way how things are or by "the order of things" (where the latter refer to the set of assumptions of a metaphysical theory and so depend on the theory).[46] For example, if A = A and 2 + 2 = 4 are propositions the (respective) truth of which is determined by the order of things, they will be necessarily true. And if A = B and "George Bush is the President" are not determined by the order of things, they will be true in some and false in other possible worlds.

Now we are in a position to comment on the attitude of the ancient Chinese thinking toward the principle of identity and on the issue whether the *Yinyang/Yao-gua* implicit *logic* has any intentional or modal features. First of all, we have to remember that the principle of identity considered in logic and formulated above in this section has nothing to do with the identity of things over time or change; the only claim that it makes is that two co-referential terms can replace each other without distorting truth value or meaning in any context in which one of these expressions appears. Taking into account that Chinese thinking is always contextual and that *Yinyang philosophy* considers the world as dynamic and undergoing change, we are committed to conclude that *Yinyang* thinking would not accept the principle of identity. Further, as long as classical Chinese *philosophy* does not involve explicit logic or philosophy of language in the modern sense of these disciplines, it does not deal with the issue of intentionality. On the other hand, the *Yinyang/Yao-gua* Model has an obvious structural similarity with possible world semantics. In order to show this, let us consider a natural reconstruction of the *Yinyang-Xiantian gua* arrangement in terms of possible worlds.

Let P_i, P_m and P_e designate the propositions "the bottom *yao* is *yang*," "the middle *yao* is *yang*," and "the upper *yao* is *yang*," correspondingly. Then, in virtue of the two-valued nature of *yaos*, $\neg P_i$, $\neg P_m$ and $\neg P_e$ will mean correspondingly "the bottom *yao* is *yin*," "the middle *yao* is *yin*," and "the upper *yao* is *yin*." For the purpose of building reconstructions for trigram arrangements no other propositions are needed. We will correlate a possible world with each trigram, so that our possible worlds will be named after corresponding *guas*: *Kun*, *Zhen*, *Li*, *Dui*, *Qian*, *Xun*, *Kan*, *Gen*. The truth-function is defined on all pairs <world, proposition> as follows in table 9.6.

What we have now at table 9.6 is actually a system of Leibniz's binary codes (see table 9.5); this seems to be the most natural reconstruction of the *Yinyang-Xiantian* Model by means of modern non-classical logics, the reconstruction in which 1 or "truth" designates *yang*, and 0 or "falsity" designates *yin* (of course, alternatively it could be defined the other way around, 1 for *yin* and 0 for *yang*). To complete our reconstruction, we would have yet to define a binary relation of accessibility on the set of possible worlds. Let us remember that the *Yinyang-Xiantian* arrangement is itself a model that can symbolize different things: compass directions, seasons in a year, stages of development in a day cycle or in a life cycle, and so on. However in the most general case of the model itself, we have no other choice but to define the relation of accessibility as all-inclusive; that is, we assume that every possible

Table 9.6.

	P_i	P_m	P_e
Qian	0	0	0
Dui	0	0	1
Li	0	1	0
Zhen	0	1	1
Xun	1	0	0
Kan	1	0	1
Gen	1	1	0
Kun	1	1	1

world is accessible from every other one. In such possible world structure, nothing (from the list of defined propositions and their negations) is necessary and everything (from the same list) is possible.

Classical Chinese *philosophy* sees the world in terms of co-existence and harmony of polar opposites, *yin* and *yang* being the paradigmatic exemplar of these. Accordingly, if there is any modal metaphysics behind the *Yinyang/Yao-gua* implicit *logic*, this is the metaphysics of diversity of combinations of polar opposites, assembled in trigrams or hexagrams and revealing themselves in *Wanwu*.

The psychologist Richard Nisbett has done some interesting empirical work to ascertain whether what this book calls the Contextual-dyadic Mode and *Yinyang/Yao-gua* Model of reasoning still have residual influence upon those exposed to them even today in the twenty-first century, and in spite of their persistent exposure to the globalized model of logic ultimately resting on the principles of excluded middle and non-contradiction. To this end, he and his team devised some very ingenious tests to determine the ways in which the two different world-views may lead people to perceiving the world differently. Nisbett cites the student called Kaiping Peng (who had alerted him and in that sense introduced him to Chinese *philosophy*) in what may be regarded as Peng's outline of that *philosophy*. This summary chimes in remarkably well with the analysis and assessment proffered by this book. Peng has articulated three principles:

> *The Principle of Change*: "The world is not static but dynamic and changeable. Being in a given state is just a sign that the state is about to change." (Nisbett, 2005:174) (This book shows that this principle is grounded in the *Yijing*.)
> *The Principle of Contradiction*: " . . . opposites complete each other and make each other up. Taoists see the two sides of any apparent contradiction existing in an active harmony, opposed but connected and mutually controlling" (Nisbett, 2005:175). (This book has attempted to show in detail how this is articulated and developed largely within the *Daojia* tradition, and which appeared to have inspired Bohr to invoke the notion of complementarity to characterise quantum reality.)
> *The Principle of Relationship, or Holism*: "As a result of change and opposition, nothing exists in an isolated and independent way, but is connected to a multitude of different things. To really know a thing, we have to know all its relations . . . " (Nisbett, 2005:175). (This book has attempted to pull all the strands of the argument behind the *philosophy* of *Wholism* in chapter 10.)

Nisbett and Peng (2005: 175–176) continue: "The three principles . . . are related. Change produces contradiction and contradiction causes change;

constant change and contradiction imply that it is meaningless to discuss the individual part without considering its relationships with other parts and prior states." We cannot agree more as the entire book is structured on that premise.

By way of concluding this section, let us make the following main points:

1. As ancient Chinese *philosophy* regarded the Contextual-dyadic Mode of Thinking to be foundational, it had ignored what in Western philosophy is a very important branch, namely, formal logic, for the obvious reason that formal logic is necessarily a-contextual.
2. This did not mean that it ignored logic altogether as it implied and used a *logic* which appears to bear remarkable resemblance to what today, since the last half century or so, is called fuzzy logic. Fuzzy logic is a form of many-valued logic (unlike classical logic which is two-valued) based on the notion of vagueness. *Yinyang/Yao-gua* implicit *logic* based on the eight trigrams may be said to be many-valued, founded on the notions of change, on process and not thing-ontology (from the *Yijing*), harmony of polar opposites to form a *Whole* (from *Yinyang* as well as the *Yinyang/Yao-gua* itself).
3. Classical Western philosophy, in the main, is based on thing-ontology (a static, not a dynamic universe); such an ontology goes well with a logic which adheres to the three principles/laws of thought (attributed to Aristotle), namely, identity, non-contradiction and excluded middle.
4. *Yinyang/Yao-gua* implicit *logic* could be said to challenge all three principles, not so much by denying their relevance *tout court*, but by implying that they (especially the principles of excluded middle and non-contradiction) are of limited applications only, in certain specific contexts, and not all contexts. On the other hand, the principle of identity is irrelevant as it is context-free and ahistorical. In that sense, *Yinyang/Yao-gua* implicit *logic* (as well as fuzzy logic and other non-classical logics) can plausibly claim to be a more comprehensive *logic*/logic than classical two-valued logic, as in nearly all contexts, the world displays fuzziness, paraconsistency, and modal plenitude.
5. One could argue that Bohr relied on *Yinyang philosophy* and its implicit *logic* when he realised that light exhibits wave-particle duality.
6. The *Yinyang/Yao-gua* implicit *logic* has a remarkable structural similarity with possible world semantics of modal logic and can be naturally reconstructed in terms of possible worlds.
7. Behind the *Yinyang/Yao-gua* Model, can be found modal metaphysics of diversity of combinations of polar opposites assembled in trigrams or hexagrams and revealing themselves in *Wanwu*.

Xiang Mode of Thinking

We have argued that the Contextual-dyadic Thinking may be said to be peculiar and perhaps even unique to Chinese culture and civilization. We next must say something about another mode which plays a uniquely important role in that culture, that is the *Xiang* mode (*Xiang* Thinking for short), superbly exemplified by the *Yao-gua* of the *Yijing*.

It is obvious that Chinese culture/civilisation is an extremely logocentric one. In the private sphere, nearly every educated person in the long history of China would have scribbled down some events observed, some thoughts entertained, some poetry about landscape and matters which had touched them greatly; in the public domain, official archives and records existed plentifully and still remain in impressive quantities in spite of the great losses endured during wars, changes of regime, invasions, uprisings and upheavals, and ideological struggles of one kind or other in its long variegated history. Hence, it may be surprising to those outside the Chinese tradition to hear that Chinese culture itself celebrates another mode of expression which is totally non-linguistic, namely, *Xiang* Thinking. Such a logocentric culture, nevertheless, also embraced the non-linguistic—may be these two modes of expression are themselves manifestation of *Yinyang* cosmology and metaphysics, that everything (*Wanwu*) in *Yuzhou* occurs and must be understood within the *Yinyang*/dyadic framework of complementary contraries. The *Yao-gua* of the *Yijing* was traditionally said to have been invented by Fuxi who according to today's scholarship was a mythological ancestor; but whoever those ancestral peoples might have been, it looks as if they invented the *Yao-gua* Mode of conveying information at a time which predated the emergence or even perhaps coincided with the first phase of the emergence of writing in China, when it would make sense to capture the essence of a thing or state of affairs through a process of abstraction (later this would be qualified), producing an "image" or "picture" of it.

However, *Xiang* Thinking, in some aspects, is not entirely alien or unknown in the Western context. Maps are used and a map is actually no more than a *xiang*. (Maps were/are common both to the Chinese and Western traditions of geographical knowledge.) On a detailed map, mountains/hills are marked in terms of their contour lines. A walker would know at a glance where the steep slopes are (where the contour lines are very close to one another), where the lowlands lie, where the valleys are, where the rivers flow (as these are clearly shown too). All these bits of data/information are captured by the map; maps are nothing but an instantiation of *Xiang* Thinking (in some respect). One could also claim that all icons are forms of *Xiang* Thinking—the dove stands for peace, so does the olive branch. The use of symbols is confined to specific items, unlike maps which stand for orderly relationships between various things. Hence, maps are closer to the *Xiang* mode as the ancient Chinese used it to encapsulate relationships between various natural processes at work, to highlight regularities and patterns which could be found in natural phenomena—in a word, it was to establish theoretical/systematic knowledge.

The character *xiang* looks like this: 象. In today's dictionaries, two entries are given under this character—the first meaning is "elephant."[47] The second entry in turn gives two meanings, the first of which relates to "(outward) form," "look/appearance," "image" (basically, what the eye takes in when looking at something), the second to "copying." In the context of the *Yao-gua*, the second entry is clearly relevant. Could there be a link between *xiang* as elephant and *xiang* as in the *Xiang* Mode of Thinking as found in the *Yijing*? Let us explore this possible link.

The first type of script to emerge in the history of Chinese writing is said to be pictographic (*xiangxing*/象形字).[48] The various evolutions of the character *xian*/象 (when it means "elephant") are set out in figure 9.4.[49]

A: its earliest form ascertained is simply a picture of an elephant, a paradigmatic instance of what is called pictographic writing.

B 1 and B 2: the late Shang Dynsaty Oracle Bone Script—the outline of the animal had been faithfully preserved, but either version had lost its details. They have become abstracted pictures; they are still pictographic writing, even when shorn of the realistic details of A.

C: the Bronze Script; however, A is also found in the Bronze Script.[50]

D: the Lesser Seal Script (evolved from the Bronze Script).

E: the Clerical Script.

F: the Standard Script, developed in the early Han Dynasty and used for over two thousand years even today.

We can see from the above that the character, *xiang*, has most probably evolved from being a mere picture of the animal (A) to various forms of abstraction until its most distinctive feature, the trunk, was no longer preserved and became no longer immediately recognizable as the animal the character was meant to represent (C, D, E, and F).

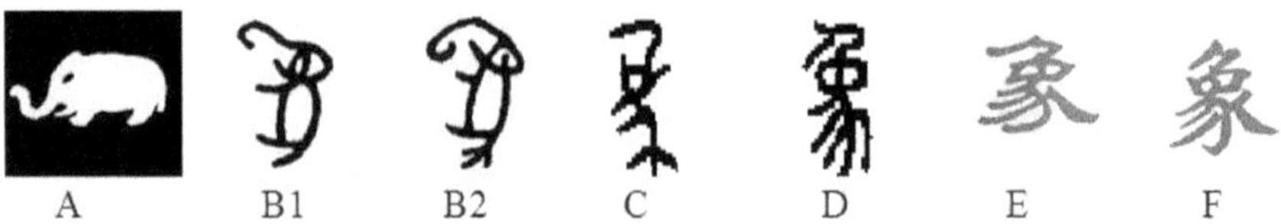

Figure 9.4. Character "xiang" in various scripts

Go back to A—at that time, people looked at the elephant, studied the beast, examining its shape and other details, then drew a picture of it, and used that as a character to stand for the animal. In the same way, and even probably around the same time or earlier,[51] people must also have pondered how to capture and embed information regarding phenomena in Heaven above and Earth below (astronomy and geography) before the advent of writing. They would also have keenly observed those natural phenomena and their processes which affected them most. As chapter 4 points out, wisdom for the ancient Chinese consisted of knowledge concerning three different domains and the relationships between them: *Tian* (Heaven/astronomy), *Di* (Earth/geography) and *Ren* 人 (Humans)—*sancai*. Indeed, the *Yao-gua* of the *Yijing* was simply an attempt to encapsulate such wisdom.

In the light of this clarification, let us now take a look at the trigrams to see how the ancient Chinese came to represent via *Xiang* Thinking their account of the respective natural phenomena presented in the trigrams:

> *Tian* (Heaven): the *gua* has three unbroken *yaos*. The ancient Chinese looked up at the sky and if they were to draw it, they would probably have drawn three curved lines to represent the layers of cloud. (Bear in mind that "three" stood for "many.") Slowly these curved lines became straight lines. Later they called the image *Qian gua*.
>
> *Di* (Earth): the *gua* has three broken *yaos*. Unlike Heaven which could not be broken up, Earth could be, as they could observe Earth's crust suddenly being broken up in eruptions over which humans had no control but also when humans ploughed up the soil, or dug holes and tunnels. (Later the ancient Chinese called the image *Kun gua*.)
>
> The ancient Chinese observed that *Tian* could be said to have three types of changes affecting Earth:
>
> (a) When the top layer of Heaven changed, the change was reflected on the surface of a largish expanse of water called *ze*/泽; the top *yao* of this *gua* is a *yin yao*, as water is *yin*. Later the ancient Chinese called it *Dui gua*.
>
> (b) When the change occurred in the middle layers,they called that fire. The *gua* has a *yin yao* in between two *yang yaos*. Fire would be associated with lightning. But whether a fire was started by lightning or by humans, fire meant danger; one must rush to put it out, stop it from spreading but if one could do neither, one must run away as fast as possible. Hence this *gua* had a middle *yin yao* which was meant to convey the information that to prevent a fire from spreading, one should create an empty space between two lots of inflammable material.[52] Later they called it *Li gua*.
>
> (c) When the change occurred at the bottom layers, nearest Earth's surface, this was wind moving, according to the *Yijing*. (In the West, one says

the trees move, not that wind moves). The *gua* has a bottom *yin yao*, with two *yang yaos* above it. Later the ancient Chinese called it *Xun gua*.

Similarly, they attributed three basic types of change to Earth:

(a) When change occurred in the bowels of Earth, they called the effects felt thunder 雷. This term was used to refer to thunder and lightning (which occurred not in the bowels of Earth) as well as to volcanic eruptions, caused by a force emanating from the depth of Earth. It was felt fitting to use a generic term to cover both types of phenomena as they were equally frightening to humans and disruptive of their existence. The *gua* has a bottom *yang yao* with two *yin yaos* above it. Later they called it *Zhen gua*.

(b) When change occurred in the Earth's crust, mountains could be said to move—mountains do move but move so slowly that their movements are imperceptible and therefore appear not to be moving at all. The *gua* has a top *yang yao* with two *yin yaos* beneath it. Later they called it *Gen gua*.

(c) When change occurred in the middle, this would involve water. The *gua* has a middle *yang yao* between two *yin yaos*. The character for water 水 is simply the *Kan gua* stood up. Water which is "alive," must have *yang qi* in it; hence the middle *yang yao* in today's scientific parlance would mean oxygen in the water. Only oxygenated water would support living organisms; "dead" or de-oxygenated water would smell, is polluting and cannot support a healthy biodiversity. Later they called it *Kan gua*.

In other words, Heaven, Earth, Water, Fire, Thunder, Wind, Mountain, and Loch/Mere/Lake stand for eight basic kinds of natural phenomena which profoundly affect humankind and which are captured by the trigrams.

As the *Yao-gua* has earlier been discussed, there is no need for repetition here except to remind the reader of some of its main features relevant to our pre-occupation with understanding *Xiang* Thinking. The information captured by it consists crucially of the following:

1. *Qi* is the basic ontological category with two modes of existence—*Qi*-in-dissipating mode and *Qi*-in-concentrating mode with the former transforming itself into the latter, the latter changing into the former in cyclic reversions.
2. *Qi* is divided into *yin qi* and *yang qi*; and the relationship between them is represented as *Yinyang*.
3. *Yin qi* and *yang qi* in reality do not and cannot exist in their respective pure states, but in varying degrees of *yin-in-yang* and *yang-in-yin*.
4. Reality is about change in the complex manner set out in 1 through 3 above.

This information above happens to be conveyed in English, but it fundamentally can be purveyed wordlessly through the *Yao-gua* of the *Yijing*, the *Xiang* Mode of Thinking. One could have presented figures/images to capture and express it without a single word, thus: — - - which constitute the basic *xiang* of *yinyang* at the level of constructing a *yao* in the *gua*; the *liangyi of Yinyang via* the *xiang* of the *Liangyitaijitu* as shown in figure 6.4; the trigrams and the sixty-four hexagrams in terms of their *yinyang* pairing at different levels *via* the *xiang* shown in figure 7.6.

If one were teaching the *Yao-gua* to people who cannot read or write, then one would simply draw the figures above on sand/paper, and talk them through the figures. If people's memory were good (as the memory of ancient peoples was), and they had understood what was said to them, then they in turn could use them to explain to others—transmission of knowledge from person to person, from generation to generation would be successfully accomplished.

Furthermore, the ancient Chinese believed that *xiang* could convey meaning, significance and information more effectively than writing. Their view would be analogous to what some people say today, that a striking photograph speaks more directly and effectively than volumes of words.[53] *Treatise on the Appended Terms, Part I* of the *Ten Wings* says: 书不尽言, 言不尽意. This author renders it as follows: "The written word cannot exhaust what is spoken, speech cannot exhaust meaning." This is followed by: 圣人立象以尽意, 设卦以尽情伪。《周易·系辞上》 which may be translated as: "The written word cannot exhaust what is spoken, in turn speech cannot exhaust meaning. Hence the wise establish *xiang* to grasp all aspects of meaning, set up *guas* to exhaust connotations." The written word cannot exhaust what speech conveys because it necessarily has to leave out crucial aspects of the spoken word such as the manner of delivery; what today we call body language is left out. Even the written and the spoken words between them do not totally permit comprehensive communication about our thoughts, our feelings/emotions to others. Hence, there is need to establish the *Xiang* Mode of Thinking. Logocentrism is not enough—the written word must be complemented by *Yao-gua* of *Xiang* Thinking. Indeed the ancient Chinese could be said to consider Xiang Thinking to be *primus inter pares*—this appeared to have been the emphasis of those who wrote the *Ten Wings*. In this context, the Latin phrase means that although writing and *xiang* modes of expressing meaning are equally important, nevertheless, the latter could even be said to take precedence. At least, historically this would be correct, as the latter would have preceded the former.

The *Xiang* Mode of Thinking and of expressing meaning rested on the ability of humans to copy Nature as well as to extrapolate from it to form an image to represent what they observe. *Treatise on the Appended Terms, Part II* writes as follows to reflect these two points: 是故《易》者, 象 也: 象 也者, 像也。*Treatise on the Appended Terms, Part I* writes: 圣人有以 见天下之 赜, 而拟诸 起形容, 象 其物宜, 是故谓 之象。This could be roughly rendered (by this author) as:

> The wise in carefully and thoroughly observing the vast flourishing diversity of *Wanwu* and states of affairs in the world around them tried to copy Nature's most basic phenomena, such as heaven, earth, water, fire, thunder, wind, mountain, and marshes/lakes, retaining their respective distinguishing characteristics in terms of form and behavior; in so doing, they managed to construct a unifying framework of the eight trigrams (and later based on these eight trigrams, the sixty-four hexagrams).

At this point of the presentation, it is relevant to emphasize two points raised by the discussion above:

1. *Xiang* Thinking and *Yao-gua* are intimately related; we find in the *Zhouyi, Treatise on the Appended Terms, Part II*, the key phrase: 易者，象也。《周易·系辞下》which could be translated as "*yi* is *xiang*."
2. There is a very important difference in the parallel drawn between *xiang* as in pictographic writing and *Xiang* Mode of Thinking as found in *Yao-gua*. The former is static; the latter is dynamic as the concept *Yi* is first and foremost about change in natural processes. The *Yao-gua* was intended to capture this fundamental dynamism between *yin qi* and *yang qi* in nature. From the "appearance" or "look" of a *gua* and its *yaos*, their positions relating to each other and so on, one can read off the dynamic interplay between *yin* and *yang*, between form and behavior/functioning, thus exemplifying that polar contrasts are complementary, not mutually exclusive, forming a harmonious *Whole*. (Remember, as shown in chapter 6, that the *Yao-gua* Model was used as a diagnostic analytical tool initially for divinatory purpose but was also applied in other domains.) This aspect of *Yao-gua* comes out very clearly in the *Ten Wings*—for instance, we find many pertinent passages of which only a very small selection are cited below to make this point:[54]

   (a) 天下之 动, 圣人 效之/"The wise make their utmost efforts to understand the processes of change and movement in nature."

   (b) 圣人 有以见天下之动, 而观其会通, 以行其典礼, 系辞焉 以断其吉凶, 是故谓之爻/"The wise through observing changes in Nature would come to know what would work and what would not; their understanding of the changes of the *yaos* in a *gua* would determine the course of rites and rituals, what is auspicious, what is not."

(c) 爻 也者，效天下之动者也/"Those who understand the *yaos* understand changes in Nature/society."

(a and b are from *Treatise on the Appended Terms, Part I* while c is from *Part II*. This author is responsible for their rough renderings into English.)

As already observed, *Yao-gua* gave meanings to the trigrams beyond that of standing for eight different kinds of natural phenomena—for instance, this *gua* with three unbroken *yaos* did not simply stand for *Tian*/Heaven (where *yang qi* resided) but was called *Qian* which could take on additional meanings, depending on the context, to stand for the sovereign in the political context, father in the familial context, head (in the context of the human/animal body) and so on, all sharing the same *xiang* of this *gua*.

Xiang Thinking was intended to encompass meanings (*yi*/意) as comprehensively as possible. It (*yi xiang*/意象) is a form of epistemology. At one level, it is a way of knowing states of affairs and phenomena—what *xiang* captured was meant to be an objective way of representing reality (or at least some critical aspects of it). But visual objectivity or at least inter-subjectivity (apprehending form/shape/outline/color) cannot capture the whole of reality; for instance, our other sense organs such as our ears, nose, tongue, skin throughout our bodies can also grasp other aspects of reality. Reality must also include meanings endowed through the individual's grasping of those aspects of that reality already touched upon. The meaning of a landscape could be different for different observers of it. Historically, the landscape of the Lake District or the Peak District in England inspired fear in the beholder—in the early eighteenth century, Daniel Defoe in his *A Tour Through the Whole Island of Great Britain*, originally published 1724–1726, recounted how the coach driver had to lower the blinds as the coach passed through such landscapes in order not to frighten the passengers; Defoe himself described the landscape as "wild barren and frightful." Yet by the time of the nineteenth century, with the emergence of Romanticism, such landscapes, under the influence of Wordsworth and others, inspired not fear, but instead awe as well as admiration for their sublime beauty, or more mundanely for being picturesque. In apprehending any segment of reality, every individual perceiver brings his/her own baggage of memories, personal associations, and cultural understanding—these subjective meanings are just as valid and authentic as the objective meanings. From the perspective of *Xiang* Thinking, the objective and the subjective are not mutually exclusive but together form a more complete *Whole*.

By way of a quick conclusion, *Xiang* Thinking could be said to encompass the following points:

1. *Xiang* could profitably be understood as a kind of picture, but not in all aspects, as *xiang* is not simply a picture, in the way the artist paints a picture of the landscape in front of him, either realistically, in an impressionistic or abstract manner. It is an attempt to capture and delineate by way of a picture what may be said to be common to various states of affairs and situations one can observe around one—in a sense, it is to seek out the commonality共性/*gongxing* behind these diversities via a picture. In other words, *xiang* enables us to grasp such a commonality behind certain diversities and it is only in this aspect that *xiang* involves abstraction.
2. The *xiang*/picture indicates a certain portion of Timespace, specifying the context in which the processes behind events take place.
3. It is an attempt to capture different aspects of reality, both objective and subjective, factual and evaluative (natural events, such as the sun shining in the sky, a river flooding its bank could be perceived to be auspicious or threatening), weaving all these into a *Whole*.
4. Although the *xiang*/picture is an abstraction (in the sense just explained), nevertheless, it is meant to capture the on-going dynamic relations between the parts and their *Whole*—*Yao-gua* is paradigmatic of the *Xiang* Mode. Indeed, *Yao-gua* may be said to be the language of *xiang*; the *Yijing* is, if you like, a *xiang* book, written in the language of *xiang*. It is because *Yao-gua* is a paradigm of *xiang* that *Yao-gua* as a set of diagnostic/analytical tools can be used in every domain, depending on the context, whether divination, *medicine*, politics, military affairs, calligraphy, aesthetics, and so on. It is, as already commented upon, an attempt to capture the commonality behind the diversities of *Wanwu*—from this perspective, *Wuxing* could be seen as *xiang*, as it, too, tries to capture the commonality behind the diversities of *Wanwu*. Ultimately *Water*, *Wood*, *Fire*, *Earth*, *Metal* embody the *qi* of *yin* and *yang* and the processes of *qi* transformation which is *Wuxing*.

Xiang Thinking, in its methodological implications, is brilliantly exemplified in CCM. As Lee, (forthcoming) will be devoted to it, no more will now be said about the matter, except to remind the reader of two points: (a) that *Xiang* Thinking penetrated/s all aspects of Chinese culture such as agriculture, the military, music, other fine arts, and so on, as *Yao-gua* of the *Yijing* and the *Zhouyi* go hand in hand with it. In Chinese painting and calligraphy, the emphasis is not on shape and form *xing*/形 but on *xiang*; drawing is called

写真/*xie zhen* (literally "writing truth"), truth is found in *xiang*, not *xing*; (b) that investigators in CCM, more than in other domains, were/are guided by leads and clues given by the reality captured by *xiang* (that part of reality which is open to direct observation) to explore that part of reality which is not available to direct observation (in the absence of high tech which has only very recently of late been made available in Biomedicine).

Conclusion

This chapter has sought to establish the following main points:

1. Chinese thinking is fundamentally Contextual Thinking.
2. It is dyadic, not dualistic.
3. Hence its uniqueness lies in combining 1 and 2 as Contextual-dyadic Thinking; as such, it did not explore/develop the binary system of thinking which is context- and content-free in the way that Western philosophy/science developed it as a formal, abstract science/technology, although it grasped it some two thousand years before Leibniz did.
4. It is also unique in its incorporation of what is a form of non-linguistic thinking, the *Xiang* Mode *via Yao-gua* of the *Yijing*.
5. Unlike classical logic in the West, it rests on an implicit *logic* which is many-valued rather than two-valued; it also appears not to embrace the principles of excluded middle, non-contradiction, and identiy.
6. *Xiang* Mode of Thinking is also an excellent example of Fact/Value *Wholism*, which will be explored in detail in chapter 11, demonstrating that unlike modern Western science, Chinese *science* embraced quite openly the so-called fact-value distinction, as its *philosophy* saw no way of eliminating/insulating values either from human lives or from the human pursuit of trying to understand the natural phenomena within which human existence is immersed.
7. This chapter, however, does not touch on what is often referred to in sinological literature as Correlative Thinking. This author feels the right place to discuss it is in the next chapter where it would be shown as an implication of a version of Wholism, to be called M-cosmic *Wholism* (short for Macro-micro-cosmic *Wholism*), and where justice could be done through establishing that its *philosophical* foundation lies in *Qi* ontology as well as the metaphysics of *Wholism*. Just to call it Correlative Thinking gives the misleading impression that it is nothing more than a quirk of the ancient Chinese who, unlike other peoples (especially people in the age of modernity), could then be regarded as extraordinary in their naïvete, being impressed by analogues between

the cosmological domain and that of human affairs in the way astrology is said to be.

Notes

1. This could be regarded as controversial, but for a reason which will soon become obvious; this author chooses to follow Kurtz, 2011 which gives a detailed discussion of the search among Chinese scholars during the last hundred years or so for fragments of texts which could be used to support the claim that Chinese *philosophy* had or must have developed logic in the European understanding of that term as formal logic. The operative phrase is "the European understanding of that term as formal logic," as it is clear that (ancient) Chinese *philosophers* had an interest in logic—it was just that their pre-occupation with it was not expressed in the same way as European philosophers (since ancient Greek philosophy) had/have pursued the subject as formal logic.

2. This author can track down one work (in English), written by the psychologist, Nisbett, 2003/2005: xix which raises this matter, claiming that even today, those brought up in and influenced historically by Chinese culture are "better able to see relationships among events than Westerners . . .", why Westerners are "so likely to overlook the influence of context on the behaviour of objects and even of people . . ."

3. For yet another interpretation, see Ziporyn, 2013. It is also important to labour the point that these other interpretations are not necessarily incompatible with the one offered here in terms of the Contextual Mode of Thinking.

4. For instance, scientific disputes are not necessarily subject to incommensurability, contrary to what some Kuhnians might wish to claim—see Lee, 1984.

5. One particular example of the presentation of syllogistic logic in an introductory text of the discipline would look like this: All Ms are Ps; S is M; therefore, S is P. This argument is valid because it satisfies the rule that the middle term (M) is distributed. One does not need to know what the terms, M, P, and S stand for or refer to, as formal logic is not interested *per se* in truth, but only in validity.

6. For a powerful account of dualism from the standpoint of feminism, see Plumwood, 1993 of which more would be said later.

7. On this ontological *volte –face*, see Lee, 2012b.

8. For a like-minded account, see *Zhang, 2008.

9. See *Han Dynasty version of Fuxi and Nüwa*, 2013 (as depicted in murals of that dynasty).

10. See *Fuxi and Nüwa*, 2013.

11. Fuxi and Nüwa were brother and sister. They realized that if they were to have progeny in order to perpetuate the human race, they must copulate. Yet they hesitated to do so initially, but later gave in to this desire under a specific condition. If Heaven were to see their act of sexual intercourse as a worthy act, it would send clouds to shield them, giving them the privacy they needed while they engaged in it. They duly ascended a

mountain; the clouds descended covering them and the mountain top. They knew then that Heaven had granted permission for this primeval act of intimacy and pro-creation. Nüwa also was the creator of human beings, literally making humans out of mud and breathing life into the clay models. She was a multi-tasking, multi-role figure.

12. According to at least one version of the myth, the gods in the sky above quarrelled and fought one another viciously. As a result, the pillar supporting Heaven collapsed and Earth was in disorder and chaos. Nüwa repaired the damage by cutting off the feet of the tortoise to support the four corners, and to use seven different colour stones to patch up the holes in the sky. Note that in this myth, those who caused damage were male and the individual who restored order was female. This could be read to reinforce the analysis pursued in this book, that the Chinese mode of thinking is consistently dyadic, not dualistic.

13. See Lee, 1975 on the jurisprudence of Legalism.

14. For a quick general account, see Theobald, 2014; for a detailed discussion especially bearing on the theme of gender identity, see Wang, 2005.

15. Note that the character *xing*/刑 in *tianxing*/天刑 is not the same *xing*/形 which may be translated in certain contexts as "shape/form", although they share the same sound and the same tone (second). Traditionally, Chinese life was regulated by natural processes of change in *yang qi* and *yin qi*, particularly, during the four seasons with the former in ascendance from Spring to Summer and the latter beginning to increase corresponding with the decline of the former. It was felt more proper to execute criminals not during Spring and Summer when life begins to renew itself with the rise of *yang qi*, but in Autumn when life forms, on the whole, tend to wind down as *yang qi* declines. Hence the Will of Heaven, so to speak, in meting out punishment to those who deserved it, would not be carried out in the first half of the year.

16. Some sinologists have recently cast doubt of their own on this matter—see Loewe, 2011. It could simply be that Dong Zhongshu appropriated the concepts of *Yinyang, Wuxing* as well as concepts from the Confucian canonical texts such as *wuchang*/五常 to create a special blend, based on his transforming polar contrasts from the dyadic into the dualistic mode of thought, which later became known as the official Han Confucian ideology. But as this author is not qualified to enter into the scholarship of this issue, the matter is simply raised here but left to rest.

17. Sometimes even those with profound knowledge, both in the theory and practice, of CCM, such as *Pan, 2012, Vol. 2: 196 can suffer a moment of departing from what this book calls Contextual-dyadic Thinking to fall back on the dualist mode advocated by Dong Zhongshu. This only goes to show how careful one must be when faced with the Dong Zhongshu's powerful legacy with some two thousand years of standing in transforming the Contextual-dyadic Mode into dualist mode of thinking (at least in the domain of social thought).

18. See *Early influences on Leibniz's account of binary arithmetic*, 2006.

19. For an image, access via "De Arte Combinatoria."

20. See *Hexagramium* Organum, 2013.

21. For an image, access via "Aristotle's Square of Opposition."

22. However, while Needham claims that such interest had inspired and impacted on Leibniz's philosophy in some way(s), Cook and Rosemont, 1981 argue otherwise, as they maintain that similarities between the ancient Chinese and Leibniz's own concepts were nothing more than isomorphism (this claim will be looked at later in this section), that the latter's real interest in the Chinese was the practical missionary one of rendering the eventual conversion of the Chinese to Christianity an easier task. If what Cook and Rosemont maintain is correct, it would follow that Leibniz was in reality a closet Jesuit (figurist) at heart in spite of his own Protestant faith. (Figurism was the view that all cultures and civilisations were descended from the Judeo-Christian tradition and any pre-Christian histories already contained intimations of future Christian teachings.)

23. For an image, see *http://www.shanghaidaily.com/sunday/now-and-then/Bagua-and-the-sequence-of-64-hexagrams/shdaily.shtml* Accessed September 14, 2016.

24. The binary system operates with 2 as base; hence it expresses all numbers as a combination of the digits 0 and 1, rather than using the ten digits 0 through 9 in the normal base 10 system. It is a place value system and uses powers of 2: 2, 4, 8, 16, 32, 64, etc.

Table 9.7.

Decimal	*Binary*	*Example: The Binary Number 110100101 is Equivalent to:*
1	1	
2	10	1 x 256 = 256
3	11	1 x 128 = 128
4	100	0 x 64 = 0
5	101	1 x 32 = 32
6	110	0 x 16 = 0
7	111	0 x 8 = 0
8	1000	1 x 4 = 4
9	1001	0 x 2 = 0
10	010	1 x 1 = 1
		411

25. Shao Yong said the *Xiantiantu* was Fuxi's. For a recent account of the complex issues in the history of Yilogy, see *Guo and Guo, 2005 who imply that the claim might not be so preposterous in the light of archaeological finds such as the jade tablet/含山玉版 found in 1987 (Hanshan county, Anhui province/安徽含山), dated to the Neolithic Dawenko/大汶口 Culture as early as c. 5,600 years ago. Another

artefact also found in Anhui province is the six-hole earthenware ball/六孔陶球, belonging to the Xuejiakang Culture/薛家岗), with patterns on the surface. These artifacts have been interpreted as three dimensional versions of the trigrams—according to this line of thinking, the first set of trigrams, traditionally attributed to Fuxi, was not two-dimentional but three-dimensional in character. Although their dates fall short of that postulated for Fuxi who was alleged to have lived sometime during the mid-twenty-ninth century BCE, they are dates of around five thousand years ago.

26. See *Explanation of binary arithmetic*, 2014 (English translation).

27. See also Mungello, 1977: 36-46 for a discussion of Bouvet.

28. This scholarship is called "Arabic" not because the scholars involved were ethnic Arabs but because the language in which their scholarly discourse was conducted was Arabic (just as in the Middle Ages, the language of scholarly discourse in Westerm Europe was Latin, not French, German, English, or any other language).

29. According to some scholars—for instance *Zeng, 2010—the sequence comes from our ten fingers. *Yang* is an odd while *yin* is an even number—hence 1,3,5,7,9 are *yang*, and 2,4,6,8 are *yin*.

30. For a slightly different though related account of the philosophical differences between Leibniz and Shao Yong, see Ryan, 1996.

31. See Joseph, 1994.

32. See *Leibniz's calculating machine*, 2002.

33. This section is co-authored with Andriy Vasylchenko who is Senior Research Associate at the Skovoroda Institute of Philosophy, National Academy of Sciences of Ukraine; he has also made significant suggestions for improvement in the preceding section on Leibniz's binary arithmetic.

34. On this subject, from the standpoint of elucidating the text using the techniques of modern formal logic, see Liu & Zhang, 2013 as well as Lucas, 2005 who argue that Mohist logic could be regarded as a logic of sortal predicates. However, see Kurtz, 2011 for a detailed discussion about this kind of project in general.

35. This has not prevented a "whole industry" generated by Chinese scholars and others (since the beginning of the twentieth century) interested in the claim that Chinese logic has a history of more than two thousand years in the same way as European logic can claim such a long ancestry. Kurtz, 2011 sets out in fascinating details the sources which have created and sustained the claim for a century or so. Our interpretation of *Yinyang/Yao-gua* implicit *logic* is not intended and should not be read as a contribution toward this claim. The reasons should by now be very obvious; all the same, it may be advisable to labor two very important points of differences between those who support the claim and this account: (a) the whole burden here is to say that ancient Chinese *philosophy* have implicitly ruled out the possibility and/or relevance of formal logic as it endorsed the Contextual-dyadic Mode of Thinking to be basic and fundamental; (b) *Yinyang/Yao-gua* implicit *logic* is many-valued, a kind of logic which did not really make an appearance until the arrival of non-classical logics in the twentieth century, whereas the ancient Chinese analogue of (implicit) multi-valence was embedded in the *Yijing* itself. Hence, this interpretation is more in

keeping with what Kurtz, 2011: 363 advocates in the epilogue of his book: "Rather than continue the forced chase for theoretical fragments, it seems to me, an alternative approach to Chinese logic could scrutinize argumentative practices and try to recover the implicit and explicit standards of validity embodied in them." The *Yijing* and in turn the *Zhouyi* are foundational to every aspect of Chinese culture and civilization, and in that sense an attempt to excavate their implicit *logic* could not be said to be part of "the forced chase for theoretical fragments."

36. This should not be taken to deny that in the context of applied logic, there will always be form and content at the same time when formal regularities are applied in some particular domain of investigation. We can analyze particular computing processes and make meaningful conclusions on the ground of formal analysis.

37. For accessible accounts, see Priest, 2000; Smith, (P), 2003; Restall, 2006.

38. For those who wish to have a very quick Cook's tour, see, for example, King and Shapiro, 1995; for others, see Gabbay and Woods, 2012.

39. For one account, see Edwards, 1967, Vol. 4: 414-417.

40. For those who wish to see how this is done, an accessible account can be found under *Law of Excluded Middle*, 2014.

41. There is some dispute as to Zadeh's status as its founder or creator, but as this is not germane to our pre-occupation, no more would be said about the matter.

42. See Kosko, 1993 for an accessible general discussion; also Zhang & Zhang, 2004; Hajek, 2010, 2009, 1998 for technical details. Some philosophers may be said to have paved the way. The American pragmatist, (Charles Sanders) Peirce, 1934: 513 wrote: ". . . vagueness is no more to be done away within the world of logic than friction in the world of mechanics." In 1937, Max Black used the word "vague" to refer to the lack of precision in the terms one uses in ordinary discourse—take "bald." When does one say that a man is bald? When he is absolutely without a hair on his head? When the top of the skull is smooth, but there is a fringe of sparsely distributed hair around the smooth top? Black realised that the logic of such terms is vague once he attained the insight that language is not truth-functional in the way that Russell and Whitehead in the *Principia Mathematica* claimed it was. He then wrote the paper "Vagueness: an Exercise in Logical Analysis," *Philosophy of Science* 4 (1937): 427–55; everything could be said to possess A to some degree and therefore not-A to some degree. When the degree is extreme, we put it at 1 at one end, along a scale from 0 to 1, and at the other end we put it at 0. Degrees of gradation are best conveyed via curves as curves are not abrupt steps from 1 to 0 or 0 to 1. Curves show instead that not-A is the inverse of A and *vice versa*; if curve A touches 1, not-A must touch and *vice versa*. As the curves move away from these two extremes, they get vaguer or fuzzier. Where they cross at the mid-point, the value is ½, the point where A equals not-A. In other words, Black applied vague logic to vague sets—see Kosko, 1993. The Anglo-Saxon world of philosophy ignored the paper; instead, post-war, when Wittgenstein announced his repudiation of the *Tractatus Logico-Philosophicus*, it whole-heartedly embraced "the New Testament" Wittgenstein (*Philosophical Investigations*) and his conception of ordinary language analysis in terms of language

games and the notion of family resemblances. In the meantime, the Japanese who had no such pre-occupations accepted with alacrity Zadeh's paper and by 1989 had manufactured washing machines using fuzzy logic. Black and Wittgenstein were not the only philosophers who turned their back upon the binary truth-functional view of language; even the co-author of *Principia Mathematica*, Whitehead stopped being a mathematician/logician and re-invented himself as a metaphysician advocating what today we call process philosophy, a subject already dealt with in chapter 8. See also Mohaghegh, 2000.

In non-European cultures, apart from the ancient Chinese, Buddhist logic is said to be four-valued (either/or, both/and, neither/nor, and Jaina logic to be seven-valued, each preceded by the term "syad" which means "in some ways" or "from a perspective: "in some ways it is," "in some ways it is not," "in some ways it is and it is not," "in some ways it is and it is indescribable," "in some ways it is not and it is indescribable," "in some ways it is, it is not and it is indescribable" and finally "in some ways it is indescribable." See Sattler, 2010/2011: chapter 3; Priest, 2008b.

43. Note that the number 8 works as a constitutive principle for the model (8 trigrams, 4 pairs of polarities) if and only if we code the trigrams by simple fractions with the denominator 7.

44. It is sorely tempting to call it "informal logic;" the temptation must be resisted, using instead the term "implicit *logic*." "Informal logic" is bespoken as it is often used to refer to that advocated by the "New Testament" Wittgenstein. Wittgenstein repudiated the main thesis of the *Tractatus Philosophicus*, when he realized that ordinary language is not truth-functional, and that it does not correspond "one to one" with the "world out there." Instead of challenging binary logic, which underpinned the truth functional view of language, and developing an alternative which could do greater justice to ordinary language, he took the "linguistic turn" in *Philosophical Investigations*. By so doing, mainstream Western philosophy did not go down the route indicated by Max Black in his 1937 paper as already pointed out. "Implicit" has the advantage of being the contrast of "explicit"—formal logic in the West is explicit, spelt out, systematized, whereas the implicit *logic* discussed here is simply embedded in the *Yinyang/Yao-gua* Model of reasoning.

45. For an introduction to contemporary modal metaphysics, see Loux, 2006: chapter 5.

46. The principle of modal plenitude articulated here is inspired by Priest's "principle of freedom" (Priest, 2005: 106), formulated within his metaphysics of modal noneism and actually is an extrapolation from the latter to the wider scope of metaphysical theories.

47. In those times, the climate of China and its ecosystems were very different; elephants were plentiful.

48. For a quick accessible account of the history of Chinese writing, see Lee, 2008.

49. Adapted from *Chen, 2006: 40-41.

50. Scholars still debate whether the Bronze Script was simultaneous with the Oracle Bone Script or indeed, even preceded it. The Bronze Script was the script

used when characters were inscribed on bronze vessels of which the Shang produced many which are both exquisitely beautiful and complex objects.

51. As evidence to date does not permit scholars to draw any firm conclusion, one can only postulate plausible hypotheses regarding them.

52. Chapter 11 looks at Fact/Value *Wholism*, citing this *gua*.

53. A young Vietnamese photographer took a photo of a girl injured, fleeing in terror from the chemical (napalm) dropped upon her and fellow villagers. This image, published in the Western media, was so powerful that some think that the tide in the Western world against the U.S. government in the Vietnam War could be dated from its publication.

54. *See Liu, 2008: 59–64; also *Pan 2012, Vol. 2: 2–9.

CHAPTER TEN

Wholism in Chinese Terms

The preceding chapters have commented that *Wholism* is endemic to Chinese culture and civilization, whether one is examining the Chinese mode of grasping the world *via Yinyang*, the components of each *gua* (as trigram or hexagram), the *Yao-gua* Model itself, Chinese process *philosophy*, the *Xiang* Mode of Thinking, or the human being as understood in CCM yet to be looked at, in detail, in the sequel to this volume. It is time to spell out in somewhat greater detail what *Wholism* in Chinese *philosophy* amounts to. Let us first give a quick summary about "wholism" as generally conceived in philosophy today. Its metaphysical/methodological contrast is commonly called Individualism/Reductionism—so it is best to approach the matter *via* this pair of contrasts.

A brief word of clarification regarding how the term "wholism" is used in this chapter/book is called for. It could be used within a Reductionist as well as a non-Reductionist philosophical framework. This author proposes to use "wholism" when referring to the former, and "Wholism" to the latter. Regarding the latter, in conformity with the convention adopted, the Chinese variety will be referred to as "*Wholism*" and the non-Chinese version as "Wholism." (Parts of chapter 11 overlap with this material).

Individualism/Reductionism consists of the following theses constituting wholism:

Wholes can be reduced to parts without loss or residue whether from the semantic, logical, methodological or metaphysical standpoint.

1. Metaphysical: wholes are not real and do not exist; their parts are real and exist; wholes are no more than sum of their parts. In visiting, say, the University of Oxford, once the visitor had been shown each and every one of the individual colleges, the libraries, the laboratories, the lecture theaters, the teaching rooms, the administrative buildings, the recreational buildings/facilities including the playing fields, the boat houses, the punts, and so on, s/he had completed the visit, that is, to say, s/he had seen all that is the University. At the end of this tour, should the visitor then ask the host: "Thank you for what you have shown me, but where is the University?" This according to Ryle, 1949 is to commit a category mistake. In this context, it is to hold that the whole is more than the sum of its parts.
2. Methodological: to understand wholes and how they function, one only needs to understand their parts, their functions and the relations between them. Engineering, for instance, enables one to construct a whole using certain elementary components; reverse engineering enables one to deconstruct a whole into its elementary components. This ability to engineer a whole from the parts and to deconstruct a whole into its parts takes the mystery out of wholes, which then reinforces the metaphysical point that wholes are no more than the sum of their parts.
3. Logical: an exhaustive list of propositions about the parts entails propositions about wholes; the two sets of propositions are logically equivalent. It is like saying "2 + 2 = 4" or that the average couple in Britain has 2.3 children. While one can shake hands with and say hello to Tom, Dick, or Harry and their respective wives and children, one cannot meet Mr. and Mrs. Average and their 2.3 children as these are mere statistical constructs arrived at by laboriously adding up the married/co-habiting couples in the UK at any one moment in time, the number of children between them, then divide the second set of figures by the first. Mr. and Mrs. Average and their 2.3 children are not flesh and blood individuals like one's neighbors.
4. Semantic: to replace statement(s) about a whole with an exhaustive list of statements about its parts involves neither loss of meaning nor content.

In contrast, Wholism is the negation of the above, as Wholes cannot be reduced to their parts without loss or residue.

1. Metaphysical: while parts are real, the Whole which is constituted of the parts is also real, albeit at a different level of existence. A famous

football team is real and exists over and above the individual team members to whom you can be introduced. A team-member such as the goaler, no matter how good his specific skill cannot be said to constitute the team—a team (in the standard game) must have eleven members, each playing a certain role who interacts not only with one another but also with the opposing team/members. One also talks about the team spirit/ethos, which is something more than simply who kicks what according to the rule books. One particular member of the team may be transferred out and another footballer bought in, but the team remains the team. Hence, for these and similar reasons, the Whole is said to be greater than the sum of its parts, or more accurately that the Whole is "over and above its parts, and not just the sum of them all" (Mitchell, 2012: 171).

2. Methodological: to understand a Whole and how it functions, one must understand not only how each part functions, but also all their functions and the complex inter-relationships between them.
3. Logical: an exhaustive list of propositions about the parts does not entail propositions about the Whole; the two sets are not logically equivalent.
4. Semantic: one cannot substitute statements about a Whole with an exhaustive list of statements about its parts without loss of meaning or content.

Chinese *Wholism* was/is compatible with these theses of Wholism. One must point out straightaway that the ancient Chinese did not spell out their metaphysics in an explicit fashion, though one could say that their thoughts implied them. As Chinese *philosophy* differs from Western philosophy in spite of commonalities (in some aspects) between them, it is best to alert the reader to these differences by writing the Chinese version as "*Wholism*" and the Western non-Reductionist version as "Wholism."

The above account holds true because Wholes are said to possess emergent properties, which are new or novel characteristics not displayed by their constituent parts. H_2O, the molecule for water, which is made out of two atoms of hydrogen and one atom of oxygen is commonly cited to illustrate this point. From knowledge about the respective properties of the oxygen and hydrogen atoms, one could not predict the properties of water. All complex systems exhibit emergent properties. It is held that consciousness is an emergent property of brain activities; that biological laws (at the level of the organism) cannot be irreducibly explained in terms of laws of chemistry and physics.[1] Wholes are also said to exhibit downward (or more appropriately systemic) causation upon their parts—an aspect which will be looked at later in slightly greater detail in chapter 11.

Wholism in Chinese *philosophy* goes beyond the above as it is embedded in process- not thing- ontology. Furthermore, it may be systematically grasped at several levels of understanding starting from the most foundational or most basic and to which other levels are related. This may be set out as follows:

1. The most foundational is that of *Qi*, *yin qi* and *yang qi* and *Yinyang*.
2. Cosmological: *Tian* and *Di*/Heaven and Earth.
3. *Yao-gua*: *Qian* and *Kun*/Heaven and Earth with two aspects: (a) the natural/cosmological (*Wanwu* and reproduction), and (b) the social/political (*sangang*/three bonds).
4. Timespace (Astronomy and Geography).
5. Humans and its relation to the cosmological: *sancai*.
6. Concept of *Tianren-heyi*/*Tianren-xiangying*, derived from 2 and 4.
7. The individual human being as the being whose health or illness is the subject of understanding in CCM.

Qi Wholism: Yin Qi and Yang Qi, Yinyang

Yinyang as the most fundamental instance of *Wholism* in Chinese *philosophy* does not need to delay us for long here, as the subject has already been thoroughly explored in earlier chapters especially in 3, 5, 6, 7, and (sections of) 9. We simply need to summarise quickly the main points to remind the reader of them:

1. *Yin* and *yang*, though polar contrasts, do not obey the principle of excluded middle; instead they necessarily co-exist, interacting intimately with each other as *Yinyang*. Within *yin* is *yang* and within *yang* is *yin*. The most potent *xiang* to represent this *Wholism* is the *Liangyitaijitu*—figure 6.5.
2. As polar contrasts, they are to be understood not as dualistic/hierarchical pairings, but as dyadic complementary pairings within the larger Contextual-dyadic Mode of Thinking. The most potent figure to represent this aspect is that of the Fuxi and Nüwa Pro-creation Myth—figure 9.2.
3. The complex inter-relationships between *yin* and *yang* within the *Yinyang-Wuxing* framework are responsible for the existence of *Wanwu* and their sustainability. The most potent *xiang* for these aspects is the *Houtiantu* but it should also be studied in connection with the *Xiantiantu*.

4. *Tian* and *Di*, with *yang qi* primarily associated with the former and *yin qi* primarily associated with the latter. The most potent *xiang* for *Tian/Di Wholism* via 1 are the *Qian gua* and the *Kun gua*, with the *Qian gua* occupying the South position and the *Kun gua* occupying the North position. *Yuzhou* and *Wanwu* would not endure if the complex set of inter-relationships between *yang qi* and *yin qi* fails to obtain—as *yang qi* rises while *yin qi* descends, the most potent *xiang* for this is figure 7.3. This point is also made via two hexagrams: if pure *yang/Qian gua* were the top *gua* in the hexagram, and the pure *yin/Kun gua* the bottom *gua*, the two *qis* would never meet, and ecological (and other) disasters would ensue. The correct position is the *Qian gua* at the bottom and the *Kun gua* at the top—the *yang qi* would rise to meet the *yin qi* as it descends, forming a co-operative functioning, enduring, and sustainable *Whole*. Such a hexagram is therefore auspicious and is called the *Tai gua* 泰卦while the inauspicious is the *Pi gua* 否卦.

Divination apart, the most cited use of the *Yao-gua* set of analytical tools was, of course, its application in the political domain, where as we have seen, the identification of the *Qian gua* with the Ruler and the *Kun gua* with Officials or the Common People were established. However, it is wrong to infer from the prominence of this usage that *Yao-gua* was exclusively applied in this domain, outside of divination—it bears laboring the point that as a set of methodological/analytical tools, it was applied in all domains of activities in Chinese culture, including, amongst others, also prominently, the military and the *medical*. From this perspective, the claim made by some sinologists that the foundation of CCM rested on nothing but the analogy of the *medical* with the political domain would appear to be misleading.

Macro-micro-cosmic *Wholism*

We have earlier touched upon this theme. Chapter 6, in explaining why a *gua* has three *yaos*, has implied the notion of *sancai*三才– the Three Powers are Heaven/*Tian*, Earth/*Di* and Humans/*Ren*, with the bottom *yao* standing for Earth, the top *yao* for Heaven, and the middle *yao* for Humans, that true wisdom on the part of Humans consisted of understanding their position in relationship to the other two powers, that without these, Humans would not exist, never mind flourish. This point can be made via any *gua*. For the sake of illustrating its *xiang*, let us take the *Qian gua* which has three unbroken *yaos*: the bottom/first yao is Earth, the middle is humankind and the top/third is Heaven.

This brief encapsulation of the meaning of the Three Powers in turn touches upon another crucial concept in Chinese *philosophy*/culture, namely, *Tianren-xiangying*/*Tianren-heyi* which literally means: Heaven, Earth (in this context, the reference to Heaven includes Earth as well), and Humankind form a harmonious *Whole*. Heaven and Earth constitute *Yuzhou*, the Macrocosm while Humankind constitutes the Microcosm in relation to the former, but also as part of it. This author, therefore, calls this version of *Wholism* "Macro-micro-cosmic *Wholism* (or M-cosmic *Wholism* for short). As *Qi Wholism* is fundamental—it provides the basis for M-cosmic *Wholism*—*Wanwu*, which includes Humankind, embodies both *yin qi* and *yang qi* with the two interacting in an intricately co-operative manner to ensure existence and flourishing. As *Wanwu* share the *qi* of Heaven and Earth, it would seem reasonable to postulate that there is a correspondence between the Macrocosm and the Microcosm, as *Qi*-in-dissipating mode of the former would also occur in the latter; similarly, the same would hold for *Qi*-in-concentrating mode in both Macrocosm and Microcosm. (Regarding the latter, Chinese *philosophy*/*medicine* took Humankind as representative case of *Wanwu*.) Sinologists call this "correlative thinking" (Graham, 1986) or "correlative cosmology" (Fruehauf, 2009). However, this author prefers to use M-cosmic *Wholism* to emphasise that the concept of *Tianren-xiangying* draws attention to the point made just now that *Wholism* in Chinese *philosophy*/*medicine* is ontologically founded on *Qi*-in-dissipating as well as *Qi*-in-concentrating modes as demonstrated in chapter 3.

Ontology, in particular, *philosophy* in general, has methodological implications which CCM exploits in depth. It suffices here to mention just a few examples to illustrate the point. *Tian*/Heaven is above/*shang*/上, Di/Earth is below/*xia*/下—hence in the human being, the head is *Tian*, the feet are *Di*, as the head is the highest part of the human person. According to Chinese cosmology/*philosophy*, humankind stands out amongst all the other organisms, and is considered to possess a unique kind of consciousness—humankind is *Wanwu zhi ling*/万物之灵. It is very important not to misunderstand this last nostrum through understanding it in terms of anthropocentrism as found in Western philosophy, as the Chinese celebration of the human intellect has severe limits, unlike its Western counterpart. Take large four-legged animals. Humans could not hope to compete with them for speed in running/sprinting as their strength lies in their four feet which are firmly planted on the ground—they are *Di*-endowed organisms and the greater part of their *yang qi* is found in their four legs. No matter how hard competitors may try to improve records of running feats at the Olympic Games every four years, they cannot hope to out sprint the cheetah, to run faster or at least as fast as the horse. The heads of all these other animals point toward the ground. On the other hand, humans are *Tian*-endowed organisms—bipedalism means that our heads point upward/Heavenward. The *yang qi* in us is more in our head than our two feet. (Unlike human adults, the *yang qi* of children lies in their feet/legs, hence their constant running, rushing about whereas by maturity, the *yang qi* has moved upwards to the head—indeed, as we pass our prime, declining into old age, the *yang qi* slowly dissipates until at death, it has left us altogether.) This clearly shows that quadrupeds and bipeds each have their respective excellences, bearing out the *axiom* that every explanation, every assertion must be understood within the Contextual-dyadic framework. It follows that humans are not superior in every respect to other animals, although it is correct to observe that they excel in the use of language, their ability to formulate abstract thoughts, to create metaphysical systems, to postulate hypotheses which could be empirically tested (the basis of doing science of any kind/description), and so on. M-cosmic *Wholism* did/does not endorse anthropocentrism as understood in Western philosophy and its civilization—the latter claims humans to be superior, *tout court*, theologically by way of an immortal soul, in secular justifications by way of possessing language, ability to do science (especially science of the Modern variety) which permits them to use the technology generated by science to control and dominate Nature. This way of looking at and understanding the world is typical of the Dualistic-hierarchical Mode of Thinking endemic in modern Western philosophy, but is totally alien to the Chinese Contextual-dyadic Mode as their ontology-*cum*-methodology does not license understanding phenomena independent of context.

To labor a critically important point—humankind, in order to exist and to flourish, must necessarily live and work within a world where *yin qi* and *yang qi* interact in a complex manner (with Mutually Engendering and Mutually Constraining relationships), producing a harmonious *Whole*. This aspect of M-cosmic *Wholism* will be explored in greater detail a little later under Ecosystem *Wholism*/Wholism.

Another example of the concept of M-cosmic *Wholism* are two phenomena which CCM considers to have something to do with the moon.[2] Take the notion of *mai*/脉. As Lee, 2017b will make clear, ascertaining *mai* is a very important diagnostic tool in CCM. As a step to understanding its meaning, let us deconstruct it in terms of some of the various scripts in which the character has been written in the history of the Chinese language. All versions (at least the Lesser Seal, Clerical, Standard scripts, the last including today's *fanti* and *jianti*) have as radical/*bushou* the character 月 which refers to the moon. The difference between *fanti* as used in Taiwan/Macao/Hongkong today and *jianti* as used in Mainland China (which is now the official script of the language at the UN) lies in their respestive right hand components, as shown below.

脈 脉

月 here is taken to refer to the moon [3]—the moon in Chinese culture is quintessentially *yin* and more specifically is associated with water, according to the *Huainanzi*: 水气之精者为月《淮南子· 天文顺训 》. In other words, in this line of reasoning, one could even say that the moon is nothing more than the *qi* of water. The meaning of 永 is permanent/lasting; in the world of natural phenomena, the ancient Chinese regarded the flow of its mighty rivers (namely the Yellow River and the Yangzi River) to stand for the idea of permanence. The right hand component of the character in *fanti* means tributaries. The right hand components of the respective *jianti* and *fanti* character for *mai* involve water.

The moon one sees in the sky itself has no light; its light is nothing but the light reflected by the Sun; hence the moon is *yin*, dark, without light as its light comes from the relationship between three heavenly bodies, the Sun, Earth, and Moon. In terms of CCM and Chinese astronomy, moonlight is simply an indication of the retreat of sunlight/*yang qi*, and the different phases of the moon also reflect the changes in *yang qi* in the context of the relationship among these three heavenly bodies. Suppose today to be four days ahead of the fifteenth day of the lunar month, one would then notice that Moon begins to wax until full moon would appear on the fifteenth itself, which would indicate that Moon's *yang qi* is at its greatest. In the cycle of Moon, the ancient Chinese also held that it could be divided into four periods found in the Earth-Sun relationship during the year, comparable to Spring, Summer, Autumn, and Winter. In the lunar cycle, according to a Han text called *Zhouyi can tong qi/* (魏伯阳·《周易参同契》), full moon could be said to be equivalent to Summer (represented by *Qian gua*), third quarter half moon the equivalent to Autumn, new moon to Winter, the first quarter half moon to Spring.

The ancient Chinese linked the changes of the tides to the phases of Moon, pointing to the linkage between Moon and water. Water is *yin*, therefore, is calm, without movement. The ability of water then to move (as in high tide) must be due to the influence of *yang qi*, which is at its greatest at full moon, but which is at its weakest at new moon. *Au fond*, it is the changes in the relationship between *yin qi* and *yang qi* which brought about high and low tides. Today's scientific explanation of the phenomenon is not all that different except that Modern Science does not rest on the discourse of *Yinyang*, but uses notions such as gravitational attraction.

Having sorted out this kind of astronomical phenomena in terms of the changing relationships between *yin qi* and *yang qi*, how would the ancient Chinese explain *mai* in the human person under M-cosmic *Wholism*? *Mai* involves blood and its flow through the human person. Remember blood is a liquid and is salty; so is sea water; a large expanse of Earth's surface is covered by water, but water/liquid also constitutes the major part (70 percent) of the human body. Blood, like water is *yin*; *yin* stands for calm, not movement. So why should *mai*—a pulsating movement—occur? Today's Modern Science explains the pulse via the fact that the heart is a muscle which is capable of contracting and expanding. The ancient Chinese did know about these movements, but nevertheless, did not rely on them to explain *mai*—ultimately, for them *mai* was accounted for in terms of the changes in the relationship between *yin qi* and *yang qi*. It could be encapsulated as 阳加于阴谓之脉 translated (by this author) as: "*mai* is the outcome of *yang* acting upon/being added to *yin*"). This means that when the Chinese physician ascertains the patient's *mai* in the process of diagnosing the patient's illness and its conditions, s/he is actually exploring the precise relationship between *yin qi* and *yang qi* in the individual, exactly as the *Neijing* says: 脉以侯阴阳/*mai yi hou Yinyang*. As everything in *Yuzhou* embodies *Yinyang*, then clearly whatever happens in the Macrocosm and in the Microcosm would be subject to *Yinyang*; M-cosmic *Wholism* embodies this most fundamental *Law of Nature*, the law of *Yinyang*.

The next phenomenon related to Moon is menstruation in (human) females which generally occurs between the onset of puberty and the onset of menopause (which CCM puts at age forty-nine), when they are capable of reproduction. One expression for referring to menstruation is 月经/*yuejing*, that which happens regularly every month. In English, the period is called "menstruation," based on the Latin "mensis" for "month;" in French common parlance, "period" is "les règles," literally meaning rules (hence regularity). The Chinese term, therefore, captures very neatly the idea of a regularity of nature as well as that this regularity comes round once a month. The *Neijing* in *Suwen* says: 月事 以时下《素问· 上古 天真论》which makes it clear that the occurrence of the period as well as the interval between periods is governed by a *Law of Nature*, and that the interval is a month (roughly twenty-eight days, give or take, in general two to three days on either side of twenty-eight). Moon (in this context, the Macrocosm) does its cycle of waxing and waning within a lunar month, with the full moon occurring once in the cycle—in the female body (that is, the Microcosm), the period also occurs once a month. Chinese researchers have also found that there is evidence that success in reproduction is greater when the woman's onset of the period occurs during the full moon, that success is much less in those females whose onset is further away from the period of the full moon. Today's science talks about the hormonal cycle which in the female appears to coincide with the lunar monthly cycle.

Timespace *Wholism* (Astronomy and Geography)

Several of the preceding chapters (2, 4, 5, 6, and 7) have referred to the notions of time and space in ancient Chinese cosmology/*philosophy*. The purpose of this section is, in one sense, simply to remind the readers what these are (but without boringly repeating the details) in order to see them as part of a larger theme, namely, that of Timespace *Wholism*. Before doing so, it may be appropriate to talk briefly about how space and time are understood in the Western tradition of science and philosophy, and in particular, to explain why in the opinion of this author, it is appropriate to talk of Timespace in the Chinese tradition and not Spacetime as the Western tradition has it.[4]

For more than two thousand years in the Western tradition, space and time were understood as absolute space and absolute time.[5] Aristotle adhered to them; geocentrism—that Earth stood still while Sun and other planets revolved around it—was the order of the day, until Copernicus published his heliocentric view in 1543.[6] Geocentrism went well with our common-sense intuitive idea of space—it was as if space was a kind of box with objects in it but the box was fixed to Earth at its center. Inside such an imagined box, one could, in principle, find out precisely where each object was via a system of grid, such as the latitude-longitude system, with its location "fixed" for good, as it were. Within such an imagined grid system, one would know where each object (including the Sun in our solar system, the other planets, the stars) could be found at which location. Although Copernican heliocentrism in principle undermined such a "picture" in terms of absolute space and absolute time, nevertheless, people continued to live with it. Furthermore, such a picture was even bolstered up by a universally acclaimed great scientist, if not the greatest in the history of Modern Science, Newton (1642–1727) who discovered the famous laws of motion which were premised on absolute space and time. Who could doubt the relevance of those laws, when all engineering (before the age of electromagnetism), and even today, all forms of engineering involving macro-sized objects rely on them? Hence, this picture was not seriously challenged until the nineteenth century, which ushered in the era of "field" physics.

The nineteenth century discovered electromagnetism via the experimental physicist/inventor, Michael Faraday (1791–1867) and the mathematical physicist James Maxwell (1831 -1879). Maxwell's great contribution to science, sometimes hailed as the "second great unification in physics" (the first being that of Newton), consisted of formulating a set of equations which encompass electricity, magnetism, and optics (light), demonstrating via mathematics that these three are all manifestations of the same phenomenon, namely, the electromagnetic field—electric and magnetic fields travel through space as waves which move at the speed of light. On the theory side, his work opened up a new era in physics, laying down the foundations for what today we call Relativity and quantum physics. Einstein himself acknowledged that Maxwell's achievements to be the most profound and fruitful since Newton's.

Scientists realized that light (an electromagnetic phenomenon) did not appear to obey Newton's laws of mechanics governing the behavior of matter. The crisis then facing physics was: how to reconcile Newton with Maxwell? Numerous physicists such as George F. FitzGerald (1851–1901) and Hendrik A. Lorentz (1853–1928) attempted to sort out this conundrum but the solutions were not good enough to pull physics out of the crisis, until Einstein realized that if the FitzGerald and Lorentz's account of light (that it appeared to travel with the same velocity, whatever the speed of its source) were true, then two conclusions would follow: (a) the speed of light and the laws of physics must be the same for all uniformly moving observers, regardless of their state of relative motion, (b) from it would follow that space and time could no longer be considered separately, independent of each other. This meant that space and time could be "transformed" from one into the other when the speed of light remained constant for all observers. The final conclusion pointed to the revolutionary view that (i) space and time are relative, meaning that they depend on the motion of the observer measuring them, and (ii) that light is even more fundamental than space and time. This then forms the basis of Einstein's theory of Special Relativity published in 1905. In this way, the notions of absolute space and absolute time were no longer regarded as fundamentally viable, holding for the entire universe, after more than two thousand years of scientific dominance.

However, Einstein himself did not go further to say that space and time be replaced by the notion of a single four-dimensional Spacetime. This task was left to Hermann Minkowski (1864–1909), a teacher of Einstein, who in a colloquium in 1908 uttered these words: "The views of space and time which I wish to lay before you have sprung from the soil of experimental physics, and therein lies their strength. They are radical. Henceforth space by itself, and time by itself, is doomed to fade away into mere shadow, and only a kind of union of the two will preserve an independent reality." (Minkowski, 1908) The four dimensions are: space provides three and time is 1-dimensional.

Spacetime is also called the "Space-Time Continuum" as both space and time can be subdivided without any limit in size or dimension. Every object is located along what is called its world-line linking its past to the future, allowing its spatial location to be ascertained at every instant in time. In the usual two-dimensional diagram in the form of a lightcone to represent Minkowski's four-dimensional spacetime,[7] everything within the cone is physical reality where nothing travels faster than the speed of light; nothing outside the cone is accessible as one would have to go faster than light in order to reach it.

The concept of Spacetime in the Western tradition, strictly speaking, is just little over a century old, as it is commonly dated from Einstein's Special Relativity of 1905, followed by his General Relativity (1907- 1915).Should one be keen to look into history, one would find some precursors, even going back to the Ancient Greeks and on to thinkers in Modern European history of science such as Galileo and others.[8] General Relativity embodies Einstein's insight that gravity itself comes from some property of Spacetime, as it does not depend on the properties of matter, but the curvature of Spacetime itself. In the Newtonian universe, space and time are not only absolute but also flat; under Einstein's theory of General Relativity, space and time can be stretched and warped, pushed and pulled by matter. Gravity is felt at its maximum when Spacetime is most curved and weakest (even vanishes) where Spacetime is flat. He said: "matter tells spacetime how to curve, and curved spacetime tells matter how to move."

In the Western tradition of philosophy and science, thing-ontology (even in spite of all the post-Newtonian sciences, such as electromagnetism, relativity, quantum physics) remains stubbornly dominant. Thing-ontology and absolute space go well together. Newton's three laws are called laws of motion, but they are, in the main, about the movement of one thing moving through space (from one location to another) bumping into another thing along the way and so on. In this sense, under absolute space, absolute time is implicated because there is a link between motion and space—motion is understood in terms of speed, and speed can be readily measured in miles/kilometers per minute/hour. Motion is simply the distance traveled through space within a specific duration of time. Even today, we still understand and grasp our macroscopic world via a thing moving through space within the thing-ontological framework; hence it might be plausible to argue that even in the concept of Spacetime, space is considered to be *primus inter pares*. In this context, it simply means that although under Spacetime, both time and space are considered to enter equally into the concept, nevertheless, it remains the case that space, historically and ontologically, remains dominant, and time is a recent add-on.

In contrast, on the subject of time and space, the Chinese tradition differs both historically and ontologically. Chinese *philosophy* and *science* implicitly adhered to process-ontology, where the concepts of process and event were key. Chapter 8 also strenuously argues that the Chinese tradition did not ignore the concept of thing or thing-hood, as *Qi* which is the most fundamental ontological category exists in two modes, *Qi*-in-dissipating and *Qi*-in-concentrating modes. In that sense, time and space were never conceived of separately and independently of each other, as in the Western tradition until the beginning of the last century. Chapter 9 argues that Chinese thought is *au fond* Contextual-dyadic Thinking; in referring to things in space (*Qi*-in-concentrating mode), one was necessarily also referring to events/processes in time (*Qi*-in-dissipating mode). A thing, which is *Qi*-in-concentrating mode, is defined as we have earlier seen, in terms of properties such as solidity, hardness, impenetrability, properties which instantiate in turn those of stability and permanence. Each thing occupies a certain portion of space; it is a physical object which can be located in space—for instance, London can be found at 51 degree latitude north and 0 degree longitude. However, as the *Yijing* tirelessly points out, the basic meaning of *yi* is "change;" behind the solidity, stability of *Qi*-in-concentrating mode is *Qi*-in-dissipating mode. Change involves processes/events which in turn necessarily involve the passage of time. However, when all is said and done, although the two modes exist, inter-linked inextricably one with the other (Em-ism as set out in chapter 3), it remains correct to observe that *Qi*-in-dissipating mode is *primus inter pares* with *Qi*-in-concentrating mode, that process is *primus inter pares* with thing. Hence, this author is in favor of using the term "Timespace" to mark the difference between the modern Western notion of Spacetime. Time stepped ahead of space, although they were both equals because, ultimately, *Qi*-in-dissipating mode transforming into *Qi*-in-concentrating mode as well as *Qi*-in-concentrating mode transforming into *Qi*-in-dissipating mode are processes which, *ex hypothesi*, involve time.

Furthermore, chapters 4, 5, 6, and 7 have tried to show the centrality of time in the Chinese tradition through its notions of the passage of time in the diurnal cycle/*zhouye jielü*, in the annual cycle of the four seasons/*sishi jielü*—these processes are basically about the ascent of *yang qi* (that is also to say, the corresponding retreat of *yin qi*), its rise to its maximum followed by its decline (that is also to say the corresponding increase of *yin qi*). Time for the ancient Chinese is measured in terms of the passage of such natural processes—the day is divided into twelve *hours*, each *hour* corresponding to two hours in today's globally used twenty-four-hour clock system, each ancient Chinese hour reflecting the natural processes out there in *Yuzhou*. Let us take a look at the hour called 子时/*zishi* which corresponds to the period between the last hour of the (modern) day which is about to end (11:00 p.m./23.00h) and the first hour of the following day (1:00 a.m./01.00h). The term *zi* literally means "child;" in this context, it means the hour in which a new day (analogous to a child) is born. It marks that period of time when *yin qi* of the night, having reached its maximum, is just set to decline, and *yang qi* of the new day is correspondingly set to increase/emerge. 子时 is the first *hour* in the Twelve Earthly Branches/地支/*dizhi* system of time reference. For the ancient Chinese, a year/岁/*sui*, is simply that period of time in which Spring is succeeded by Summer, then Autumn and finally Winter. A person is a year older when s/he has lived through one cycle of the four seasons. Recall that in chapter 4, the deconstruction of the character 时/時 has revealed the intimate link between time and space; as the traditional form (*fanti*) of the character—時– is more detailed in bearing out this intimate link, we have concentrated on deconstructing it. Just to remind the reader, the deconstruction shows that: (a) the radical on the left stands for "sun," (b) the right hand component is itself constituted of two components (i) the top 土is the character for "the ground" in this context and (ii) the bottom character 寸 refers to the distance "traveled" by the Sun in the course of a day, a year as marked by the gnomon on Earth/ground. The radical could then be interpreted to refer to time and the two sub components on the right to refer to space and the character itself to refer to the link between time and space.

For the ancient Chinese, astronomy is about the passage of time, the sun rising, followed by it setting, the moon waxing followed by it waning, the daylight hours getting longer (after the Winter Solstice) as the hours of darkness became correspondingly shorter until at the Summer Solstice the daylight hours are at their longest. The astronomers, from the earliest days, could not help but notice that the ascent/descent of *yang qi* and the corresponding decrease/increase of *yin qi* in the course of a day, of a year on Earth had a lot to do with the positions of the heavenly bodies relative to Earth—for instance, in chapter 4, we saw that the Neolithic peoples in China noticed that time and space were linked and were not independent of each other—when the handle of the Great Bear pointed East, it was Spring, when it pointed South, it was Summer, when it pointed West, it was Autumn, when it pointed North, it was Winter. Heaven and Earth were linked in this way—it looked as if terrestrial time (the four seasons) was linked with astronomical space, the handle pointing to the four compass points (geographical space). In the diurnal cycle, terrestrial time (morning/noon/twilight/night) was also linked with astronomical time and space, the Sun rising in the East just above the horizon, then ascending to the sky right above the horizon at noon, before descending toward the West, until it disappeared altogether beneath the horizon at the end of twilight and onset of night.

The intimate/inseparable relationship between time and space (Timespace) can be vividly displayed in the Chinese word for "existence"—this is a two-character word,[9] 存在/*cunzai*. Note that the two characters share something in common, but what is of interest here are those components which differ—the first character contains the component 子, while the second 土. We have already commented on 子, that it refers to the first hour in the Chinese 12-hour day. This shows very clearly that the first character 存 is about time. As for土 in the second character, it refers to earth/Earth, to space/geography. In other words, the existence of *Wanwu* is a phenomenon which necessarily exists within the Timespace framework, as existence is indeed about Timespace. Heaven/time/astronomy and Earth/space/geography make up the framework for understanding the existence of *Wanwu*. The Ten Heavenly Stems and Twelve Earthly Branches/天干地支/*tiangan-dizhi* system of reference in the sixty-year cycle of the calendar bears testimony to the very notion of Timespace in Chinese *philosophy* and *science*.

In the *Yinyang/Yao-gua* system of thinking, each of its sixty-four hexagrams stands for a segment of timespace/时空/*shikong*; every segment occurs within a certain context, and when the context changes, the segment of timespace changes, that is, the *Yao-gua* changes. For instance, in the domain of humans and human affairs/人事/*renshi*, the context changes all the time; a change in context entails a change/modification of mind, behavior in accordance with three major considerations—what is advantageous from the time point of view (天时/*tianshi*), what is advantageous from the space point of view (from that of geography/location/地利/*dili*), and what is in accordance with harmony with fellow human beings/人和/*renhe*. The insight embodied in such a system can be said to have been caught in very general/partial terms by the nostrum in English which says "when in Rome, do as the Romans do." It is also expressed within the Confucian tradition by the following story (whether apocryphal is not to the point) about a disciple who was very upset over an altercation he had with a man at the gate who insisted that there were only three seasons in the year, not four. The disciple asked the Master to adjudicate the dispute, to which Confucius was reported to reply: "Did you not notice that the being/man at the gate was all dressed in green?" This shows that it/he was a being born in Spring, lived through Summer but died during Autumn. Such a being clearly would not know about Winter and to it/him, naturally, the year had only three seasons. In other words, the respective contexts of its/his existence and our existence make it quite clear that one cannot determine "right" or "wrong" independent of context. It follows that epistemologically speaking, there is no such thing as absolute truth/falsehood, that the distinction between what is objective and what is subjective cannot be meaningfully made independent of context. The general meaning of the (*Zhouyi*-derived) dictum 仁者见仁, 智者见智, 各得欲见, 各取所需/*renzhe jian ren, zhizhe jian zhi, ge de yu jian, ge qu suo xu* may be translated (by this author) thus: "One sees in any given situation what one is looking for, what one needs." Confucius himself has said: 勿意, 勿必, 勿固, 勿我 (*wu yi, wu bi, wu gu, wu wo*) which may be translated as: "In understanding a situation or state of affairs, do not simply interpret it without due regard to meaning/evidence, do not adhere to a viewpoint as if logically it was the only possibility, do not be stubbornly constrained by the perspective of any one view, as each epistemological standpoint has its own boundaries and therefore limitations, and finally, one should not confine oneself solely to the egocentric starting point." In other words, be open to evidence, avoid dogmatic certainty, pay due respect to understanding the claims of others, do not succumb to epistemological egocentrism—in short, this is Confucian epistemology in a nutshell, which goes to reinforce what chapter 9 affirms, namely, that Contextual Thinking is basic to the Chinese Mode of Thinking, a mode which both the *Daojia* and Confucian traditions agree upon.

Ecosystem Wholism/*Ecosystem Wholism* and "Ecosystem Science/*Ecosystem Science*"

We have already made numerous remarks in earlier chapters about this theme; here is the place to bring them together as well as to elaborate more systematically. Again a quick word of clarification is called for with regard to the terms themselves. Their Chinese form will be referred to in italicized fonts while the non-Chinese version will be written in roman font.

What is this academic discipline called Ecology which instantiates what this book calls Ecosystem Wholism. Ecology became accepted as a science in the way understood today only after the Second World War, especially through the work of Eugene Odum.[10] It may be defined as that branch of science which studies the relations and interactions between organisms and their abiotic environments as well as among the organisms themselves, at the level of communities, populations, ecosystems both at local and global scales. An ecological community may be defined (albeit simplistically) in terms of a group of actually or potentially interacting species of organisms living in the same place—one well-known type of possible interaction is of course the prey-predator relationship, another is mutualism. A population in ecological literature refers to a group of individuals of the same species inhabiting the same area—for instance, the Arctic supports a population of polar bears. Ecology concentrates on population rather than on the individual organism in a population for the simple reason that scientists/society have neither the economic nor technological resources to study individual organisms, even very large ones such as polar bears. Instead, they focus primarily on characteristics of population: distribution (the area in which the population exists); abundance or size of the population; its rates of growth, birth, and death; spacing and dispersion, emigration and immigration (as animals are mobile while seeds of plants can spread via wind, water, mobile animals), predator-prey relationship; disease which can affect population growth either directly by killing off the young before they can even reach reproductive age or by affecting the reproductively mature animal through undermining their health and, thereby, their reproductive performance. (See Berryman and Kindlmann, 2008.)

The notion of an ecosystem may be spelled out as follows:

1. Ecosystems do not come labeled as such; the scientific investigators have to identify and delimit them for the purpose of their study at hand. This does not mean that they are simply theoretical fictions with no bearing to reality on the ground. Some have clearly identifiable boundaries (such as a meadow, or an estuary), others are not so obviously the case. Some can be very big, such as Antarctica or the Arctic, others infinitesimally small in comparison, such as a handful of soil.
2. Any ecosystem, such as that of Yellowstone Park or the Gobi Desert, occupies a certain portion of time and space which has a historical dimension both in terms of time and space. Neither Yellowstone nor the Gobi had existed from time immemorial, nor historically would the space they each commanded be necessarily identical to that they each now respectively occupy. It is sometimes possible, though not frequently, to ascertain the precise beginning of an ecosystem, such as suddenly springing up a small island in the middle of an ocean as a result of an undersea volcanic eruption.
3. An ecosystem evolves, changing all the time—at time t_1, a particular constituent predominates, at time $t_{2,}$ that item may have retreated somewhat, its predominant position taken over by another. In a shoreline ecosystem at t_1, large cliffs stand out, but at t_2, some of the cliffs might have collapsed into the sea below, generating a new landscape with changes for the ecosystem, even to the extent of perhaps creating two related but different ecosystems.

4. Over time, one ecosystem may evolve into a distinctively different ecosystem. Of all geological formations, lakes are said to be the most ephemeral as they evolve and change the quickest. A lake would shrink (for a variety of reasons such as climate change or excessive extraction of water by humans), would dry out completely, eventually evolving into a meadow. Inland seas also shrink, such as the ongoing shrinkage of the Aral Sea.
5. An ecosystem may be defined in terms of all the organisms of each species living in community interacting with other communities as well as with all the abiotic factors in their habitat. As far as the latter is concerned, the dynamics of an ecosystem involve three key abiotic processes which cannot be caught simply by population processes and phenomena: these are energy flow, hydraulic flow, chemical cycling with which the population interacts. In an ecosystem, the complex interplay between the numerous variables operating within it determines the characteristics of the population in question.
6. Every ecosystem is necessarily an open system. It is in principle an open system as ultimately it requires input from outside Earth, that is to say, from Sun, as we have seen, to supply it with sunlight (energy) to maintain it. It cannot violate the laws of thermodynamics.
7. Every ecosystem must be grasped as a Whole; an ecosystem Whole cannot be understood in a Reductionist manner. This Whole has properties which are different from, not simply the sum of the properties of all the constituent parts. Let us briefly look at this implication of Ecosystem Wholism by considering a handful of soil. The soil consists of both biotic (usually micro-organisms but also macro-organisms such as worms which are visible to the naked eye) as well as abiotic elements, such as water, air, and chemicals (pH content, etc.). The character of the soil (such as its texture) cannot be accounted for solely in terms of the properties of each of its constituent components—it may be said, therefore, to be an emergent property of the whole system, born of the complex interplay between all the variables involved in that handful of soil and the micro-climate of which it is a part.
8. This complex interplay may be displayed through considering a hypothetical potential creation of an ecosystem: first, a hair-line crack occurs in a rock, conceivably produced by a difference in temperature between day and night, summer and winter (A); next, water (B) enters the crack, turning into ice in the winter, thereby enlarging the crack in the process; a seed in the following autumn floats by, lodges itself in the crack and the following spring begins to grow (C); C together with

> B cause A to widen, which in turn permits more water and ice to enter, giving more space for C to grow by widening the crack still further and thereby allowing more rain and frost (B) to enter and erode it, and so on. These processes of change and development show that the causal paradigm at work is dynamic, historical, reciprocal (with both negative and positive feedback), synergistic, multi-factorial and non-linear, to be further explored in chapter 11.

This book wishes to contend that the understanding of the ancient Chinese with regard to the notions of *Yuzhou*, *Wanwu*, *Qi* in its two modes of existence and operation, *qi* as *yang qi* and *yin qi*, of *yin* and *yang* as *Yinyang*, of the *Yao-gua* Model as an analytic tool, the marriage of *Yinyang* and *Wuxing* to produce complicated relationships of which there are two main modes, the Mutually Engendering and Mutually Constraining modes, and so on may be said to constitute *Ecosystem Wholism* and the *science* based on it as an instance of what this author calls "ecosystem science" both in the larger and narrower senses of these two concepts. Earlier chapters of this book which explore the *Zhouyi*, the *Laozi* amongst other texts, the *Yao-gua* Model of the *Zhouyi* (see chapters 3 through 7) have already discussed the wider sense (especially in chapters 5 and 6 which look at the *Yinyang/Yao-gua* Model with regard to systems thinking, as well as in chapter 7 of the *Yinyang-Wuxing* Model). So, here, we shall confine our remarks only to the narrow sense.

Let us begin by reminding readers that the terms *Yuzhou* and *Wanwu* were used in such a way as to be inclusive of the abiotic and the biotic. One must also point out straightaway that the ancient Chinese tended to focus more on the latter in general and on humankind in particular when they discussed the relationship between it and the abiotic domain, for several reasons: (a) one could infer that organisms are singularly good exemplars of process-ontology—recall that Whitehead, the twentieth century philosopher of process philosophy in the Western tradition called it the "philosophy of organism;" (b) the ancient Chinese were also greatly impressed by the fact that here on Earth is life; no ancient texts could be found which said that they also believed life obtained in the other heavenly bodies known to them, in particular, Moon, Sun and the other planets such as Mercury, Venus, Mars, Jupiter; (c) furthermore, as an earlier section in this chapter has argued, the ancient Chinese had regarded humankind to be significant because of the unique type of consciousness humans possess. Recall, too, that humankind is one of the three powers/ *sancai*, which alone, of all the organisms on Earth, could grasp the relationship between itself and the other two. (This aspect will also be further explored in chapter 11 under the rubric of the fact-value distinction.)

We have also seen earlier in this chapter that they perceived humans to be Microcosm while the other members of *Yuzhou* and *Wanwu* constituted Macrocosm. Macrocosm included both the abiotic and the biotic domains; Microcosm dwelt within Macrocosm (necessarily participating in the same *Qi* in either mode of *Qi*'s operation); Microcosm and Macrocosm in turn constituted M-cosmic *Wholism*.

In other words, the analysis given above of the ancient Chinese cosmology and ontology may be said to satisfy all the prerequisites of Ecosystem Thinking, as set out under our brief discussion above of the discipline today called Ecology.

Another way of grasping that the ancient Chinese discussion of *Yuzhou, Wanwu* embody the notions of *Ecosystem Wholism* and *Ecosystem Science* is for us to return to the theme of the *Yijing*, where the key concept of *yi* means change; these changes follow a pattern and so could be said to constitute *Laws of Nature* which themselves do not change, while regulating change itself. We have seen ecosystems are dynamic systems, changing all the time, yet the changes within an ecosystem leading ultimately perhaps even to the evolution of a different ecosystem can all be understood and explained, as changes for the ancient Chinese occurred within a sustainable framework which embodies Cyclic Reversion—life on Earth would, hence, continue and flourish. Today, given our understanding of cosmology, relativity physics and deep astronomy, Modern Science does not talk of Cyclic Reversion; instead, it talks about the Sun in our solar system continuing to power us with energy until ultimately, our star depletes its energy in about another seven billion years. The Sun's core has hydrogen; every second, 600 million tons of hydrogen are converted into helium, generating 4×10^{27} Watts of energy. The Sun has been generating energy like this for roughly 4.6 billion years. Without such a source of energy from the Sun, no life on Earth, as we know it, would be possible. In the language of the ancient Chinese and within the discourse of their *science*, unless the daily rhythm of Sun rising in the morning/setting in the evening occurs and re-occurs (*zhouye jielü*), and the annual rhythm of the four seasons occurs and re-occurs (*sishi jielü*), *Wanwu* on Earth would no longer occur. Ecosystems would no longer be a feature of Earth. *Yang qi* and *yin qi* must intertwine if life on Earth is to endure—this can be interpreted as evidence that the ancient Chinese implicitly recognized Earth as an open system, with Sun as the source of *yang qi*. In other words, it would be correct to observe that *Wanwu* would only evolve and endure because ultimately the system is a Sun-driven one, as chapter 6 has already shown in some detail. One must immediately qualify this remark by reminding the reader that for the Chinese, although *yang qi* undeniably powers life enabling it to continue and evolve, year after year, generation after generation, yet that *yang qi* must be complemented by *yin qi* to form a harmonious *Whole* as *Yinyang*, in the absence of which, no life is possible on Earth. (See also chapter 5 about the necessary intercourse between *yin qi* and *yang qi* as essential condition for the perpetuation of *Wanwu*.)

So far, we have been pointing out some similarities between ancient Chinese and modern ecological thinking via the notion of ecosystem. Let us now turn to an aspect of the former which the latter does not focus on, at least not explicitly. This is the *Yao-gua* as well as the *Yinyang-Wuxing* Models as analytical-*cum*-explanatory tools as set out in chapters 6 and 7 which enabled the ancient Chinese to go beyond using the *Yijing* as a divinatory text and to generate *scientific* thinking and *sciences* of which a very well worked-out example could be said to be CCM. What we would like to draw attention to, here, is the aspect of what may be called "Ecosystem-nesting." A simple example would be the following: every cell in the human body may be regarded as an ecosystem, exemplifying *Ecosystem Wholism* and therefore Ecosystem Thinking. Recall that the *Yao-gua* Model as analytical tool may be applied at any level of the state of affair under study. Hence let us imagine the application of the model to the level of the cell in the human person. The cell may then be called *Ecosystem* 1. However, cells make up tissue—we can in turn regard the tissue of a certain part of the person, such as those of the muscles as an ecosystem, call this (larger) *Ecosystem* 2. Tissues make up an organ—liver tissues make up the organ which is called the liver. Here, one must straight-away add that as far as CCM is concerned, an organ is not simply the liver that one can point to in anatomy drawings or inside a corpse on a table stretched out in a pathology lab. It is an organ-system that one is talking about in CCM. (We raise this to warn readers of this crucial difference but here is not the place for detailed exploration of this notion.) We can call this organ-system *Ecosystem* 3. One organ-system is related to the other organ-systems in the human person—the ensemble of organ-systems/(*wuzang-liufu*/五脏六腑 may then be regarded as *Ecosystem* 4. *Ecosystem* 4 is part of another, *Ecosystem* 5, consisting of the entire individual person including bones, various liquids, secretions and so on. In turn, this *Ecosystem* 5 may be related to another, *Ecosystem* 6, which consists not merely of the cells, tissues, organ-systems, and so on, but also these in the context of *qi* (*yang qi* and *yin qi*), the so-called meridians *jingluo* (经络), conveying *qi* and infusing it in every part of the human person, the emotions/feelings/thoughts experienced by the human person. Human agency takes place only in the context of *Ecosystem* 6, not at the levels below. However, *Ecosystem* 6 itself is part of another, *Ecosystem* 7, as human agency can only occur and be sustained when there is clean air/water, protective clothing/shelter against the weather, and nourishing food. Furthermore, such a human agent does not operate as Robinson Crusoe—the human person has to be sustained by other fellow human beings to whom s/he is related as family/tribe/clan/ethnic grouping/local communities/citizen/even stranger in the wider context—this would constitute *Ecosystem* 8. *Ecosystem* 8 in turn forms part of *Ecosystem* 9, consisting of such a community of human beings together with all the plants/animals/rivers/valleys/mountains in which the community finds itself. To cut a long story short, finally all these ecosystems would not survive/endure, as has been pointed out ad nauseam unless *Ecosystem* 9 is embedded in, say, the largest of all the foregoing ecosystems, *Ecosystem* 10 which includes Earth (and *Wanwu* on it), Earth's relationship to Heaven (Sun, Moon, the other planets, the Milky Way), that is to say *Yuzhou*. (However, please note that ancient Chinese medical texts do not talk about 1 and 2 but deal explicitly or implicitly with what this author calls *Ecosystems* 3 through 10.)

The above clumsily drawn-out account is an attempt to demonstrate what is meant by "ecosystem-nesting" in Chinese *philosophy* and *science*. Perhaps a more elegant way of putting the matter is to present the information via *xiang* in terms of concentric circles or a nest of boxes, with the smallest ecosystem at the center—see figure 10.1.

In this ecosystem nesting of concentric circles, their respective pairings with the human being are as follows:

1. Cell
2. Tissue
3. Organ-system (such as Spleen-stomach/脾胃)
4. All organ-systems (wuzang-liufu/五脏六腑)
5. Entire material parts and total functioning of the person including emotions
6. Qi in Yuzhou (macrocosm) as well meridians operating in the person (jingluo 经络)
7. Immediate external environment in which person lives (air, water, food, shelter, climate . . .)
8. Social/cultural environment in which person lives (tribes/ethnic groups/polity)
9. Larger physical/social environment in which person lives (plants/animals/humans/rivers . . .)
10. Cosmological environment in which person lives (Sun/Moon/Earth/Stars/Planets)

The nearest approximation to such a model which this author can think of in modern Western medicine occurs in epidemiology (see Lee, 2012b), and for this reason, could be said to be an Ecosystem Science (see Lee, 2012a) which

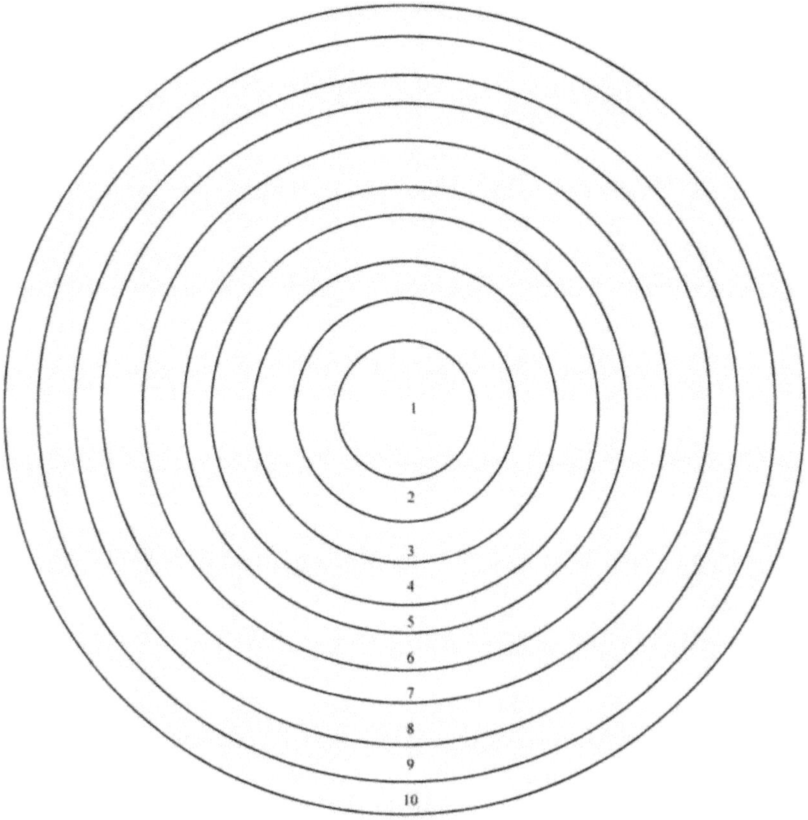

Figure 10.1. Ecosystem-nesting in terms of concentric circles

would increasingly become the norm, according to this author, of science in the twenty-first century—see chapter 11 for further elaboration of this point. Let us then talk briefly about the history and the science of epidemiology.

Epidemiology is like ecology, as it is that branch of Modern Medicine which deals not so much with the individual patient *per se* as in clinical and laboratory medicine but with population. In ecology, the population consists of plants and animals as already explained above; in epidemiology, the population is about the nature and distribution of diseases within a human population, and across human populations through immigration and emigration (just as plants and animals do, moving across regional, national and international boundaries). A slightly more expanded account may be found in Bhopal, 2008: 3: " . . . epidemiology is the science and practice which describes and explains disease patterns in populations, and uses this knowledge to prevent and control disease and improve health."

The truly outstanding instance in the last six decades is the establishment of the link between smoking and lung cancer—as a result of this impressive series of research, governments in many parts of the world, from the 1990s, had begun to ban smoking in public space, as a public health measure. This work began with the publication in 1950 in the *British Medical Journal* of an article ("Smoking and Carcinoma of the Lung") reporting the results of their research (a case control study) on the subject by Austin Bradford Hill (1897–1991) and Richard Doll (1912–2005).[11] However, its findings, on the whole, did not convince the medical community that the link could be construed as a causal one. It took another study, involving 40,000 British doctors whose health was monitored for twenty years, to provide convincing evidence on this score.[12]

It is generally claimed and accepted that the research of Bradford Hill and Doll has transformed epidemiological research, putting it on an impeccable scientific footing from the methodological point of view; that Doll's substantial findings cover not only the tobacco/lung-carcinoma link, but also between other substances such as asbestos and cancer, radiation and leukaemia, alcohol and breast cancer, as well as establishing that smoking increases the risk of heart disease. Their work in demonstrating that tobacco is a crucial factor in the production of lung cancer leading to the ban of smoking in public space and other measures to discourage smoking, has "probably prevented the premature deaths of millions already and . . . may well prevent tens of millions more."[13] Doll is said also to be the most distinguished epidemiologist from the twentieth century.

John Snow (1813–1858) is normally credited with being the founding father of epidemiology for his work during the cholera epidemic in London in 1854, thirty years before Koch (1843–1910) discovered in 1884 that the infectious causal agent was the *vibrio cholera*. One may also cite Ignaz Semmelweiss (1818–1865) in Vienna who, in 1847, carried out his investigation which appeared to be methodologically similar to Snow's, thereby demonstrating that puerperal fever was infectious as well as contagious and that its incidence was reduced significantly when medical staff were told conscientiously to wash their hands, after visiting the mortuary and touching the cadavers, before tending to patients in the maternity ward.

Epidemiology often uses the so-called model of the Triangle of Causation, in terms of three major variables (figure 10.2). In the case of smoking and lung cancer, an analysis could be worked out as follows:

Host would include the smoking habits of the individuals, their genetic inheritance, state of their health, their nutritional status.

Agent would include the carcinogenic nature of the many chemicals found in tobacco smoke, of which nicotine is only one.

Environment would include whether the space in which the individuals dwell consist of smokers, even if they themselves do not smoke, whether the space is enclosed or not, and so on.

These three variables mutually work upon one another, as indicated by the two-way arrows in the diagram below. Hence the final outcome would depend on the complex interplay between all the sub-variables under the three main variables of the Triangle of Causation model.

If one were to adapt the concentric model of ecosystem-nesting as earlier set out, then the Triangle of Causation could be represented in terms of three concentric circles as shown in figure 10.3.

This *xiang*, in one sense, represents better the reality of the relationship between the three variables of Agent, Host, and Environment. As the concepts of *Ecosystem Wholism*/Ecosystem Wholism and Ecosystem-/*Ecosystem*-nesting make clear, the functional relationships within each ecosystem/*ecosystem* as well as between ecosystems/*ecosystems* are a mutually interactive one. A greatly simplified outline in some (but not every) detail would look like this:

1. The sub-variables listed under Host ecosystem would mutually reinforce one another, producing an effect which is greater than the sum of the effects of each sub-variable. This would hold true of each set of sub-variables listed under Agent ecosystem and Environment ecosystem. (This point will be further explored in chapter 11 under the related notions of non-linear causality in general, and synergism in particular.)

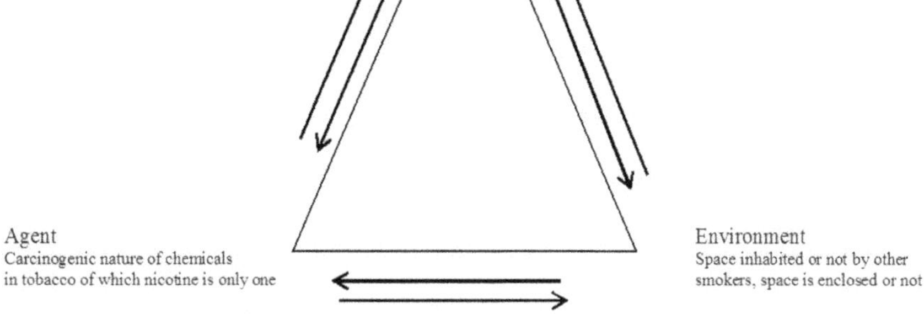

Figure 10.2. Epidemiological triangle of causation

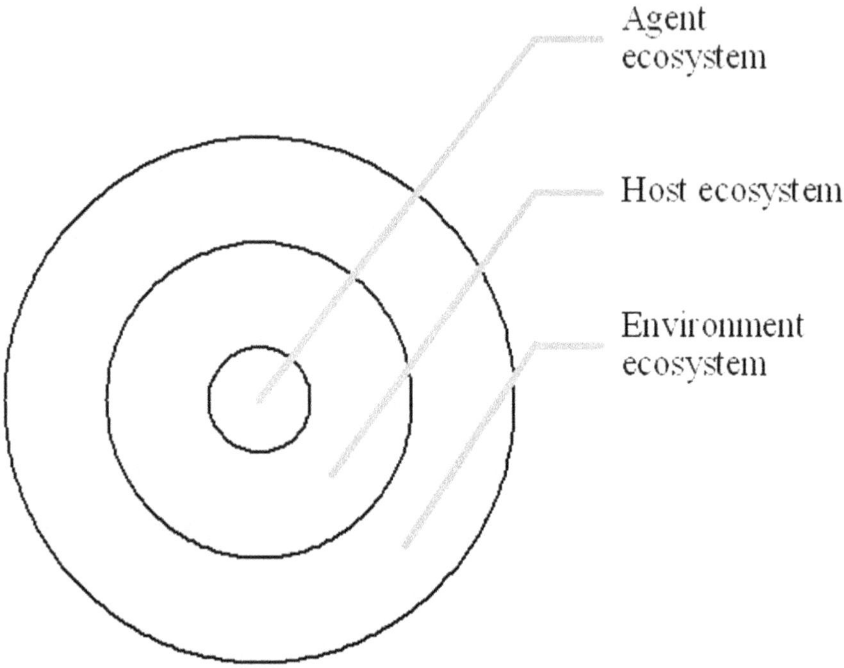

Figure 10.3. Epidemiological model of causation in terms of concentric circles

2. The Agent ecosystem mutually interacts with the Host ecosystem—for instance, the carcinogenic variables act upon the genetic inheritance to bring about lung cancer manifesting itself in the individual; the chemicals of tobacco may act to suppress the appetite, thereby affecting the nutritional/health status of the Host, which in turn could make the Host more open to the carcinogenic nature of the chemicals in tobacco smoke.
3. If the space is occupied by fellow smokers (Environment ecosystem), this might reinforce the behavior of the Host and vice-versa, as well as reinforcing the effects of the Agent upon itself. In other words, the largest identified ecosystem of the three can affect the other two smaller ones. If the space occupied by Host and fellow smokers is enclosed, this would have the effect of reinforcing the carcinogenic effects upon the Host.

Conclusion

This chapter has identified for fuller comment four forms of Chinese *Wholism*: *Qi Wholism*, Macro-micro-cosmic (M-cosmic) *Wholism*, Timespace *Wholism*, and *Ecosystem Wholism*. All four forms bear out the following features which can be found in ancient Chinese texts, either explicitly or implicitly:

1. Chinese *Wholism* is necessarily non-Reductionist in character (as opposed to the wholism understood, in the main, within the modern Western philosophical tradition).
2. It occurs within the framework of process-ontology based on the two modes of *Qi*, *Qi*-in-concentrating mode and *Qi*-in-dissipating mode, on the mutual interaction between *yang qi* and *yin qi* as *Yinyang*. In this respect, one may even argue that *Qi Wholism* and Timespace *Wholism* are more foundational than the other two forms of *Wholism*.
3. It also occurs within the analytical/explanatory framework of the *Yaogua* as well as the *Yinyang-Wuxing* Models, emphasizing change and interactive relationships between variables identified at any level of the analysis of a state of affair/situation.
4. From within such a framework, the four *Wholisms* identified in this chapter necessarily follow.
5. These four *Wholisms* also point to systems thinking in general (which can be found of late in the development of Modern Science), as well as Ecosystem Thinking and Ecosystem Science in particular (which can be found also of late in Modern Science, such as Ecology and for about a century and a half in Modern Medicine, such as Epidemiology).
6. However, one form of *Wholism* which may be called Fact/Value *Wholism* will be deferred until the next chapter which discusses at some length the fact/value distinction as it exists, so distinctively in modern Western philosophy.
7. Yet one other form of *Wholism* has been deliberately left out of the discussion here, and, indeed, in this volume—it is the *Wholism* of the person. The person is at once a *Whole* embedded within a nest of smaller as well as larger *Wholes*. As such a person is the concern of CCM, its exploration is best left to its sequel volume rather than this one.
8. It may be fitting to quote again from Bohm, 1980: 11 whose insight as expressed below appears to chime so well with this author's interpretation of *Daojia* thinking in Chinese *philosophy*:

   The new form of insight can perhaps best be called *Undivided Wholeness in Flowing Movement* [= holomovement].

Notes

1. One cannot do justice to this notion here—for a brief and accessible account, see O'Connor and Wong, 2012.

2. The discussion closely follows *Liu, 2003: 170-174, 306-307.

3. Strictly speaking, 月 could also stand for "flesh" 肉. However, scholars in this context have preferred to read 月 to stand for the moon—see *Liu, 2003: 170.

4. This subject is too vast to do it even a smidgeon of justice; the literature on the subject is correspondingly vast. Here, one can only modestly suggest a very few which this author has, amongst others, recently consulted: Overduin, 2007a, 2007b; Oldenwald, 2013a, 2013b; diSalle, 2009; *Spacetime*, 2014; Cox and Forshaw, 2010.

5. It may be relevant to point out that although for Newton space and time had nothing to do with each other, nevertheless, this did not prevent physicists after the appearance of Einstein's relativity theories to try to re-cast Newtonian physics as a kind of Spacetime theory—see Hoeffer, 2009: 668-690.

6. Heliocentrism was not totally new, as in the Western tradition, Aristarchus of Samos (c310 BCE—230 BCE) had already postulated such a hypothesis. Nor did Copernicus himself entirely desert Aristotle—he thought that the planets moved in circles around the sun (in our solar system), not in ellipses as Kepler later (seventeenth century) established.

7. URL= http://www.pitt.edu/~jdnorton/teaching/HPS_0410/chapters/spacetime/, accessed October 13, 2014.

8. For a truly brief but succinct account, see Overduin, 2007a.

9. It is a myth that in the Chinese language, all words are one-character words—see Lee, 2008.

10. For a brief account of ecology, see Stewart, 2008. For a detailed account, see McIntosh, 1985, Golley; 1996. For a discussion on whether the ecosystem concept is surplus to requirement in the twenty-first century, see O'Neil, 2001. For a quick account of Odum's life and work, see *Odum*, 2014.

11. See Doll and Bradford Hill, 1950. German scientists, in 1939, had already raised such a link but probably because of the war and political reasons, nothing came of this earlier publication. Other small-scale investigations after WWII also confirmed it. In 1950, the results of a larger-scale study in the U.S. (involving 601 patients) strengthened the claim even further. Doll's and Bradford Hill's case control study, conceived and begun in 1947, involved twenty London hospitals; the lung-carcinoma group as well as the control group (which consisted of patients with diseases other than cancer) each numbered 709 participants, with a male/female gender break down as 609/60 in each group. In the former group, the figure of non-smokers among the men was 0.3 percent and 31.7 percent among the women; in the latter group, men non-smokers were 4.2 percent and women non-smokers were 53.3 percent. It followed that a significant and clear relationship between smoking and carcinoma of the lung emerged, no matter which measure of tobacco smoking was used. This much larger-scale study, consequently, ruled out exposure to tarmac or car fumes, but not tobacco smoking, as being implicated in lung carcinoma.

12. The first results were reported by Doll and Bradford Hill, 1954; Doll and Peto, 1976; Doll, Peto and Boreham, 2005. See also Boyle, 2005.

13. See Peto, 2005 which is a celebration of Doll's lifetime achievements.

CHAPTER ELEVEN

Implications of Wholism/*Wholism* for Science/*Science*, Methodology and Ontology

This chapter deals first with two implications of *Wholism* as identified in ancient Chinese *philosophy* and *science*, namely, the notion of causality as well as how it engendered a *science* to accommodate both facts and values within its epistemological framework, which in turn made it possible to establish a subject which today is called "ecosophy." The exploration of the first theme is conducted via an initial discussion of it in the context of modern philosophy in order ultimately to cast light on Chinese *Wholism*/ontology and its implications for causality—it would explore the link between linearity and non-linearity as causal models respectively and wholism/upward causation/Reductionism, on the one hand and Wholism/*Wholism*/*systemic causation*/ *irreducibility*, on the other.

Causality—Humean Linearity and Non-linearity

A brief account[1]of the notion of causality used mainly in modern philosophy and Modern Science is called for. It is Humean in roots—it can be found in the empiricist philosophy of the Scottish Enlightenment thinker, David Hume, whose analysis of the notion of cause[2] is in terms of constant conjunction or uniformity of sequence. Of two events, X and Y, X is said to be the cause of Y if it is the case that whenever X occurs, Y follows.[3] However, this analysis as it stands baldly is flawed as, for example, lightning and thunder may always occur the one very soon after the other, but this does not mean that lightning is the cause of thunder; there may be a third factor which is responsible for both lightning and thunder (known in medical literature as the *confounding factor*). In other words, scientists cannot straight-forwardly adopt the Humean analysis but must enrich it to render it relevant to their investigation.

One way of doing so is to use what may even be called the gold standard version, which understands cause in terms of joint necessary and sufficient conditions. To say that X is a necessary condition of the occurrence of Y is to say that in the absence of X, Y would not occur, and to say the X is a sufficient condition of Y is to say that in the presence of X, Y would occur. To say that X is both necessary and sufficient for the occurrence of Y is to say that X is the cause of Y. If one were to say that *Helicobacter pyloris* is the cause of stomach ulcers, this means that if the bacterium were absent, the patient would not have stomach ulcers but if the bacterium were present, then the patient would have such ulcers. This account of cause in a medical context would not be very helpful; instead, the notion of cause is best regarded as bound up with the criterion of controllability, singling out a condition from the set of jointly necessary and sufficient conditions which the scientist/physician can control—see Lee, 2012b.

Sometimes the Humean account is presented in another way, namely, the "billiard ball" model. The player with the cue sets a ball on the billiard table moving along a certain path, which then runs into and hits a second billiard ball causing it to move, and so on. The model reflects well the world occupied by macro-sized objects within thing-ontology and a framework of absolute space as set out by Newtonian mechanics.

In other words, the notion of cause rooted in Humean empiricism within Newtonian absolute space would possess two distinctive but related features which merit some detailed examination in this chapter, namely, that cause is linear and monofactorial. They could be summed up in the dictum "one cause, one effect." Basically, one is saying, as already indicated, that only two events/things are involved—A and B, A as the identified cause and B the identified effect. This relationship may be represented thus:

$A \rightarrow B$

In the billiard ball model, the first billiard ball (A) hitting the second billiard ball (B) is then the cause of the motion of the latter (B), its effect; in turn, the second billiard ball may hit a third ball, imparting motion to it and so on; however long the chain of events, the pattern will always conform to the linear model with the causal arrow always pointing in one direction only:

$A \rightarrow B \rightarrow \ldots N$

This model remains the dominant model in all the Newtonian sciences. Lee, 2012b has attempted to show its application in one domain, namely,

Modern Medicine, especially in its monogenic conception of disease. It may be summed up by the dictum "one bacterium, one disease"/"one virus, one disease"/"one (offending) gene, one disease." The classic studies involved Koch's (1843–1910) discovery in 1882 of the tubercle bacillus as the cause of tuberculosis for which he was awarded the Nobel Prize in medicine in 1905 and Warren and Marshall's discovery of the bacterium, *Helicobacter pylori*s as the cause of peptic ulcer a century later in 2005. In genetics, Down's Syndrome (Trisomy 21) is caused by an extra chromosome 21, resulting in the embryo having a total of 47 chromosomes instead of the normal 46. This leads to the developmental features associated with Down's Syndrome.[4] However, in Modern Medicine, this model, in spite of its triumphal successes is not above criticism. It fails to apply universally—take phenylketonuria (PKU). This disease is an autosomal single gene disease,[5] which results in the body's inability to produce an enzyme necessary to metabolize the amino acid phenylalanine (which forms about 15 percent of the proteins in most natural foods), to turn it into tyrosine; the amino acid accumulates in the brain, leading to brain damage and the presence of phenylketones in the urine. However, evidence shows that early diagnosis together with a diet low in phenylalanine can stop the occurrence of brain damage.[6] PKU clearly demonstrates that one can, at best only pick out a combination of factors (single faulty gene,[7] failure of early diagnosis/dietary advice, and hence exposure to a diet high in phenylalanine) that may be said jointly to constitute the cause in terms of necessary and sufficient conditions. This in turn serves to demonstrate that the monofactorial model of cause has its limits. If cause is not mono- but multi-factorial, then linearity also suffers from similar limitation.

Multi-factorial causation looks like this:

$$X_{1,2,3} \rightarrow Y$$

Multi-factorial causation, and not monofactorial linear causation, in real life, may be said to be the norm rather than the exception. This is true, as we have already seen, in the domain of medicine, with epidemiology leading the way, though with no official acknowledgment from bodies such as the Nobel Prize Committee in medicine—see Lee, 2012b.

Multi-factorial, non-linear causation differs from the Humean monofactorial, linear model in the following important respects:[8]

1. Is reciprocal, involving negative and positive feedback possibilities—see chapter 7.
2. Involves synergism.

The simplest of reciprocal relationship obtains when only two variables are involved, such as X and Y; their relationship may be represented as follows:

$$X \leftrightarrow Y$$

The following very simple example illustrates this point: When agent A acts on B, producing an effect on B, B in turn can produce an effect on A. A—either a human or an animal—finds itself itching in a part of the body; to ease the itch (B), A scratches B; A's scratching, far from easing the itch, increases it, as scratching makes the skin react with greater ferocity than in the absence of such intervention; when itching intensifies, A resorts to scratching it even harder, and so on, until the skin becomes so raw and so bloody that A could no longer scratch B. A very well-known more complex example is found in the nature/nurture controversy, as to whether genetic inheritance is more important in accounting for intelligence or that education within a certain familial/social/cultural environment is more important. A third way, which is both more fruitful and more correct is to construe the relationship as one of reciprocity,[9] namely, that the two variables mutually affect each other in a dynamic fashion. Genetic endowment on its own may not produce the effect expected without the intervention of other variables from the environment—a child may have innate musical talents but without being exposed in any way to music, s/he would have no means to develop that genetic endowment. With exposure and teaching, the child's musical talents would improve. As these improve, s/he would be inspired/encouraged to work even harder which in turn would improve those talents even further, and so the virtuous spiral would continue. A non-virtuous, degenerate spiral could also occur when, for instance, school and family perceive a child to be stupid, leave her/him unstimulated and neglected; as a result, s/he would indeed be stupid and remain so. In other words, genetic endowment should not be perceived as a "thing" which one can simply find located in a gene. This also shows that Humean linearity finds a ready home within the framework of thing-ontology, whereas the natural home of reciprocal causality is within the framework of process-ontology.

A more elaborate account of reciprocal causation would involve more than one variable X in its causal relationship with Y, and may be represented as follows:

$$X_{1,\,2,\,3} \leftrightarrow Y$$

An example to illustrate this has already been invoked in chapter 10, the imagined case of the hairline crack on the surface of a rock, leading to the eventual establishment of a flourishing new ecosystem.

Not only is the Humean monofactorial linear model unable to accommodate reciprocal causal relationships, it also ignores the phenomenon of synergism. Synergism is an aspect of Wholist/*Wholist* Thinking—"one is concerned with the simultaneous interacting effects of two or more kinds of input, where each kind of input acts to intensify the effects of others" as understood by Ehrlich, Ehrlich, and Holden, 1973: 217, who cite two instances to illustrate the concept. The first concerns polluted city air which contains both sulphur dioxide and various carcinogenic particulate matter. Sulphur dioxide can impair the capability of the lungs to eliminate these particles, thereby ensuring that they spend a longer time in the lungs to cause more damage to the person. Their joint effect is synergistic as the total damaging effect exceeds the sum of the individual effects if each were present separately in the body. The second example concerns the effect of oil spills on DDT on the surface layer of the ocean where many marine organisms spend a considerable amount of their time. DDT is not very soluble in water but is very soluble in oil. As a result, marine organisms would be exposed to far higher concentrations of DDT than would otherwise be the case if the oil spill had not happened. The combined effects of DDT and oil are calculated to be greater than their individual effects taken separately but when added together.

Two states of affairs obtaining at the same time and space have emerged as an important aspect of synergistic understanding of causation. The temporal aspect (together with other entailed aspects) may also be explored via the proverbial nostrum "the last straw which breaks the camel's back." Assume that a straw weighs 1g and that the camel can normally bear a weight of 50kg. The camel can carry a bale of 50,000 straws. Up to the loading of the 50,000th straw, the animal stands firm; yet it collapses when the 50,001st straw is added. On the Humean linear model, such a phenomenon is neither foreseeable in principle nor intelligible, since it presumes that small causal changes will also produce small changes in the effects generated. On the non-linear model embedded within Ecosystem Wholism/*Ecosystem Wholism*, it can be both foreseen and explained. This is because, according to the linear model, the causal impact of each straw is regarded in isolation from the causal impact of the other straws piled on the camel's back. Each straw in isolation would be expected to produce no untoward effect on the camel. Yet the 50,001st straw, which weighs exactly the same as each of the others preceding it, has the dramatic effect of making the camel collapse. This cannot be explained by a linear understanding which regards causes and effects to be merely additive or subtractive, ignoring cumulative causes and effects. Such a linear orientation fails to recognise that the causal impact of the 50,001st straw on the camel's back is not the same as the causal impact of the 1st, 2nd, or 50,000th straw. The total causal impact on the camel of 50,000 straws is not simply the sum of the causal impact of each preceding straw taken separately and in isolation from other straws, which explains why the camel collapses with the addition of that proverbial last straw.

The linear understanding of causes and effects to be merely additive/subtractive may be further elaborated as follows. For the sake of the argument, imagine an old-fashioned weighing machine called a spring, with a hook attached at one end so that one could hang the objects to be weighed on it. When an object is put on the hook, the spring is depressed while a pointer on the front of the spring is calibrated to show the weight of the object as 2.5 kg, 1.2 kg, and so on. When more such objects are attached to the hook, the pointer is calibrated to show the total weight of all the packages; and as a package is removed from the hook, the pointer shows the weight of the packages but minus that of the one removed. The pointer moving down or up the scale is the effect of each of the packages attached to the hook of the spring—in other words, the weight of each package causes the spring to depress by so much and the pointer to move down the scale. As packages are either added or removed from the hook, the effect is demonstrated either in an additive or subtractive manner. This then demonstrates that the cause-effect relationship embedded in the notion of linearity is either additive or subtractive.

Indeed, on the non-linear model, the camel could collapse even well before the 50,000th straw was loaded on to its back if we understand cause not merely in terms of an event but also of standing conditions, which are part of the systemic boundaries of the phenomenon under study. In such a case what is causally relevant is not simply the fact that straws are being piled on to the camel's back, but also that these straws are being piled on the back of a particular camel with its own specific conditions of health, age, and state of exhaustion, which may be said to constitute the standing conditions. How much a camel can bear depends on its general physiological conditions at the time it enters the causal equation.

It follows that the camel-straws relationship must be regarded as a Wholistic/*Wholistic* system which is dynamic, not static. Although factors such as exhaustion, hunger, disease, and old age would not on their own distress the camel, acting together synergistically, the distress could be magnified several times over, so that even before the 50,000th straw was piled on to its back, it could collapse. In contrast to the linear account where the impact of each straw is constant and unchanging, irrespective of the state of the camel, the non-linear alternative is historical and dynamic. The latter regards the straw and its causal impact to be part of the standing conditions and systemic boundaries which produce causal effects. What constitutes the effect at time t_1 can be part of the cause at time t_2. This explains why the state of the camel bearing 50,000 straws at t_1 together with the 50,001st straw causally bring about the collapse of the camel at t_2.[10]

The difference between synergistic and non-synergistic conceptions of causal thinking may be schematically represented as follows:

Non-synergistic mode of thinking: $X_1 = n$, $X_2 = n$, $X_3 = n$; 3X (input) = 3n (output)

Synergistic mode of thinking: X = n; 3X at t_1 (output) $_>$ 3n (input separately added up)

Or:

X_1 at $t_1 = n$, $X_{1\,+}X_2$ at $t_2 = 2n+2$, $X_{1\,+}X_{2\,+}X_3$ at $t_3 = 3n+5$

This dimension to causal thinking ignored by the linear model further justifies the view that the latter belongs to a framework which is bounded by Newtonian absolute space in which macro-sized objects move about according to Newton's laws of mechanics. On the other hand, non-linear thinking takes into account this more complicated causal dimension and is therefore more appropriate for the post-Newtonian Spacetime framework.

Foregoing chapters have amply demonstrated that ancient Chinese *philosophy*, as implied by the texts examined, subscribed to multi-factorial, non-linear causality. This inference is justifiably drawn given that the whole implied burden of these texts appears to advance inter-relatedness between variables as shown in the concepts of *Yinyang*, *Wuxing*, Mutually Engendering and Mutually Constraining Modes within *Wuxing*, the models of *Yinyang/Yao-gua* as well as *Yinyang-Wuxing* respectively as a set of analytical tools. One can perhaps say that non-linear thinking was/is endemic to the Timespace framework of ancient Chinese *philosophy* and *science*.

Increasingly, non-linear thinking is establishing itself as a mode of thinking which can no longer be side-lined to play second fiddle to linear thinking in today's world of science. For instance, in the medical domain, the study of cancer appears ready to embrace the multi-factorial, non-linear approach instead of the simplistic "engineering approach" (for instance, "excising" the offending bit of tissue or certain genetic material) behind linear thinking. So let us briefly look at the changing conceptions in the study and understanding of cancer as a medical phenomenon in the last few decades. First, one must realise that cancer is not one disease entity. There are about two hundred different types of cancer—lung cancer in which the inhalation of tobacco may play an important role is not the same as melanoma in the leg which involves over-exposure to the sun. A carcinogen is something that can help to cause cancer. Tobacco smoke is a powerful carcinogen, but not everyone who smokes gets lung cancer. So there must be other factors at work such as genetic predisposition. The BRCA 1 and BRCA 2 breast cancer genes are examples of genetic predisposition; women who carry one of these faulty genes have a higher chance of developing breast cancer than women who do not. This does not mean that a person born with one of these genetic mutations will definitely get cancer. In any case, most women with breast cancer do not have a mutated BRCA 1 or BRCA 2 gene. Less than 5 percent of all breast cancer is due to these genes. So although women with one of these genes are individually more likely to get breast cancer, most breast cancer is not caused by a high risk inherited gene fault.[11]

Second, age appears to play a clear role as most types of cancer become more common with age. Changes which render a cell cancerous take a long time to develop; there have to be a number of such changes within a cell before the cell becomes cancerous. These changes can happen by accident when the cell is dividing. Or they can happen because the cell has been damaged by carcinogens and the damage is then passed on to future cells when that cell divides. The longer we live, the more opportunities there are for genetic mistakes to occur in our cells.

Third, cancer, increasingly establishes itself as the dominant disease in the world's population, especially in economically advanced countries which have by and large eliminated infectious diseases, but now are prone to cancer which is caused in the main by certain lifestyle factors and stressful conditions of living in general.

Fourth, it is very important that cancer is now perceived to be part of epidemiology rather than simply clinical medicine. As a result of the kind of understanding just mentioned, the *World Report on Cancer* (WHO, Stewart and Wild, eds. 2014) highlights the fact that the rising incidence of cancer is preventable by changes to lifestyle choices such as cutting back on smoking, and excessive alcohol, or sugar consumption.

Fifth, what is most significant from the perspective of this book is that one should appreciate that the relationship between these several causal factors mentioned above are not related simply in a straight-forward linear manner. For instance, eating an excessive amount of red meat (processed) could put one at greater risk of incurring bowel cancer; but eating an excessive amount of sugar and sugared foods can cause obesity; that obesity could increase cancer risk. In other words, cancer ought to be studied within the framework of "Ecosystem Wholism" and "Ecosystem Science."

From the above very brief account of the changing perspectives in the study of cancer, one may be justified in inferring that this epidemiological/ ecosystem approach brings Modern Medicine closer to CCM, as the latter had/has always been nothing but an *Ecosystem Science*.

Let us end this section with an example from the history of science to illustrate the difference between linearity and non-linearity. It is taken from the dispute about fermentation and how to understand this phenomenon in terms of those who upheld Reductionism and non-Reductionism respectively. This debate may be understood also in terms of their respective linear and non-linear representations of the causal pathways involved.[12] The Reductionists endorsed the linear representation in terms of chemical reactions, but non-Reductionists including Schwann and Pasteur held that fermentation processes involved another level, the physiological level. They argued that the processes occurred within a special context, that these chemical reactions took place in living cells. Later research bore out that the non-Reductionists were correct—it turned out that the component reactions are linked with one another at multiple levels, such linkages constituting a system whose behavior is different from what could be expected from simply studying the reactions as separate, isolated chemical reactions. In other words, there is an organization in the cell creating a system—the fermentation system—which controls the chemical reactions taking place at a level below. The debate about fermentation had long died down, but what clinched the argument against Reductionism is therefore a more adequate understanding of the causal processes involved. Today we can say that that understanding could be cast in the form of talk about emergence as an aspect of Wholeness in the context of non-linearity as opposed to linearity as causal models.

Emergence/Downward Causation and Systemic Causation[13]

We need to raise briefly the problem of the twin concepts of emergence/downward causation (which may more appropriately be replaced by the encompassing concept called systemic causation). Vintiadis, 2014 defines emergence as: " . . . a property is emergent if it is a novel property of a system or an entity that arises when that system or entity has reached a certain level of complexity and that, even though it exists only insofar as the system or entity exists, it is distinct from the properties of the parts of the system from which it emerges." Today, this notion is prominent in the philosophy of mind (where mental properties of the person are said to be emergent from properties at the level of chemistry/neuroscience which can impact on properites at these lower levels of organization.[14] Historically, it can be traced back to Mill, 1843: book III, chapter 6, section 1 in which he distinguished between "homeopathic effects/laws" and "hetereopatic effects/laws"—the former is about wholism, the latter about Wholism/*Wholism*. The term "emergent" was coined by another philosopher G. H. Lewes, 1875: 412, who wrote:

> Every resultant is either a sum or a difference of the co-operant forces; their sum, when their directions are the same—their difference, when their directions are contrary. Further, every resultant is clearly traceable in its components, because these are homogenous and commensurable. It is otherwise with emergents, when, instead of adding measurable motion to measurable motion, or things of one kind to other individuals of their kind, there is a co-operation of things of unlike kinds. The emergent is unlike its components insofar as these are incommensurable, and it cannot be reduced to their sum of their difference.

Lewes used "homogeneous" and "commensurable" instead of "homopathic" and "incommensurable" instead of "heteropathic." In this passage, he also referred to the notion of irreducibility of the "emergent" to "the sum" or "the difference" of the components of "the emergent."

By the end of the nineteenth century, the scene had already been set in the philosophy of science for the link between emergence and causation or ontology and causality. However, the fortune of emergence rose and fell in the following century; it reached its nadir with the claim that it was killed by science rather than philosophical mistakes (McLaughlin, 1992: 72–74, 89–90), by Einstein's special and general relativity theories, particle physics and quantum mechnics, Mendelian and later molecular genetics/biology. Such demise was premature, as by the 1990s, in quantum mechanics, there has appeared a new assessment of the subject which has implications for Wholism/*Wholism*;[15] molecular geneticists/biologists have also toned down their original "gung-ho" faith in Reductionism (Lee, 2005); on other fronts, science even before 1990 has advanced on different lines, developing new theoretical approaches such as systems thinking which includes complexity theory. Information theory and technology have made computer simulation possible—see Deacon, 2006, 2012). All these give a new lease on life to emergentism/ontological Wholeness. One should also point out that emergence may mean different things in different contexts, and that the emergent properties of the system/Whole are synchronic or diachronic, with the tracking of the latter being more complicated than in the former, but which shows more clearly that emergence is an aspect of Wholeness/downward causation embedded in process-, not thing-ontology.

We next look at two examples to illustrate how scientists themselves may argue for Wholeness/emergence/downward causation. The first comes from the study of genetics which involves diachronicity, and hence is not lab- but field-based. Any particular sequence of bases in the DNA constituting the development of DNA coding is the outcome of an evolutionary process leading to an adaptation of the organism to its particular ecological niche. Take the case of the polar bear in the Arctic with specific genes in its genome causing its fur to be white as opposed to the brown bear in the Canadian forest with another set of specific genes in its genome causing its fur to be brown. In either case, the specific sequence of bases in their respective genomes is the result of the organism adapting to its environment. Ellis, 2006: 90, writes: "This is a classical case of top-down action from the environment to detailed biological microstructure: through the process of adaptation, the environment (along with other causal factors) fixes the specific DNA coding. There is no way one could ever predict this coding on the basis of biochemistry or microphysics alone."

The second is from quantum physics, about a phenomenon called "decoherence" which has emerged as a "hot" topic since the 1990s, whose technical details this author cannot pretend to comprehend. (The lay person may find Schlosshauer, 2007 and Bacciagaluppi, 2012 accessible.) Leggett, 2002 has pointed out that although the term is new, the matter is not, as its importance has been recognized for several decades, since the early 1960s. It bears critically on the role that Wholeness/ontology of Wholes plays in the understanding of phenomena at the quantum level of observation, in a context where two quantum states are said to interact with the "environment."[16] (As what follows is entirely non-technical, and like all such extremely simplistic accounts, it is liable to misunderstanding the physics involved. Hence, readers beware, there is a very large "Health-warning" label on it!)

A minority of physicists feel obliged to grapple with the relationship between quantum and classical physics. Einstein was uncomfortable with it, and yet, so far attempts to "tame" it have not proved successful. This is because it appears to have paradoxes built into it, such as that pointed out in 1935 by Schrödinger in his thought experiment that a cat could be both dead and alive (but without us knowing which) until we opened the box to find out. Such seeming "absurdity" arises because quantum physics invokes the principle of superposition regarding the motion of a state of any atomic system (composed of bodies with specified properties such as mass, moment of inertia interacting according to certain specified laws of force). A state of a system may be characterized as an undisturbed motion permitted by theory and experimental apparatus. According then to the principle of superposition, certain rather peculiar relationships exist among states of a system such that though the system is in one state, it is also the case that it is (partly) in each of two or more other states. This cannot be understood in terms of concepts familiar from classical physics.

It turns out that in some experiments such as the two-slit experiment when, say, electrons are sent through a screen with two narrow slits, and the electrons then hit a second screen, the predicted interference term is not found.[17] When the disappearance of the interference term is said to occur spontaneously, it is considered that the suppression of interference lies in some interaction of the electron with the environment (the environment could be other particles with which the electron could have become entangled)—this is referred to as "dynamical" or "environmental" decoherence. It could be said that under such conditions "quantumness" has been suppressed, and quantum coherence no longer holds. Bacciagaluppi, 2012 writes: "(t)here are situations . . . in which interference effects are artificially or spontaneously suppressed. The theory of decoherence is precisely the study of (spontaneous) interactions between a system and its environment that leads to such suppression of interference."

The above has led some to wonder if the relationship between classical and quantum physics is really similar to that between classical physics and relativistic mechanics. In the latter, it turns out that classical physics is a limiting case in relativistic mechanics. Physicists in general agree with Einstein that it is so, because the velocities of objects studied by classical physics are so much smaller compared with the value of *c* (the constant of light) in empty space. Under such circumstances, it can be said that Newton's laws of mechanics are comparable to those of special relativistic mechanics as they can be derived mathematically from the latter as a limiting case; under such circumstances, special relativistic phenomena like length contraction and time dilatation disappear, and the relativistic expression of momentum agrees with Newton's second law. However, the relationship between classical and quantum physics may not be analogous to the above, in spite of the fact that physicists do not deny that classical notions can be derived from quantum concepts. What a minority of physicists are impressed with is that "the elements of classical physics emerge through an irreversible process called 'decoherence,' that is to say quantum objects acquire classical properties only through interactions with their natural environment as a consequence of the holistic features of quantum theory," according to Joos, 2006: 53. This shows then that the relationship between quantum and classical physics is not a straightforward one of bottom-up causation. Joos, 2006: 71, writes:

> The properties of the 'ordinary' objects of our experience—precisely those that we call macroscopic—are now seen not to be inherent in these objects. Instead, they emerge from, or are created by, irreversible interactions with the environment. In this way the local classical properties with which we are so familiar have their origin in the nonlocality of (entangled) quantum states. The properties of the interaction decide which properties become classical . . . It should be evident by now that classical properties can be seen to merge from the quantum world only after decoherence has properly been taken into account. No classical notions are needed at the fundamental level. The robust-

ness of certain quantum states—these that survive under the influence of the environment—defines what we typically call "classical."

And, "We do not need classical notions as the starting point for physics. Instead, these emerge through the dynamical process of decoherence from the quantum substrate." (Joos, 2006: 77)

Joos appears to infer from this line of development that the standard relationship between classical physics (higher-level phenomena) and quantum physics (lower-level phenomena) is being overturned—it is not so much that the former may be reduced to the latter, but that, more radically, even within the domain of the so-called lowest level, the quantum level, emergence and downward causation have raised their disquieting heads.

As this discussion is not meant to pronounce on the matter of the so-called transition from the quantum to the classical, it simply confines itself to observing that when a predicted effect does not occur, but an effect different (or the opposite) from that predicted occurs instead, and if the observed effect cannot be explained as the simple sum of the effects of each of the components of the system of interest, then one could plausibly infer that the system of interest exhibits Wholeness. This is a more minimal claim than the transition claim from quantum-to-classical. If true decoherence does occur and cannot be denied, then it is time that we pay serious attention to the ontological aspect of quantum mechanics, not merely in terms of process-ontology but also of Whole and Wholeness. Maybe Wholism can be found to apply in any domain of scientific enquiry (just as the *Yao-gua* Model as a set of diagnostic/analytical tool is similarly held to apply).

Emergence as an aspect of Wholism in physics is found not only in quantum mechancis but also in the physics of the macro-world such as in condensed matter systems involving superconductivity and superfluidity, as pointed out in Leggett, 1987:141.[18] This means that the Reductionist program which, in spite of obvious successes in the history of science, might not obtain in all scientific contexts of investigation.

We next return to the theme about the link between causality and ontology, between emergence/downward causation and Reductionism on the one hand and on the other, relations of causation via systems thinking in terms of the latter's following characteristics:

1. Systems thinking tells us that a system is hierarchical structuring plus its functionings.
2. What takes place at a lower-level can lead to phemomena at a higher level, to characteristics not possessed by phenomena at a lower-level. This kind of bottom-up causation does not provide a basis for Reductionism.

3. Bottom-up causation is not the only causal relationship at play, as there are top-down, side-to-side (same level) relationships, not to mention those between neighbouring systems. These relationships may also involve diachronic (time-delayed) as well as environmental processes. An example comes from biology illustrating intra-systemic and inter-systemic causal relations—figure 11.1 below.

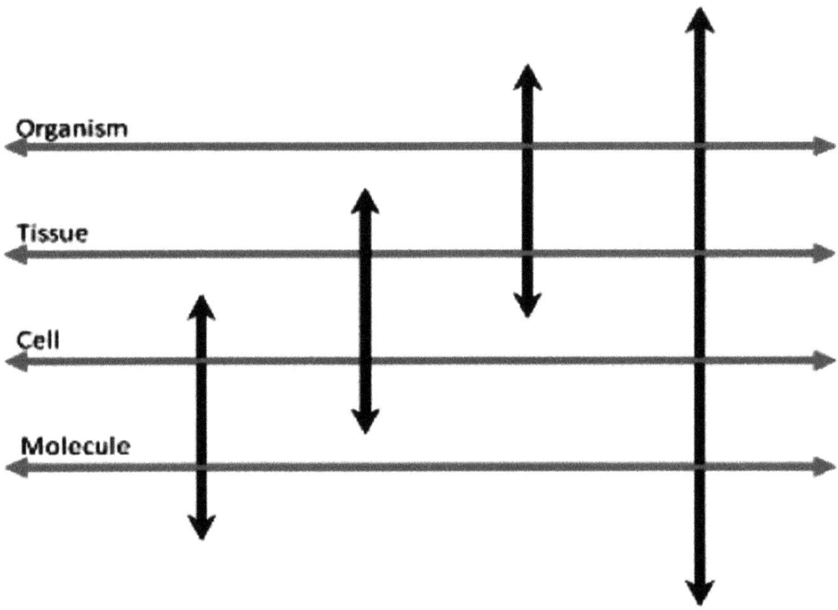

Figure 11.1. Biology: causal relations

(The above figure is borrowed from Van Osten who, however, may not endorse the precise way which it is employed in this context by the author.) The arrows are bottom-up, top-down, side-to-side, across levels (i.e., across the sub-systems) within the system as well as beyond the system of interest to other systems. The network of relationships in such a system which is what Prigogine would call dissipative structures (structures "at the edge of chaos") is diachronic, entangled as well as wide (Silberstein, 2006: 207). It is wide because emergentism of the kind of Whole one is interested in, here, concerns open systems; such a system must have "relationships" with its neighbours, the neighbours in turn with their neighbours. We can use another image to illustrate a related point, such as the ring of concentric circles in figure 10.1. If we were to take the molecule as the system under study, then we note the respective levels of the atom and the molecule and the bottom-up/top-down relationship between them, but the system also has relationships with its own members, other molecules as well as with another system, namely the cell. In turn one cell is linked to other cells and the cell system to the tissue system which in turn is connected with the organ system and that to the organism which must be open to yet other systems, such as the social/cultural, and larger natural environment.

4. There are causal relationships which are non-linear, involving negative and positive feedback mechanisms as well as synergistic effects.

   A caveat must be entered here for a more nuanced understanding between linearity/non-linearity and emergence, as pointed out by Leggett, 2014 (private correspondence). Controversy could arise because experts could disagree about the respective definitions they each proffer concerning the key terms involved such as "non-linearity" and "emergence" which, in turn, raises a problematic issue about the relationship between them. Leggett has commented that depending on the definitions of "non-linearity" and linearity proffered, the conclusion would be different. According to Bishop (2006)'s definition of non-linearity,[19] sound waves in a crystalline solid (to stay at the level of classical physics) are an instance of a linear dynamical system; yet all the same, many would regard such a system to be an example of "emergence." This line of reasoning would show that emergence could occur without non-linearity. Leggett has also pointed out that there are instances in both classical and quantum physics which, if one were to follow Bishop's definition, would be non-linear but, in which, one would be able to make exact predictions, such as exemplified by the quantum-mechanical theory of the hydrogen atom. How then should one categorise the behavior of the hydrogen atom—does it count as displaying "emergent" behavior? All such conceptual issues would have to be clarified, discussed at greater depth by others more qualified than this author. The important point to emphasize here is this—authors cited are not necessarily endorsed as correct in all aspects, but crucially because they have articulated a point of view which must be addressed and the issues behind it further explored and examined.

5. Such a complex web of causal relationships presupposes Wholism/*Wholism*.
6. Systemic causation as understood above renders emergence and downward causation non-mysterious, denying room to vitalism (in accounting for the emergence of the living systems from non-living ones), without

resorting to Cartesian dualism (in the case of mental phenomena in conscious living beings), or epiphenomenalism (which holds that while mental events are caused by physical events in the brain, they themselves have no effects on any physical events).

7. It explains why lower-level phenomena cannot completely explain many higher-level phenomena; it forms the basis of the claim by emergentists (or Wholists) that lower-level phenomena provide only necessary but not sufficient conditions for the occurrence of higher-level phenomena.
8. Newtonian science presupposes absolute space, occupied by particles/bodies which are extended in space interacting with one another according to Newton's laws of motion. The spectacular achievements of this kind of science over the last few centuries have ensured the dominance of thing-ontology. Developments of science during the last hundred years have shown that this ontology cannot accommodate their extraordinary findings. What is required is process-ontology which so far in the Western tradition has only been systematically articulated for at most several decades ago, such as the attempt of Whitehead.
9. A new philosophical framework has to be forged to accommodate the post-Newtonian sciences and their findings which would embrace process-ontology and non-linearity.

We turn next to considering how the theses listed above under systemic causation would apply to Chinese *Wholism*. This does not need to detain us for long as one can say that they are all compatible with *Wholism* as set out in the chapters in this book so far. However, more particularly, one may point out:

1. Chapter 8 argues that Chinese *philosophy* for about three thousand years has presupposed process-ontology, although, it also argues that Chinese *philosophy* does not ignore thing-ontology altogether, given that its most fundamental mode of thinking is not dualistic but Contextual-dyadic.
2. Chapter 3 demonstrates that *Qi* is its fundamental ontological category, that *Qi* manifests itself as *Qi*-in-concentrating mode as well as *Qi*-in-dissipating mode, that the two inextricably co-exist mutually transforming each other, that the latter though not ontologically prior to the former, could be said to be *primus inter pares*.
3. Chapter 4 argues that the notion of *Ziran* is autopoiesis and autopoiesis is *Ziran*, which means that *Ziran*/Nature is self-ordering at any level we epistemologically/methodologically care to distinguish; that *Ziran* implies process-ontology.
4. Chapters 5 shows that the most foundational *philosophical* text in the Chinese canon, the *Yijing* is concerned with change in Nature, with

the claim that *Yuzhou* is dynamic, not static in character. It is not the flux standardly ascribed to Heraclitus—it can take on stability under certain circumstances (*Qi*-in-concentrating mode) but such a mode also operates at the "edge of chaos," what Prigogine and Stengers call "dissipative structures" (see Chapter Eight) or what the Chinese call *Qi*-in-dissipating mode always hovering by *Qi*-in-concentrating mode—the tension between the two modes permits interactions of a very complex kind to take place which may result in the appearance of novel structures, properties and functioning.

5. Chapter 6 demonstrates that the *gua* and its three *yaos* constitute a paradigmatic illustration of Chinese *Wholism*; relative to the *yaos*, the *gua* is at a higher-level (the system level or *Whole*) and the *yaos*, its components, are at a lower-level; as the "quality" of the *yao* (in changing from a *yang yao* to a *yin yao* and *vice versa*) alters, the *gua* changes—analogous to bottom-up causation. However, the "quality" of the *gua* itself appears to exert constraint/influence on the "quality" of the *yaos*—analogous to top-down/downward causation. The structure/organization/composition of the *Qian gua* (which consists of three *yang yaos*) once achieved would in turn ensure that one of the *yaos* would change from *yang* to a *yin yao*. It has also argued that the *Yao-gua* Model, although originating as a divinatory tool ended up by being a set of diagnostic/analytical tools which was/is used in nearly all domains of Chinese culture including *science*, *medicine*, military strategies, just to mention a few.
6. Chapter 7 shows that *Yinyang* constitutes *Wholism*, a harmonious *Whole*, driving forward the kind of changes discussed in point 5 above. It also demonstrates that the *Yinyang-Wuxing* Model can be used to explain the complicated causal relationships between the components of a system, as well as how the system itself can be driven forward in a certain direction—the discussion uses ecological examples to illustrate this aspect. The Mutually Engendering and the Mutually Constraining cycles of *Wuxing* may be seen as the Chinese analogues of negative and positive feedback controls in non-linearity.
7. Chapter 10 sets out the various forms of Chinese *Wholism* which are all compatible with the theses listed under systemic causation.

One may summarize the discussion above in terms of the following theses:

1. Causality is not a notion which can be understood independent of the philosophical framework in which it is embedded. Different frameworks endorse different models or understanding of causality. In the

history of philosophy and science, there are two major contrasting models, that which may be called Humean, the other (for lack of a more convenient term) non-Humean.

2. The Humean model of causality is linear, monofactorial; the non-Humean model is non-linear, multi-factorial. The causal effects under the former are additive or subtractive (the total effects of the whole are simply the sum of the causal effects of its parts), but under the latter, they are more than merely additive/subtractive (the total effects of the Whole are more than the sum of the effects of its parts); synergistic effects occur as a result of these various factors inter-acting with one another.
3. Under non-linearity, novel structures, effects and functionings could emerge at higher-levels of organization in a non-mysterious manner, dispensing with the need to advocate a dubious force (in the case of living systems) such as vitalism.
4. The linear model may be said to have arisen out of the world-view behind Newtonian science which presupposes absolute space; in turn the model reinforces Newtoninan science itself. On the other hand, the non-linear, multi-factorial model increasingly is emerging in post Newtonian science which presuspposes Spacetime during the last hundred years or so. However, the history of Chinese *philosophy* and *science* consistently, though implicitly only, invoked/invoke the non-linear, multi-factorial model presupposing Timespace.
5. A world-view based on Newtonian absolute space is committed to thing-ontology, while a world-view based on Spacetime (and Timespace) is committed to process-ontology.
6. Thing-ontology in turn is embedded in wholism which understands the part-whole hierarchical structure aggregatively (chapter 10), in terms of decomposing exhaustively the whole into its parts, at each level of organization, until the lowest level is reached, the level occupied by fundamental elementary particles. It is, therefore, necessarily Reductionist in character—the whole is no more than the sum of its parts. It also follows that causation could only be bottom-up, never top-down.
7. In contrast, process-ontology is about events, about the relationships between events which generate a configuration/pattern. It is necessarily historical and dynamic in character. It is embedded in Wholism/*Wholism*, where the Whole/*Whole* is simply that pattern of events operating at a higher-level of organization but which can and does have an effect upon a lower-level of organization. It is, therefore, necessarily

non-Reductionist in character; it endorses a suite of complex relationships: bottom-up, top-down, side-to-side, inter-level, intra-level, inter-systems relationships. In a word, it amounts to claiming that complex causal relations obtain at any and every level of analysis and organization of the system which is under investigation, as well as between that system and other systems.

8. However, the discussion in this section on non-linear causality within the Wholist/*Wholist* framework has left out one very significant aspect of systemic causation, namely, the relationship between ontology and epistemology which is raised by the question: in what sense could one know the effects of systemic causation and that such effects could be said to be real? As this question must be raised and addressed in Lee, 2017b in order to meet the fundamental criticism that certain key concepts in CCM are considered by skeptical critics not to be "real," and therefore do not "exist," we shall delay exploring this matter until that volume which discusses key notions such as that of *jingluo*/经络 (often translated as "meridians" or "channels," but which this author prefers to leave untranslated), a network said to exist, permitting the circulation of *Qi* thereby ensuring the continuing existence and maintenance of the individual person.

Fact/Value Wholism

A defining characteristic of Modern Science, since its emergence four centuries ago, is its objectivity, of which quantification is a part. Its identity being defined by objectivity, its investigation of the world is necessarily confined to that which can be ascertained by the five senses understood in a literal manner or when these senses are mediated via instruments of one kind or another, such as a thermometer or today's high tech instruments, such as PET or TOM machines. Under the philosophy of empiricism, whatever cannot be thus ascertained is not "real" and should be excluded from the domain of science, and as such matters are disreputable, they are to be labelled "metaphysical" in the abusive sense of that term, meaning "unintelligible"/"nonsensical."

Values in aesthetics (beauty), in morality (good/evil, right/wrong) are not matters which could be ascertained empirically in the way just outlined and thus sanctioned as objective matters; instead, they are labeled subjective. To warrant the label/imprimatur of "scientific/objective," one must systematically purge values from one's investigation of the empirical world. The slogan could well have been: "stick to facts, eliminate all values."

The requirement that objectivity is a defining, if not the sole, defining characteristic of Modern Science does not exhaust the case against the unfitness of values to enter scientific discourse. It is reinforced by two other strands of thought, both of which could be traced back to Hume; one rests on logic/philosophy of language and the other on ontology.

Take the case from logic. Hume had detected that a so-called logical gap exists between the premises and the conclusions of inductive arguments. One has laboriously observed that individual men around us and in human history died no matter how long they lived—Alexander the Great, Hitler, Confucius. Call this set of evidence (p_1 –p_n). One is emboldened by it to conclude that all men are mortal (Q). Is this form of reasoning rational? Not really according to Hume and Humeans, because the logical operator "all" in Q means that Q includes not simply those who have died, those dying right now; Q goes beyond p_1 –p_n to events in the future, covering those not yet dead, and even those not yet born. This entails that accepting p_1–p_n as correct but denying Q is not self-contradictory. As this maneuver does not lead to self-contradiction, this in turn means that a logical gap exists between evidential premises and conclusions, which leaves modern philosophy with the so-called problem of induction.[20] However, this gap only exists because inductive logic is not deductive logic. The relationship between premises and conclusion is logically tight only in the case of deductive logic. According to this light, inductive reasoning/logic is judged to be "inferior"/"sub-standard" compared with deductive reasoning/logic.

Following Hume, one would say that an analogous gap holds between the premises in a moral argument and its conclusion. People, in general, confidently assert that, other things being equal, assaulting others is morally wrong (Q). What evidence can one cite in favour of Q? That violence means inflicting pain on the victims (p_1). However, one can admit p_1 to be correct, but go on to deny Q without committing any self-contradiction. The relationship between premises and conclusion is obviously not a deductive one; hence it, too, like inductive reasoning, may be judged to be "defective"/"sub-standard."

Given the gap between premises and conclusion in such a type of argument, skepticism follows—we cannot know that injuring others (other things being equal) is morally wrong. The skeptics observe that the phrase "is morally wrong" is misleading as it is cast in a form which makes it look as if it is a descriptive assertion analogous to "is square," "is green." The conclusion in a moral argument does not describe any state of affairs which can be ascertained by the five senses but is prescriptive in character—it tells us that we ought not to injure others. Humeans call this the "is"/"ought" gap—what one ought to do does not deductively follow from what is the case, as description is not the same as prescription (or that the descriptive use of language is not the prescriptive use of language). On such a view, prescription is free-floating and cannot be tied down to what the world is like as a matter of fact. As moral values pertain to prescription not description—moral "ought" language does not describe the world, it prescribes our conduct. In the case of description, what is the case and what is not the case can be settled by ascertaining by means of the five senses; it is, therefore, possible to hold that factual beliefs may or may not be rationally held. Today, it would be irrational to deny that the earth is round, given the large array of evidence available for asserting that the earth is not flat (however, in spite of the fact that the long list of evidence all the same does not entail the conclusion that the earth is not flat). With prescription, as no facts of the case could logically (either deductively or inductively) undermine it, rational considerations are neither here nor there. Hence moral values are, to Hume and those in modern Western philosophy who follow him, irrationally or non-rationally held.

Such moral scepticism is reinforced by appealing to an ontological consideration about the nature of the human individual. Western philosophy, ever since Plato, tends to divide the self into three parts. These are the cognitive faculty (the Intellect which ultimately in today's understanding is the brain, where reason is said to reside, rendering deductive reasoning in particular possible), the volitional faculty (Will), and the emotional part that handles what in old-fashioned language is called the Passions. Only the Intellect is concerned with reason (in today's language of neuroscience, it is the brain and its synapses which are in charge); the other two components have nothing to do with reason, and so are non-rational, if not irrational. Hume (1987 edition: 415–416) has notoriously written:

> Thus it appears, that the principle, which opposes our passion, cannot be the same with reason, and is only call'd so in an improper sense. We speak not strictly and philosophically when we talk of the combat of passion and of reason. Reason is, and ought only to be the slave of the passions, and can never pretend to any other office than to serve and obey them.

and

> it is not contrary to reason to prefer the destruction of the whole world to the scratching of my finger.[21]

In other words, Hume's moral psychology is such that we are driven to act by our Passions/emotions alone which are non-rational if not irrational, thereby rendering moral deliberations and decisions subjective. Values are tied up with Passions which together are the drivers of moral action. They can "do what they please," so to speak, and hence one's prescriptions for action may ignore, have nothing to do with what the world and other people are like, which constitute matters of fact. Strictly speaking, a person cannot be called mad (in the sense of going deeply against reason) if that person were to choose to kill another—or even a million people—for five pence, as his/her own Passion alone for that five pence dictates to him/her how s/he ought to act.

Let us pause quickly to observe about how Chinese culture normally understands the role of reason, and whether within it the dichotomy between Reason and Passion so clearly made under moral scepticism in modern Western philosophy occurs. Take a look at the two-character word in contemporary Chinese for "reason"—it is 情理/*qingli*. The second character *li* on its own means reason/principle. Why then is there a need to add another character in front of it? One superficial way of answering the question is to say that in its long history of development and evolution, the Chinese language has a tendency to use increasingly two-character rather than one-character words—see Lee, 2008. This may at best be a partial explanation, as in this case, the use of *qing* is telling. On its own 情 means feeling/sentiment/affection. In other words, the word 情理/*qingli* stands as perfect evidence that Chinese culture does not recognize the dualism so characteristic of modern Western culture between Reason and Passion. Instead, Chinese culture recognizes that Reason is informed by appropriate and/or appropriate degree of Passion/emotion (as the context dictates), that Reason and Passion are not in conflict, though opposable, and can even be said to form a harmonious *Whole*. This relationship between Reason and Passion embodied in *qingli* is also found in a *gua* which embodies 理, 象 as well as 数 *shu* (numbers as numerology)—the first in this context may be rendered as Principle, while the second, *xiang* rendered as picture/image (see chapter Ni9ne) also embodies feelings or sentiments. While Reason/Principle bids one (especially one who occupies high status/office) to be humble, humility itself would elicit approbation, respect, appreciation, and even love from others—this is the "content/message," for instance, of the 地山谦卦/*dishanqian gua* (where 地 stands for lower places, and hence the more lowly in life, and 山 stands for mountains/hills, and hence the higher strata in society.) Hume who "prefer(s) the destruction of the whole world to the scratching of my finger" is, according to the Chinese view, acting "contrary to reason;" Hume would be acting unreasonably/irrationally if he were to choose in the way he had set out. A person making such a choice would be profoundly unbalanced, unhinged, sick or pathological at the very least, if not a total moral monster. Conduct this thought experiment: suppose a very powerful politician in the world with his finger on the nuclear button is about to press it to destroy the world because his little finger suffers from some slight discomfort if he did not press that button. Would you "buy" Hume's argument or would you and others overpower him to prevent him from carrying it out? Would he not be considered to be unhinged, and therefore unfit for office? If this were your response, could it be more than merely your subjective preference for compassion over mild personal discomfort? For Hume, Reason is totally divorced from feeling/sentiment/affection; for the Chinese, built into their understanding of reason are feelings/sentiments/affection. The former is dualistic, the latter dyadic.

The kind of deep-seated scepticism about moral values provided by the powerful Humean strand in modern Western philosophy serves to reinforce the requirement that the "scientificity" of science can only be guaranteed by a systematic elimination of values from its domain. Ancient Chinese *philosophy*, on the other hand (Chapter Nine) has never been mesmerised by the power of deductive logic in the way that Western philosophy has. (See also Lloyd, 2015.) Chinese *philosophy* has no room for a branch of philosophy called "formal logic;" it relied on implicit *logic* to underlie and guide its thinking. Ancient Chinese *philosophers* were just as keen not to be incoherent and inconsistent as philosophers in other philosophical traditions, but its Contextual-dyadic Mode of Thinking made it incompatible with the pursuit of formal logic.

Chapter 9 has pointed out that Western dualistic thinking is hierarchically ordained such that only humans have intrinsic value while other non-human beings only have instrumental values for humans. Under extreme anthropocentrism, the only beings with moral values in the world are human beings; furthermore, moral skepticism has even gone further to say that humans create or construct their own values as they see fit, according to their feelings/desires/passions and as these are non-rational if not irrational, humans can simply endow anything in the world with any value/disvalue they please. Nature has only instrumental values for us, because we happen to find Nature useful to us. What was useful may no longer now be useful—horse-drawn carriages were very useful as a mode of transportation in by-gone eras, while today, automobiles have replaced them in our list of useful items. What makes the change in the chart of utility turn around? Technology in a word, and what makes technology itself change (from the mid-nineteenth-century)? Science—for details, see Lee, 1999.

Ironically, at the heart of Modern Science itself since the seventeenth century (a science which we have just seen must expel values from its remit of investigation in order to lay claim to scientificity) lies a key value, that is the value of using science and technology to control Nature for human benefit—see Lee, 1999, 2005, 2012b, as Nature itself has no intrinsic/moral value but only instrumental/use value for humans. So far, our science and technology are not yet ingenious enough to enable us humans to dispense with Nature in the sense of seeing (macro-sized) Nature as a storehouse of resources—oil, plants, water and other natural kinds—for our industries and our economy; Nature would, then, continue to have instrumental value for us. In particular, to those wedded to this stance, the claim that Nature may itself possess intrinsic/moral value irrespective of whether it has instrumental value to us is one which makes no sense.

In contrast, according to the Chinese world-view, values are endemic in the universe, in *Wanwu*, including in us, humans. Chapter 9 in exploring the *Xiang* Mode of Thinking has argued that *Yao-gua* quite explicitly incorporates values into the model itself—for instance the *Li gua*, as *xiang*, conveys the information that fire is a dangerous phenomenon, that we must use an effective method to contain and/or eliminate it. Creating a fire-break is not only a scientific/factual/efficacious mode of containing a fire, but also that we, humans, only bother to use our brain power to work out such a technique because we perceive fire to constitute a danger to our lives and our property—values, in such context, invariably pervade and impregnate thinking.

Chapters 4 and 10 have reminded us that humans, indeed, are different from other animals as their type of consciousness is somewhat different, permitting us to use language to a very high level of abstraction such as in scientific theorizing, in philosophical speculation. Chinese *philosophy* did/does not appear to imply anthropocentrism, although it acknowledges the uniqueness of human consciousness by saying that it is 万物之灵/*Wanwu zhi ling* which entails not so much the right to control and subdue Nature for its own benefit but more a duty to ensure that *Wanwu* (including humans) should thrive and flourish. Recall, too, that Chinese *philosophy* upholds the notion of the three powers/*sancai*—Heaven/Earth/Humans which together constitute a harmonious *Whole*, *Tianren-xiangying*. Unlike in modern Western philosophy, there is no implication of humankind lauding it over Heaven and Earth because of its unique kind of consciousness via its science and its technology. Instead, as the *Daojia* tradition emphasises, humankind, as one of the three powers, must nevertheless follow Nature/*Ziran*/Heaven and Earth, *Ziran* being obviously all-encompassing with humankind, as part of it, being constrained by it. Contrary to anthropocentrism, a dominant strain of modern Western philosophy, which implies humankind to be the "master" of Nature, and Nature its "slave," Chinese *philosophy* holds the opposite view, that it is Nature /*Ziran*/Heaven and Earth which are "superior" and we, humans are "subordinate" to them. (It may be helpful here to remind readers that chapter 4 has emphasised that *Ziran* should not be straight-forwardly equated with Nature; literally, it means "self-bringing forth"/ "self-engendering." Hence this author proposes that it be translated by "autopoiesis" in the Greek meaning of the word. *Ziran* primarily refers to processes—see chapter 8; as a noun, it refers to *Yuzhou* and *Wanwu* within it and in that context, the term "Nature" in English is invoked.)

This, in turn, implies that if humankind is intrinsically valuable, so, too, would Nature, its *Wanwu*. It also implies that while respecting Nature's superiority, humans, all the same, like the rest of *Wanwu*, are entitled to use some of Nature to provide a flourishing home/habitat for themselves; humans, unlike the rest of *Wanwu*, given their unique type of consciousness, are capable of being aware that they have an obligation not to act in such a way as to destroy the intrinsic value residing in *Wanwu*/Nature itself.

Is it intelligible to argue that *Wanwu* is intrinsically valuable? Lee, 1999 has attempted to mount a positive answer to that question. Very briefly, in this particular context of enquiry regarding ancient Chinese *philosophy*, for such an attempt to make sense, it must touch upon the following:

1. The notion of trajectory for each domain of *Wanwu*, each type of *Wanwu*.
2. The distinction between "valuable by themselves," "valuable for themselves," and "valuable in themselves."
3. Recognized-articulated values and mutely-enacted values.
4. Three theses of teleology: external teleology, intrinsic/immanent teleology, extrinsic teleology.
5. The notion of independent value.

Wanwu covers two basic domains, as we have reminded the reader on numerous occasions: the abiotic and the biotic. The former is inorganic and purely physical—such as air, rivers, or mountains. The latter includes all organic life; one may also distinguish plants from animals as plants on the whole are rooted in the ground, do not move and have no consciousness, whereas animals move/swim about, and at higher levels possess a central nervous system, and feel pain. At a level even above that on the evolutionary scale, they possess not only consciousness but also self-consciousness—the last group may include not only humans but also chimpanzees. This means that the trajectory followed by each category and sub-category of *Wanwu* is different. Take some simple examples: a mountain is geologically stable and may last thousands of years; a volcano explodes but may soon become extinct; a tree may last several hundred years; a male cat about fourteen years; and the world average today for a human is 67.2 years. To achieve its natural trajectory, a mountain range such as the Himalayas is not much affected by what we humans do, short of us dropping a nuclear bomb on it. The natural trajectory of a river, even a large one, could be affected by our diverting, digging, dredging it. The natural trajectory of plants depend on the activities of large mammals (such as elephants) and of course humans. The lifespan of a cat cared for within a human household depends on the sustenance and maintenance provided by its owners including vet services and medication. The trajectory of a human depends on a whole host of factors such as economic considerations, the availability, not merely of food, but wholesome food, favorable environmental conditions, access to medical facilities, exposure or otherwise to activities and circumstances that involve violence such as military/terrorist enterprises, not to mention emotional instability.

Given the differences so far commented on, it is not surprising that the notion of intrinsic/moral value cannot be applied in a blanket manner—human beings are "valuable in themselves" as they are beings with not only consciousness but also self-consciousness as well as the capability of abstract reflection and theorising. Plants and (non-human) animals are "valuable for themselves" as they are organisms, even if not all possess consciousness to any extent. Plants, though without consciousness, nevertheless, embody what one may call an intrinsic/immanent teleology—an acorn, if left undisturbed, will grow into an oak sapling, develop and mature into an oak tree, which in turn produces acorns by way of continuing the reproductive processes of the oak species. The oak, like all plants, can take steps to search out more sunlight by growing upward under certain circumstances, close up the pores on its leaves in order to reduce transpiration, shed its leaves in the autumn in order to preserve resources for growth next spring. An animal, such as the squirrel hoards nuts during the autumn as food for the winter; the polar bear gorges itself before settling down into the hibernation mode during the winter. Organisms, depending on the species, have their own rhythm of life during the four seasons, ensuring that their reproductive facilities are not damaged, ensuring the continuity of their own species.

The abiotic and the biotic as well as the sub-divisions of the latter, then, possess their own respective kinds of value. In the case of entities belonging to the inorganic and the organic domains (apart from humans) which lack consciousness altogether or fail to possess it to the same level as that of human consciousness, their values are simply embedded in their existences, their trajectories. Hence it may be appropriate to say that the intrinsic values they possess are "mutely-enacted," whereas the intrinsic value which humans possess is "recognized-articulated value." We can recognize that fellow human beings are "valuable in themselves" and we can, through language, articulate these values in moral philosophy. We can also at the same time observe and infer that other organisms embody in their existences/trajectories intrinsic values but as they are exhibited and "lived," we can call them "mutely-enacted" and beings which possess them are "valuable for themselves." We also are capable of distinguishing the domain of the abiotic from the biotic, and can observe and infer that such entities possess a value which has nothing to do with us humans, that they come into existence, exist, and go out of existence, entirely independently of humankind; for this, we can appropriately say that they are "valuable by themselves," that they possess independent value.

Although Chinese *philosophy* did not quite work out explicitly the arguments set out above, this is not to say that what it says is incompatible with such an attempt to render their world-view more comprehensible to those who stand outside it. Unlike a strident tendency in modern Western philosophy, it implicitly rejects anthropocentrism by acknowledging that other *Wanwu* each have their own place in Nature, leading their own respective lifestyles/trajectories, each displaying intrinsic values appropriate to its own domain. In the case of organic life, it implies the thesis of intrinsic/immanent teleology. Furthermore, it implicitly rejects the view that Nature exists solely for the benefit of humankind (the thesis of external teleology). As it exhorts humans to follow Nature/*Ziran*, it also thereby rejects the thesis of extrinsic teleology, that it is the destiny of humankind to subdue, control and conquer Nature/*Ziran*/*Wanwu* using science and its generated technology to do so. As a member of *Wanwu*, we are entitled like the rest of *Wanwu*, to carve out a home for ourselves within which we can flourish, but we are not morally entitled to make over Nature/*Ziran*/*Wanwu* in order to be the lord and master. Given our peculiar type of consciousness, we have a moral duty to ensure that the rest of *Wanwu*, too, would have appropriate homes within which to exist and to flourish.

In other words, in a nut-shell, the *Daojia* tradition constitutes an "ecosophy," a term coined by the Norwegian Deep Ecologist, Arne Naess in 1972.[22] This, however, is not to say that Naess's vision and the Chinese one are identical, even though they overlap. It may be handy to borrow the term "ecosophy" from Naess (not its contents) to use it to refer to a world-view which celebrates humankind's involvement with the rest of *Wanwu*, as part of *Wanwu*, yet also apart from the rest of *Wanwu*, given that humankind does possess a very peculiar type of consciousness, unique in *Wanwu*. Unlike Naess's Deep Ecology which sees humankind simply as part of Nature/*Wanwu*, or the dominant strand in modern Western philosophy which champions anthropocentrism holding that humankind is apart from Nature/*Wanwu*, Chinese *ecosophy* is more nuanced. It rests on an acknowledgement that humankind is both part of Nature/*Wanwu* and yet also apart from Nature/*Wanwu*. After all, this book has argued that the fundamental mode of thinking in Chinese *philosophy*/culture is Contextual-dyadic, in which polar contrasts such as "part of Nature," "apart from Nature" may complement rather than merely confront each other thereby forming a harmonious *Whole*.

The salient points raised in this section may be summarized as follows:

Modern Science, generated within the framework of modern Western philosophy, is defined in terms of objectivity/facts/description which cannot and should not be contaminated by values which are considered to be subjective/irrational/non-rational/prescriptive, if its claim to "scientificity" is to be maintained. In contrast, ancient Chinese *science*, generated within the framework of Chinese culture in general and the *Daojia* tradition of *philosophy* in particular, does not recognize the "is"/"ought" or the Reason/Passion dichotomy. Instead, Chinese *philosophy* appears to embed values even at the heart of Reason; furthermore, its *ecosophy* celebrates value in all domains and sub-domains of *Wanwu*, and charges humankind as *Wanwu zhi ling* with a duty and responsibility to ensure that all *Wanwu*, encompassing diverse trajectories, are able to engage in their own existences, flourish in their own homes or habitats.

Chinese *philosophy* does not endorse the so-called fact/value distinction; it holds that values are necessarily embedded in the search for knowledge, such that epistemology cannot simply be exclusively concerned with the establishment of so-called "objective" empirical facts. Hence it follows that its *science* (such as CCM) embodies both facts and values, and that, the "objective/subjective" distinction between Reason and the Passions (as understood in the Western tradition) is questionable. As further evidence of this claim, take the word 道理 *daoli* which translates as "Reason." This word has two characters—as already observed, the second character *li* may be translated as "rational principle." What role, then, does the first character play in this word? Its role is to declare in no uncertain terms, that according to Chinese *philosophy*, *Reason* is not simply a cognitive matter but also a moral matter. *Reason* must also conform to the *Dao*. (Chapter 4 explores the *Dao* cluster of concepts.) This section has already discussed the word *qingli* in order to show that for the Chinese, Reason and Passion are not dissociated but always go together. The deconstruction of both *qingli* and *daoli* go to show a systematic linkage between concepts in Chinese *philosophy* which Western philosophy systematically sunders. This constitutes a key difference in the two world-views—for the latter, science is, therefore, value-free but for the former, *science* (including *medicine*) cannot be value-free.

Conclusion

This chapter has dealt with three main methodological differences which flow from the respective philosophies standing behind Newtonian science and Chinese *science*. The first is tied up with their respective understanding of the notion of causality—two different models are identified, the Humean/linear/monofactorial model in the former and non-linear/multi-factorial in the latter. It is correct to note that while post-Newtonian science today departs from linearity, Chinese *science* is premised on non-linearity and has done so for more than two thousand years.

The second is to demonstrate a close link between linearity and non-linearity respectively with what are traditionally discussed in terms of emergence and downward causation but which this book prefers to call systemic causation, a more comprehensive notion.

The third concerns their respective stances regarding the fact/value distinction. Science, as conducted within the framework of modern Western philosophy, must expunge all values in its investigation before the activity could merit the label "scientific;" in contrast, Chinese *philosophy/science* regard values as intrinsic to all forms of intellectual inquiry, and hence that it is neither possible nor desirable to expunge them, thereby, whole-heartedly embracing Fact/Value *Wholism*.

Notes

1. Here, the explication given is deliberately kept non-technical partly for lack of space.
2. For details, see Beebee, 2006; for more general discussion see Beebee, Hitchcock and Menzies, 2009.
3. For a full-dressed philosophical account, see, for example, Dowe, 2000.
4. See *Down Syndrome*, 2014.
5. "Autosomal" means that the condition does not involve sex chromosomes.
6. See Bhopal, 2002: 134.
7. PKU involves a single genetic defect which leads to a specific metabolic disorder. This should not lead to the oversight that the genetic defect constitutes only a necessary, but not also sufficient, condition of the manifestation of the specific metabolic disorder in the bearer of the genetic condition. A more severe case of failure to meet the gold standard of cause as necessary and sufficient conditions may be found in *H. pylori* as the cause of peptic ulcer—the bacterium is neither necessary nor a sufficient for peptic ulcer disease. This raises a puzzle, namely, how to reconcile

the failure to meet the gold standard with the claim that it is nevertheless the cause of peptic ulcer. For those interested in unpicking this nest of complicated issues, see Lee, 2012b.

8. See Ehrlich et al., 1973: 218 for a graph illustrating the difference between linear and non-linear effects in dose response; for a more detailed account of linear and non-linear causation by this author, see Lee, 1989b.

9. For one account regarding the relationship between genetic endowment and intelligence, see Dickens and Flynn, 2001.

10. This case of non-linear synergistic thinking is not meant to imply that the developments in mathematics and physics of late either cannot cope with non-linear thinking or that they may not themselves be forms of non-linear thinking. The point is simply to say that Modern Science since the seventeenth century is by and large Newtonian in conception, whose notion of cause is linear. That is why quantum physics raised and still raises numerous problems in any attempt, philosophically speaking, to reconcile these two very different paradigms of physics.

11. See Stöppler, 2014; also, *Causes of cancer*, 2014.

12. For these two different types of causal pathways, see Bechtel and Richardson, 1992.

13. The originator of this term is Silberstein, 2006.

14. See MacDonald and MacDonald, 2010.

15. Four Nobel Laureates (between 1977 and 2003) appear divided. Stephen Weinberg (1979) has famously pronounced that the "explanatory arrows always point downwards (1992)" while Philip W. Anderson (1972), Robert Laughlin (1998) have argued against Reductionism, with Anthony Leggett (2003) being critical about Reductionism in Leggett, 1987. Anderson, 1972 in the field of condensed matter physics, has implied a plea on behalf of Wholes and Wholeness through his misgivings about Reductionism. Earlier chapters have already mentioned another physicist, Bohm, 1980.

16. The account here is not particularly concerned with the claim that decoherence is the transition from quantum to classicality.

17. Yet as pointed out by Leggett (in private correspondence in August 2014), as a matter of fact, the late Akira Tonomura and others at Hitachi, had successfully demonstrated the interference effect in a beautifully mounted sophisticated experiment—see Tonomura, 1989.

18. "The phenomena of superconductivity and superfluidity were not, and probably could not reasonably have been, predicted ahead of their experimental discovery in various metals and in 4He respectively; indeed, for many years they constituted a major mystery. What they show beyond any doubt is that interactions between a very large number of 'elementary' particles can give rise to macroscopic effects which are qualitatively totally unexpected, effects which could never have been deduced by studying small groups of particles. Thus, however true it may be that these phenomena are 'merely' consequences of well-understood electromag-

netic interactions between the elementary particles involved, the 'merely' begs some important questions."

19. Bishop, 2008: 231.

A dynamical system is characterized as *linear* or *nonlinear* depending on the nature of the equations of motion describing the system. A differential equation system $dx/dt = Fx$ for a set of variables $x = x1, x2, \ldots, xn$ is linear if the matrix of coefficients F does not contain any of the variables x or functions of them; otherwise it is nonlinear. Roughly, a system behaves linearly if any multiplicative change of its initial data by a factor b implies a multiplicative change of its output by b.

. . . In nonlinear systems . . . (w)hen the behaviors of the constituents of a system are highly coherent and correlated, the system cannot be treated even approximately as a collection of uncoupled individual parts ("the whole is *different* than the sum of its parts"). Rather, the principle of linear superposition fails and some particular global or nonlocal description is required taking into account that individual constituents cannot be fully characterized without reference to larger-scale structures of the system. . . . the individual constituents are so correlated with all other constituents that no constituent of the system can be changed except by applying some change to the system as a whole. Such holistic behaviors are often referred to as emergent (as opposed to resultant).

The tight coupling between constituents in nonlinear systems is related to the nonseparability of the Hamiltonian, a function which corresponds to the total energy of the system and is related to its time evolution. Roughly, a Hamiltonian is separable just in case there exists a transformation carrying the Hamiltonian describing a system of N coupled constituents into N equations each describing the behavior of one constituent of the system. Otherwise, the Hamiltonian is nonseparable and the interactions within the system cannot be decomposed into interactions among only the individual components of the system.

20. Note: Hume himself was only a philosophical, not an ordinary, commonsense skeptic; he said he left philosophical scepticism behind in his study the moment he left it.

21. Like all great philosophers, their works are subject to different interpretations and are not free of controversy. This is not the place to consider the matter—for one fairly detailed but easily accessible account, see Cohon, 2010.

22. For a quick account, see Naess and Sessions, 1984.

CHAPTER TWELVE

Conclusion

This book is about the *philosophical* framework within which it is possible to make CCM intelligible, and is intended to be a companion volume to Lee, 2012b. Both pursue the theme that no science/medicine could be innocent of philosophy, that science and philosophy are not mutually exclusive (notwithstanding what positivist philosophy maintains to the contrary). It follows that as ancient Chinese *philosophy* is very different from modern Western philosophy, the two frameworks would give rise, quite unremarkably, then to very different types of *science/medicine*.

This companion to Lee, 2012b, consists of two volumes. The remit of this volume is to set out systematically the *philosophy* in general which informs or stands behind CCM, while that of Lee, 2017b is to demonstrate in detail why CCM possesses the characteristics it does in terms of that *philosophy* and its entailed methodology. This volume has strenuously attempted to establish the following:

1. Chinese *philosophy*, or that lineage—*Daojia*—examined here shows that the *science* generated within it, differs from modern Western philosophy and the science it in turn has generated for the last few centuries. The latter science may conveniently be labeled Newtonian; its ontology is thing-ontology, its notion of causality is Humean/monofactorial/linearity, and is Reductionist in character. Chinese *science* is conducted within process-ontology and multi-factorial/non-linearity (chapters 7, 8, 10, and 11). These critical differences

have served, up to now, to fuel the view that CCM is unintelligible and "non-scientific," if not pseudo-scientific. This is to judge CCM in terms of a yardstick which is appropriate to assessing Modern Medicine/Biomedicine which in the main is a Newtonian science, but not appropriate to assessing CCM. It amounts to saying that a cat is declared to be sub-standard at a dog show, when cats are judged by what dogs could do, what characteristics dogs display.

2. Chinese *science* would remain unintelligible or alien to those who are familiar only with Newtonian science. It should increasingly seem less baffling and unintelligible, as scientists working at the cutting edge of science and technology, are being confronted with phenomena which appear not to be amenable to "Newtonian" treatment. Increasingly, some of them have found it necessary to turn to an alternative framework which rests on process-ontology and which can accommodate non-linearity. Bohr, a founding father of quantum physics, was the first to turn to *Yinyang* understanding of Reality as he at once grasped that wave-particle duality in that physics could not be accounted for within the Newtonian framework of things/particles moving in absolute space. This approach was carried further in the work of Prigogine (also a Nobel Laureate). From the 1960s onward, systems thinking has appeared to reinforce such a re-orientation (chapters 8 and 5).
3. Such developments show signs of informing increasingly the way that science is pursued, transforming slowly but surely Newtonian science to become post-Newtonian, what this book calls "ecosystem science" in the larger sense of the term. This tendency leads to a greater degree of (though not total) convergence than one might have thought possible until of late, with Modern Science moving toward the Chinese model based on process-ontology, non-linearity and *Wholism* (chapters 8 and 10 in particular).
4. In the light of such a convergence, CCM could no longer be written off as "unscientific"/"pseudo-scientific"/"irrational"/"unintelligible" without, at least, a fair hearing. This author hopes that this volume (and its sequel) make such a fair hearing possible.
5. As this work maintains, a careful exploration of the *philosophical* framework within which CCM has always been conducted would show its theoretical richness with crucial methodological implications for doing *science*. More broadly speaking, it shows to those outside the tradition that a text which began life as a divinatory manual could, unexpectedly, end up by transforming its *Yao-gua* Model into a set of diagnostic/analytical tools for understanding numerous (if not

all) domains of theoretical/practical activities, forming the bedrock for Chinese culture/*science* down the ages (chapter 6).

6. To grasp Chinese understanding of process-ontology, non-linearity, one would have to go back to the meanings of the character *yi*/易, to the translation of the title of that text in English as *The Book of Changes*. Notice that the Chinese did not call that text the book of divination. Its title—the *Yijing*—shows clearly that the ancient Chinese conception of divination rested primarily on a notion which had nothing to do with gods/ supernatural beings and their hold over humankind, but on one which was/is perfectly non-mysterious, non-mystical, non-religious/non-theological, this-worldly and in that sense "naturalistic" matter called "change." Given this as a starting point, its "fate" turns out to be unsurprising, namely, that its application to divinatory matters was but one application only—after all, it sprang from the central insight that *Yuzhou* was/is constantly changing, and as we humans live in *Yuzhou* and are part of it, we ourselves and all that we do were/are subject to change, whether the activities we engage in were/are divination, rulership, military affairs, *science*, or *medicine*. As *Wanwu zhi ling*, we seek out patterns of change in the universe, in Nature, in other *Wanwu*—in this way, the ancient Chinese discovered *Laws of Nature* (chapter 5).
7. Biology: causal relations. Change is tied up with events and processes; to understand the former we must come to grips with the latter. The basic *philosophical* insight of the *Yijing* points to process- rather than thing-ontology (chapter 8).
8. Biology: causal relations. The most readily extrapolated pattern which the ancient Chinese could make from their observation of *Yuzhou* and *Wanwu* was that involving time and space which then gave them the framework of Timespace—that night follows day follows night (*zhouye jielü*), Spring follows Winter, Summer follows Spring, Autumn follows Summer, Winter follows Autumn (*sishi jielü*). Without the cyclic repetition of these *Laws of Nature*, they were convinced that no life on Earth would have been possible—the very notion of ecological sustainability (to use a contemporary term) would be undermined in the absence of Cyclic Reversion/*zhou er fu shi*. Time was/is not so much linear but cyclic, although one should not infer from this that every day, every night, every year, every spring, every summer is identical with every other day, night or season. Far from it, as two of the meanings of the term *yi* are Change and No Change, which for the ancient Chinese are not mutually exclusive (chapter 10).

9. This then leads to two very distinctive characteristics of Chinese *philosophy*. First, it did/does not regard polar contrasts to conflict with each other but instead to form a harmonious *Whole*. Both in their intellectual as well as in their moral/social lives, the ancient Chinese considered achieving harmonious *Wholeness* to be the ideal goal. Unlike modern Western thinking, which is dualistic (since Descartes, if not before), Chinese thinking was/is dyadic. As they also understood that meanings cannot be ascertained/laid down independent of context, their most fundamental mode of thinking may be called Contextual-dyadic (chapter 9). Such a mode meant that the ancient Chinese could not and did not engage with formal logic (as understood in Western philosophy), but relied on an implicit *logic*, what this work calls *Yinyang/Yao-gua* implicit *logic*. Formal logic is alien to Chinese *philosophy* as it is both content- and context-free, attaining the most extreme level of abstraction possible. *Yinyang/Yao-gua* implicit *logic* may be seen as an analogue of what today is called Fuzzy logic, a kind of non-classical logic which is many-valued, developed alongside other versions of many-valued logics in the twentieth century. *Yinyang/Yao-gua* implicit *logic* violates Aristotle's three laws of thought but does not, all the same, fall into incoherence/unintelligibility as paraconsistent logic has shown. Bohr, in his attempt to render quantum phenomena intelligible, implicitly invoked the *Yinyang* pairing of polar contrasts via his notion of complementarity as evidenced in his coat of arms which bears the *Liangyitaijitu*; at the same time, he also showed a grasp of what today we call paraconsistent logic—see chapters 8 and 9.
10. This key mode of Contextual-dyadic thinking comes out very clearly in the concept of *Yinyang*, that what is *yin* in one context may well be *yang* in another, and vice versa. Furthermore, *yin* cannot thrive without *yang* and *yang* cannot thrive without *yin*—they are yoked together as a *Whole* (chapter 6).
11. So averse was/is Chinese *philosophy* to dualistic thinking that even in the notion of *Qi* which is its fundamental ontological category, the dyadic aspect is preserved. *Qi* not only exists as two categories (*yin qi* and *yang yi*) but operates in two modes, *Qi*-in-dissipating mode and *Qi*-in-concentrating. Those used to the Western mode of thinking might be tempted to regard *Qi* under the latter mode (as part of thing-ontology) to be about Matter and therefore Materialism and *Qi* under the former mode (as part of process-ontology) to be about what they call Energy, and therefore not Matter. The ancient Chinese simply

regarded the two modes to be part of the *Whole* called *Qi*, which is neither plain Matter nor plain Not-matter (whether one calls it Energy or not) but both, what this book (chapter 3) has called "Em-ism" if one must dream up a label.

12. Their *Wholism* involves what Silberstein, 2006 calls systemic causation (which is non-linear). This is to say that (a) the components of a *Whole* at any level of analytical organization are causally linked with one another—bottom-up, top-down, side-ways, reciprocally at the intra-level; (b) a *Whole* at any one level of analytical organization is causally linked with another *Whole* at another level of analytical organization—inter-level. This is what this book has called "ecosystem science" with one system being open to another system (chapter 10).
13. The ancient Chinese, invoking *Wuxing*, identified two main modes of generating causal relationships between parts and *Whole*, *Wholes* and *Wholes* called the Mutually Engendering and the Mutually Constraining Modes which are their specific contribution to the notion of non-linearity (chapter 7). These may plausibly be understood as analogous to feedback mechanisms—negative and positive—recognized today by science in numerous domains.
14. True to the spirit of complementarity of polar contrasts endemic to Chinese *philosophy*, this work has also tried to demonstrate that Chinese *philosophy/science* appear to harmonize the empirical with the metaphysical rather than perceiving these two domains to be mutually exclusive as modern Western philosophy does (chapter 4). In the same spirit, its *science* could be said to embrace Fact/Value *Wholism* quite unashamedly, unlike modern Western science backed by its philosophy which upholds the fact-value distinction as a gold-standard of the "objectivity" of science.
15. In sum, if this book has done its job conscientiously, then it should be possible to appreciate ancient Chinese *philosophy* (the *Daojia* strands of it) and the kind of *science* it entails in their own lights.
16. The introduction has promised to discuss the interpretation followed in this work under another rubric; it is time now to redeem that promise. The alternative rubric is to see it as an attempt to answer the so-called Needham Question: "Why did the West overtake China in science and technology when China led the world up to the beginning of the seventeenth century?" Or "Why did Western Europe develop Modern Science in the seventeenth century, but not China?" For nearly five decades, many scholars have been stirred to answer this question, including Needham himself. Although many

answers have been proffered, none has proved convincing; some have argued that the question as it stands, being too general/large/vague, is unanswerable. This is not the place to review all these answers.[1] (For the most recent attempt to answer this question, see Cohen, 2015, which pursues, in the main, a historical explanation rather than a more philosophical one, as this work does.) The Question has even preceded Needham—see Sivin, 2005: footnote 8. Indeed, over the decades, it has even brought on a degree of ennui and much fatigue. Sivin, after exploring in depth the issue in its various aspects, has concluded that the Question might even no longer be posed once the focus is shifted from China where Modern Science did not arise, to Western Europe where it did from the seventeenth century onward. In this, he is right but only perhaps half-right—one must, indeed, first look at Western Europe, but having done so, one must return to China, to see where the differences lie that could explain the emergence of Modern Science in the latter and the failure to do so in the former. Doubtless, the differences between the two societies (each informed by different histories and cultural traditions) could be indefinitely identified, then examined and consequences teased from them. In the opinion of this author, a key, if not the critical difference lies in the two respective philosophical frameworks, based on the supposition/axiom that no science is innocent of philosophy, whatever the society and the period of its history one is investigating. Sivin, 2005 is right to say that "China's failure to beat England to Modern Science (is not) a failure of thought."

The brisk answer to the Needham Question is this: China could never have developed what today we call Modern Science, albeit European in origin but now globalized. To ask why China failed to develop Modern Science is to presuppose that it could, but for the intervention of certain factors which acted as impediments to such a progression. Examples of such impediments include claims as: China's cultural tradition looked down on merchants and entrepreneurs, while celebrating the literary scholarly class; it emphasized bureaucratic administration at the expense of other intellectual pursuits; the nature of the Chinese language itself; the lack of a monotheistic religion with a transcendent deity such as the Abrahamic one in Christianity. Indeed, Needham himself as well as another scholar, Ho Peng Yoke, blamed the *Yijing*[2] for having caused China to fall by the wayside in the relentless march to progress and modernity as blazoned by Western Europe from the seventeenth century onward.

This volume may be construed, if one wishes, as a detailed attempt to answer the Needham Question. The Chinese failure to develop Modern Science is not due *per se* to impediments, or so-called "inhibiting factors" such as those just mentioned, although some of the factors referred to could have played a role in discouraging scientific and technological pursuits in some respect.[3] The "failure" is primarily due to the different philosophical frameworks for science in China and Western Europe from the seventeenth century onward. Modern (Western) science with its crowning achievements in (Newtonian) physics and chemistry is a very specific distinctive kind of science with a distinctive methodology which cannot be understood independent of the metaphysics it presupposes. By contrast, Chinese *science* in general and CCM in particular, were practised within a *philosophical* framework resting on process-ontology, a dymaimc conception of Nature, *Wholism*, multi-factorial/non-linear causality which is totally incompatible with a one based on thing-ontology, a static conception of Nature, Reductionism, monofactorial/linear causality. Furthermore, as Lee, 2012b, argues, modern/Western science rests on the ontological *volte-face* regarding Nature as machine, with all that this entails in methodological terms for doing science. The Chinese, however, never suffered such drastic rupture in its *philosophical* orientation for more than two thousand years. For all these reasons, Chinese *science* would "naturally" appear alien, unrecognisable as science to Westerners who tacitly accept that nothing counts as science unless it is an identikit instantiation of modern/Western/Newtonian science.

In a nutshell, their different philosophical/methodological frameworks are at the core of the matter. One should not commit the category mistake of saying that only one can lay claim to the status of "scientificity"—to put matters more accessibly one should not judge a dog-show by the standards of a cat-show and vice versa, as it is obvious that cats are not dogs, dogs are not cats, cats are not sub-standard dogs, and dogs are not sub-standard cats. To do so is to commit Essentialism of Method.

Notes

1. Needham, Robinson, and Huang, 2004.

2. Needham &Wang, 1956: 336 writes: " . . . while the five-element (*wu-hxing* 五行) and two-force (*yin-yang* 陰陽) theories were favourable rather than inimical to the development of scientific thought in China, the elaborated symbolic system of the Book of Changes was almost from the start a mischievous handicap. It tempted those who were interested in Nature to rest in explanations that were no explanations at all. The Book of Changes was a system for *pigeon-holing* novelty and then

doing nothing more about it." It is obvious that Needham's understanding of the *Yijing* is different from that of this author. Ho, 1972 writes: " (when they) were fully satisfied with an explanation they could find from the system of the *Book of Changes* they would go no further to look for mathematical formulations and experimental verifications of their scientific studies. Looking at the system of the *Book of Changes* in this light, one may regard it as one of the inhibiting factors in the development of scientific ideas in China."

3. Confucian ideology, since its official adoption in the Han Dynasty, could have played an important role, as Confucian *philosophy* is primarily value-oriented with near exclusive preoccupation with ethical/social/political issues. A text, the *Liezi*/列子, *Daojia* in inspiration, mocked the Confucian perspective. (Some scholars say it contains material as early as the fifth to the first century BCE, but which was stitched together with other material toward the end of the third century CE; others, consider it a circa late third century CE text.) It contains a charming story about Confucius and two small children regarding the perceived distance between Sun and Earth in the course of the day. Confucius was traveling east when he met two children sitting by the roadside, hotly disputing between themselves: when is the sun nearest Earth and when furthest away? One child held that the sun was nearest in the morning, but farther away at noon, as then the sun looked so much bigger then than later in the day. Surely, what was larger was nearer, what was smaller was farther away. The second child held the opposite. In the early morning, the sun was not as hot but at midday, it really burned; surely, the hotter the sun, the nearer it must be. They approached the kindly looking sage to arbitrate the matter, upon which he scratched his head, but could not meainingfully comment. The children were not very pleased. They told him: you are supposed to be a learned man, a know-all. Why can't you answer our question as to who is right? Ah, so even you are ignorant about certain things. This entirely apocryphal story is meant to say that Confucius knew no astronomy and, more damningly, appeared not to be interested in the subject. This tale is often cited to make the point that Confucius was too preoccupied with social/moral matters to bother with natural phenomena.

References and Select Bibliography

*Items preceded by * are publications in Chinese*

Ackoff, R. (1981). The Art and Science of Mess Management. *Interfaces* 198111:1, 20–26.

Adler, J. (2002). *Introduction to the Study of the Classic of Change*. New York: Global Scholarly Publications.

Alexander, S. (1920). *Space, Time and Deity*. London: Macmillan.

Allinson, R. (1998). Complementarity as a Model for East-West Integrative Philosophy. *Journal of Chinese Philosophy*, 25, 505–517.

Ames, R. (1986). Tao and the Nature of Nature. *Environmental Ethics*, 8.

——— (2003). Yin and Yang. In Cua (2003).

Anderson, P. (1972). More Is Different. *Science*, 177, 393–396.

Atkins, P. (2010). *The Laws of Thermodynamics: A Very Short Introduction*. Oxford: Oxford University Press.

Bacciagaluppi, G. (2012). The Role of Decoherence in Quantum Mechanics. In *The Stanford Encyclopedia of Philosophy*, E.N. Zalta (Ed.). URL = < http://plato.stanford.edu/entries/qm-decoherence/>, accessed 06/05/2014.

*Ban, G. (1995). *Hanshu*. Beijing: Chinese Press.

Bechtel, W. and R. Richardson (1992). Emergent Phenomena and Complex Systems. In Beckermann *et al.* (Eds.).

Beckermann, A., Flohr, H. and Kim, J. (1992). Eds. *Emergence or Reduction?: Essays on the Prospects of Nonreductive Physicalism*. Berlin and New York: Walter de Gruyter.

Beebee, H. (2006). *Hume on Causation*. London: Routledge.

Beebee, H., C. Hitchcock and P. Menzies (2009). Eds. *The Oxford Handbook of Causation*. Oxford: Oxford University Press.

Bensky, D. (2000). Appendix F in Kaptchuk, *The Web That Has No Weaver*. London: Ryder.

Bergson, H. (1998). *Creative Evolution*. New York: Dover Publications.

Bergson's letter to William James, 2014. URL = http://www.britannica.com/EB checked/ topic/61856/Henri-Bergson, accessed 05/01/2014.

Bergson on Process Philosophy (2014). URL = http://www.britannica.com/EBchecked/ topic/ 61856/Henri-Bergson, accessed 05/01/2014.

Berryman, A. and P. Kindlmann (2008) *Population Systems: A General Introduction*. New York, NY: Springer. URL = http://www. springerlink. com/content/ g15j69/#section=205350&page=1.

Berryman, S. (2010). Leucippus. In *The Stanford Encyclopedia of Philosophy*, E.N. Zalta (Ed.), URL = <http://plato.stanford.edu/entries/leucippus/>, accessed 14/11/2013.

——— (2010). Democritus. In *The Stanford Encyclopedia of Philosophy*, E.N. Zalta (Ed.) URL = <http://plato.stanford.edu/entries/democritus/>, accessed 14/11/2013.

Bhopal, R. (2002). *Concepts of Epidemiology: an integrated introduction to the ideas, theories, principles and methods of epidemiology*. Oxford: Oxford University Press.

(The) Big Bang Theory (2013). URL = http://map.gsfc.nasa.gov/ universe/bb_theory .html ; URL = http://map.gsfc.nasa.gov/universe/, accessed 06/12/2013.

Black, M. (1937). Vagueness: An Exercise in Logical Analysis. *Philosophy of Science*, 4(4), 427–455.

Blaedel, N. (1988). *Harmony and Unity: The Life of Niels Bohr*. Berlin and New York: Springer-Verlag .

Bohm, D. (1980). *Wholeness and the Implicate Order*. London: Routledge and Kegan Paul.

———. (1976). Fragmentation and Wholeness. URL = https://philpapers.org/rec/ BOHFAW-3

Bohr, H. (1967). "My father". In *Niels Bohr: His Life and Work as Seen by His Friends and Colleagues*, edited by S. Rozenthal, Dordrecht: North Holland Publishing Company.

Bohr, N. (1934). *Atomic Theory and the Description of Nature*. Cambridge: Cambridge University Press.

——— (1961). *Atomic Physics and Human Knowledge*. New York: Science Editions, INC.

Boyle, P. (2005). Tobacco Smoking and the British Doctors' Cohort. *British Journal of Cancer*, 92, 419–20.

Burnham, H. (2005). "Leibniz: Metaphysics", URL = http://www.iep.utm.edu/leib -met/, accessed 18/11/2013.

Camman, S. (1985). Some Early Chinese Symbols of Duality. *History of Religions*, 24, 215–254.

——— (1991). Chinese Hexagrams, Trigrams, and the Binary System. *Proceedings of the American Philosophical Association*, 135 (4).

Capra, F. (1975). *The Tao of Physics*. London: Fontana/Collins.

Carnielli, W., and M. Coniglio (2016). *Paraconsistent Logic: Consistency, Contradictions and Negation*. Berlin: Springer.

Carroll, J. (2009). Anti-Reductionism. In Beebee (2009).

Carroll, S. (2016). *The Big Picture: On the Origins of Life, Meaning, and the Universe Itself*. London: Oneworld Productions.

Chan, A. (2014). Laozi. In *The Stanford Encyclopedia of Philosophy*, E.N. Zalta (Ed.), URL = <http://plato.stanford.edu/entries/laozi/>, accessed 04/01/2014.

Causes of Cancer. URL = http://cancerhelp.cancerresearchuk.org/about-cancer/causes-symptoms/ causes/what-causes-cancer, accessed 17/02/2014.

Checkland, P. (1981). *Systems Thinking, Systems Practice*. New York: John Wiley.

*Chen, J. 陈久金 and J. Zhang 张敬国 (1989). *Hanshan chutu yupian tuxing shikao*. In *Wenwu* 文物, 4, 14–17.

*Chen, Z. (2006). *The Pleasures of Discoursing the Origins of Words*. Beijing: The New World Publishing Company. 陈政《字源谈趣: 详说中国文化系列》北京: 新世界出版社.

Cheng, C-Y. 1977. Towards Constructing a Dialectics of Harmonization: Harmony and Conflict in Chinese Philosophy. *Journal of Chinese Philosophy*, 4, 209–245.

——— (2003). Qi (Ch'i): Vital Force. In Cua (2003).

——— (2006b). Philosophy of the Yijing: Insight into Taiji and Dao as Wisdom of Life. *Journal of Chinese Philosophy*, 33(3), 323–333.

Cheng, C-Y. and N. Bunnin (2002). Eds. *Contemporary Chinese Philosophy*. Malden and Oxford: Blackwell Publishing.

Chinese Astronomical Record Keeping, 2013. URL = http://www.planetquest.org/learn/chinese.html, accessed 10/11/2013.

Clayton, P. and P. Davies (2006). (Eds). *The Re-emergence of Emergence: The Emergentist Hypothesis from Science to Religion*. Oxford: Oxford University Press.

Cleveland, J. (1994). Complexity Theory: Basic Concepts and Applications to Systems Thinking. URL = http://www.slideshare.net/johncleveland/complexity-theory-basic-concepts, accessed 23/01/2013.

Close, F. (2013). *The Infinity Puzzle*. Oxford: Oxford University Press.

Cohen, F. (2015). *The Rise of Modern Science Explained: A Comparative Study*. Cambridge: Cambridge University Press.

Cohen, S. (2014). Aristotle's Metaphysics. In *The Stanford Encyclopedia of Philosophy*, E.N. Zalta (Ed.), URL = <http://plato.stanford.edu/entries/aristotle-metaphysics/ >, accessed 20/04/2014.

Cohon, R. (2010). Hume's Moral Philosophy. In *The Stanford Encyclopedia of Philosophy*, E.N. Zalta (Ed.), URL = < http://plato.stanford.edu/entries/hume-moral/>, accessed 04/01/2014.

Confirmation of Einstein's Theory (2013). URL = http://www.aip.org/history/einstein/emc1.htm#ae22, accessed 08/10/2013.

Cook, D. and H. Rosemont (1981). The Pre-established Harmony Between Leibniz and Chinese Thought. *Journal of the History of Ideas*, 42 (2).

Cooper, D. (2003). *World Philosophies: An Historical Introduction*. Oxford: Blackwell Publishing.

——— (2014). *Daoism, Nature and Humanity*. Cambridge: Cambridge University Press.

Correa, N. (2014). Translation of the *Zhuangzi*. URL = http://www.daoisopen.com/ZZ7.html, accessed 01/03/ 2014.

Cox, B. and J. Forshaw. (2010). *Why Does* $E = mc^2$*?* London: Da Capo Press.

Cua, A. (1981). Opposites as Complements: Reflections on the Significance of Tao, *Philosophy East and West*, 31 (2), 123–140.

——— (2003). Ed. *Encycopedia of Chinese Philosophy*. New York and London: Routledge.

Danto, A. (1973). Language and the Tao: Some Reflections on Ineffability. *Journal of Chinese Philosophy*, 1(1), 45–55.

**Daojia and Daojiao* (2013). (for two different accounts). URL = http://baike.baidu.com/view/6683.htm; URL = http://www.daoistcenter.org/ daojiao.html, accessed 13/08/ 2013.

Dawenkou Writing (2013). URL = http://www.chinapage.com/archeology/2000year.html;URL=http://english.people.com.cn/english/200004/21/eng20000421_39442.html, accessed 13/11/2013.

Deacon, T. (2006). Emergence: The Hole at the Wheel's Hub. In Clayton and Davis (Eds.) (2006).

——— (2012). *Incomplete Nature: How Mind Emerged from Matter*. New York: W.W. Norton.

Defoort, C. (1997). *The Pheasant Cap Master (He guan zi): A Rhetorical Reading*. New York: SUNY Press.

Dickens, W. and J. Flynn (2001). Great Leap Forward, *New Scientist*, 2287 (21 April).

DiSalle, R. (2009). Space and Time: Inertial Frames. In *The Stanford Encyclopedia of Philosophy*, E.N. Zalta (Ed.), URL <http://plato.stanford.edu/entries/spacetime-iframes/ >, accessed 10/05/2013.

Doll, R. and A. Bradford Hill (1950). Smoking and Carcinoma of the Lung. *British Medical Journal*, v. 2(4682), 739–748. URL = http://www.ncbi.nlm.nih.gov/pmc/articles/PMC2038856/, accessed 20/10/2011.

——— (1954). The Mortality of Doctors in Relation to their smoking Habits: A Preliminary Report. *British Medical Journal* 228, 1451–1455.

Doll, R. and R. Peto (1976). Mortality in Relation to Smoking: 20 Years' Observations on Male British Doctors. *British Medical Journal*, 2, 1525–1536.

Doll, R., R. Peto, J. Boreham and I. Sunderland (2005). Mortality from Cancer: 50 Years' Observations on British Doctors. *British Journal of Cancer*, 92, 426–429.

Donnelley, S. (1978). Whitehead and Jonas: On biological organisms and real individuals. In Spicker (1978).

Dowe, P. (2000). *Physical Causation*. Cambridge: Cambridge University Press.

——— (2009). Causal Process Theories. In Beebee (2009).

Down Syndrome. 2014. URL = http://kidshealth.org/parent/medical/genetic/ down_syndrome.html.

Early influences on Leibniz's Account of Binary Arithmetic (2006). URL = http://history-computer.com/Dreamers/Llull.html, accessed 18/12/2013.

Edwards, P. (1967). Ed. *The Encyclopedia of Philosophy*. New York: Macmillan.

Ehrlich, P., A. Ehrlich and P. Holden (1973). *Human Ecology*. San Francisco: W.H. Freeman and Company.

Ellis, G. (2006). On the Nature of Emergent Reality. In Clayton and Davies (2006).

Elstein, D. (2004). *Xunzi* (Hsun Tzu, c 310–220 BCE). URL = http://www.iep.utm.edu/xunzi/, accessed 18/12/2012.

Eno, R. (2010). Huang-Lao Ideology. URL = http://www.indiana.edu/~g380/4.8–Huang-Lao-2010.pdf, accessed 05/04/2016.

Explanation of Binary Arithmetic, 2014. URL = http://www.leibniz-translations.com/binary.htm, accessed 10/01/2014.

Feng, G. and J. English. (1989). *Tao Te Ching*. New York: Vintage Books; URL = http://www2. hawaii. edu/~freeman/courses/phil394/Daodejing.pdf., accessed 03/02/2013.

Fruehauf, H. (1999). On the Relation Between Medicine and Philosophy (by Zhang Xichun, as introduced and translated by Fruehauf). URL = http://www.classical chinesemedicine.org/ on-the-relationship-between-medicine-and-philosophy/, accessed 06/01/2015.

——— (2009). *Correlative Cosmology: Energetics of the First Month of Spring and Lung Function* (A collection of relevant classical sources), URL = http://www.classical chinesemedicine.org/wp-ontent/uploads/2010/03/fruehauf_ correlativecosmo-lung .pdf, accessed 23/04/2013.

Flose, H. (1986). Niels Bohr, Complementarity, and Realism. *Proceedings of he Bennial Meeting of the Philosophy of Science Association*. Vol. 186, 96–104.

Fu, C. (1973). Lao-tzu's Conception of Tao. *Inquiry*, 16, 367–394.

Fuxi and Nüwa (2007). See *Worshipping the Three Sage Kings and Five Virtuous Emperors: The Imperial Temple of Emperors of Successive Dynasties in Beijing*. Beijing: Foreign Language Press.

Gabbay, D. and J. Woods (2012). Eds. *Handbook of the History of Logic*. Amsterdam and London: Elsevier.

Geocentric and Heliocentric Systems (2013). URL = http://www2.astro.psu.edu/users/rbc/a1/ lec4n.html, accessed 14/12/ 2013.

Gibbs, P. and S. Hiroshi (1997). What is Occam's Razor? URL = http://math.ucr .edu/home/baez/physics/ General/ occam.html, accessed 06/07/2013 .

Glaser, A. (1981). History of Binary and Other Nondecimal Inventions. URL = http://www.eipiphiny.org/ books/ history-of-binary.pdf pp 31–52, accessed 08/01/2013.

Golley, F. (1993). *A History of the Ecosystem Concept in Ecology: More Than the Sum of the Parts*. New Haven: Yale University Press.

Graham, A. (1986). *Yin-yang and the Nature of Correlative Thinking*. IEAP Occasional Paper and Monograph Series, No. 6. Singapore: Institute of East Asian Philosophies.

Graham, D. (2005). Heraclitus. URL = http://www.iep.utm.edu/heraclit/, accessed 09/07/2013.

——— (2008). Leucippus' Atomism. In P. Curd and D. Graham. (Eds). *The Oxford Handbook of Presocratic Philosophy*. Oxford: Oxford University Press.

——— (2011). Heraclitus. In *The Stanford Encyclopedia of Philosophy*, E.N. Zalta (Ed.), URL = http://plato.stanford.edu/archives/sum2011/entries/heraclitus/, accessed 09/07/2013.

*Guo, Zhicheng and Guo Tao 郭志成、郭韬 (2005). *Zoujin Fuxi: pojie yixue qiangu zhi mi/* 《走进伏羲—破解易学千古之谜》,北京：光明出版社.

Haack, S. (1993). *Evidence and Inquiry*. Oxford: Blackwell.

Hajek, P. (1998). *Metamathematics of Fuzzy Logic*. Dordrecht: Kluwer.

——— (2009). On Vagueness, Truth Values and Logics. *Studia Logica*, 91(3), 367–382.

——— (2010). Fuzzy Logic. In *The Stanford Encyclopedia of Philosophy*, E.N. Zalta (Ed.), URL = < http://plato.stanford.edu/entries/logic-fuzzy/>, accessed 25/11/2013.

Hansen, C. (1992). *A Daoist Theory of Chinese Thought: A Philosophical Interpretation*. Oxford and New York: Oxford University Press.

*Hao, Wanshan/郝万山. 2011. Series of lectures on Zhang Zhongjing and the *Shanghanlun*. URL = http://video. baidu. com/v?word, accessed 20/09/2014.

Healey, R. (2009). Causation in Quantum Mechanics. In Beebee (2009).

Heisenberg, W. (1958). *Physics and Philosophy: The Revolution in Modern Science*. New York: Harper and | Brothers Publishers.

Hejazi, A. (2013). *You Must Know Guide to Systems Thinking*. URL = http://www.futuresdiscovery.com/ Newsletter/ SystemsThinking.pdf., accessed 23/05/2013.

Henderson, J. (1984). *The Development and Decline of Chinese Cosmology*. New York: Columbia University Press.

——— (2003). Wuxing (Wu-hsing): Five Phases. In Cua (2003).

Heraclitus. *The Fragments of Heraclitus*. URL = http://www.heraclitusfragments.com/Fragments.html

Hexagramium Organum, 2013. URL = http://blindmen6.tumblr.com/post/19649027526/ leibniz-de, accessed 18/12/2013.

Higgs' Bosun (2013. URL = http://www.livescience.com/23826–nobel-prize-why-not-higgs-boson.html; URL = http://www.newscientist.com/article/mg21628963.900–higgs-boson-having-an-identity-crisis.html, accessed 05/12/2013.

Ho, P. (1972). The System of the Book of Changes. *Japanese Studies in the History of Science*, 11, 23–39.

——— (2007). *Explorations in Daoism*. London: Routledge.

Hoeffer, C. (2009). Causation in Spacetime Theories. In Beebee (2009).

Hoffert, B. (2006). Distinguishing the 'Rational' from the 'Irrational' in the Early Zhuangzi Lineage. *Journal of Chinese Philosophy*, 33(1), 159–173.

Honner, J. (1987). *The Description of Nature: Niels Bohr and the Philosophy of Quantum Physics*. Oxford: Clarendon Press.

(The) Huainanzi: Its Philosophical Thoughts Concerning Nature. Beijing: Scientific Publishing Press.

**Huangdi Neijing Suwen Jiaozhu Yuyi* (2010). A. Guo (Ed.). Guizhou, China: Guizhou Education Press, Ltd, 2010. 郭靄春《黄帝内经素问校注语译》贵州教育出版社 2010年.

Humphreys, P. (2009). Causation and Reduction. In Beebee (2009).

Illari, P., F. Russo and J. Williamson (2011). *Causality in the Sciences*. Oxford: Oxford University Press.

Irvine, A. (2010). Principia Mathematica. In *The Stanford Encyclopedia of Philosophy*, E.N. Zalta (Ed.). URL = <http://plato.stanford.edu/entries/principia-mathematica/>, accessed 05/11/2013.

Jin, G., H. Fan and Q. Liu (1996). The Structure of Science and Technology in History: On the Factors Delaying the Development of Science and technology in China in Comparison with the West since the Seventeenth Century. In D. Fan and R. Cohen (Eds.), *Chinese Studies in the History and Philosophy of Science and Technology*. Dordrecht: Kluwer Academic.

*Jin, X. 靳晓日 (2013). URL = http://blog. sina.com. cn/s/ blog_598e62420100qxup.html, accessed 11/12/2013.

Joos, E. (2006). The Emergence of Classicality from Quantum Theory. In Clayton and Davies (2006).

——— (2012). *Decoherence*. URL = http://www.decoherence.de/, accessed 22/05/2014.

Joseph, G. (1994). "Different Ways of Knowing: Contrasting Styles of Argument in Indian and Greek Traditions". Edited by Paul Ernest, *Mathematics, Education and Philosophy: An International Perspective*", Volume 3 in *Studies in Mathematics Education*. Sussex: The Falmer Press.

Kalanithi, P. (2016). *When Breathe Became Air*. Oxford: Bodley Head.

Kaptchuk, T. (2000). *The Web That Has No Weaver*. London: Rider.

Kauffman, S. (1993). *The Origins of Order: Self-organisation and Selection in Evolution*. Oxford: Oxford University Press.

——— (1995). *At Home in the Universe: The Search for Laws of Self-organization and Complexity*. Oxford: Oxford University.

——— (2000). *Investigations*. Oxford: Oxford University Press.

——— (2006). Beyond Reductionism: Reinventing the Sacred. URL = http://edge.org/conversation/beyond-reductionism-reinventing-the sacred, accessed 25/05/2013.

Kelley, D. and E. Milone (2005). *Exploring Ancient Skies: An Encyclopedic Survey of Archaeoastronomy*. New York: Springer.

King, P. and S. Shapiro (1995). History of Logic. In *The Oxford Companion to Philosophy*. Oxford: Oxford University Press; URL = http://individual.utoronto.ca/pking/miscellaneous/history-of-logic.pdf, accessed 13/12/2012.

Kosko, B. (1993). *The New Science of Fuzzy Logic*. New York: Hyperion.

Kuhlmann, M. (2011). Mechanisms in Dynamically Complex Sytems." In Illari (2011).

Kurtz, J. (2011). *The Discovery of Chinese Logic*. Leiden: Brill.

Lach, D. (1945). Leibniz and China. *Journal of the History of Ideas*, 6, 436–455.

Lai, K. (2006). *Learning from Chinese Philosophies: Ethics of Interdependent and Contextualised Self*. Aldershott: Ashgate Publishing Company.

———. (2008). *An Introduction to Chinese Philosophy*. Cambridge: Cambridge University Press.

Lane, A. and K. Shipp (2000). *Systems Thinking and Practice*. URL = http://www.open.edu/openlearn/science-maths-technology/computing-and-ict/systems-computer/systems-thinking-and-practice/content-section-0, accessed 10/02/2013.

Lang, K. and J. Zhang (1999). *A Taoist Foundation of Systems Modeling and Thinking*; URL = http://www.systemdynamics.org/conferences/1999/PAPERS/PARA142.PDF, accessed 21/02/2013.

Lange, M. (2009). Causation in Classical Mechanics. In Beebee (2009).

Law of Excluded Middle (2014). *Introduction to Philosophy*. Stanford University. URL = http://www. stanford. edu/~bobonich/glances%20ahead/IV.excluded.middle.html, accessed 13/04/2014.

Lawlor, L. and V. Moulard Leonard (2013). Henri Bergson. In *The Stanford Encyclopedia of Philosophy*, E.N. Zalta (Ed.), URL = http://plato.stanford.edu/archives/win2013/entries/ bergson/, accessed 24/06/2013.

Lee, K. (1989a). *The Positivist Science of Law*, Avebury: Gower.

——— (1989b). *Social Philosophy and Ecological Scarcity*. London: Routledge.

——— (1999). *The Natural and the Artefactual: The Implications of Deep Science and Deep Technology for Environmental Philosophy*. Lanham: Lexington Books.

——— (2005). *Philosophy and Revolutions in Genetics: Deep Science and Deep Technology*, Palgrave, Basingstoke (second edition).

——— (2008). *Warp and Weft: Chinese Language and Culture*. New York: Eloquent Books.

——— (2012a). Towards Constructing Post-postmodern 21st Century Sciences: The Relevance of Classical Chinese Medicine. In B. Arun (Ed.), *Asia, Europe Dialogue and the Emergence of Modern Science: Knowledge Crossing Boundaries*. New York: Palgrave MacMillan.

——— (2012b) *The Philosophical Foundations of Modern Medicine*. Basingstoke: Palgrave Macmillan.

——— (2017a). RCTs & EBM as Gold Standards: A Trojan Horse for Biomedicine? In R. Bluhm (Ed.), *Knowing and Acting in Medicine*. Lanham: Rowman and Littlefield International.

——— (2017b). *Classical Chinese Medicine: Theory, Methodology and Therapy In Its Philosophical Framework*. Newcastle: Cambridge Scholars Publishing.

Legge Translation of the Daodejing (2012). (Ed. By Donald Sturgeon). URl = http://ctext.org/dao-de-jing, accessed 16/01/2013.

Leggett, A. (1987). *The Problems of Physics*. Oxford: Oxford University Press.

——— (2000). New Life for Schrödinger's Cat. URL = http://www.ipod.org.uk/reality/reality_ schrodingers_cat.asp, accessed 06/05/2014.

——— (2002). Testing the Limits of Quantum Mechanics: Motivation, State of Play, Prospects." *Journal of Physics: Condensed Matter* 14, R415–R451.

Leibniz, G. (1714). *The Principles of Philosophy known as Monadology*. URL = http://www.earlymoderntexts.com/assets/pdfs/leibniz1714b.pdf, accessed 11/05/2016.

——— (1975). *Explication de l'arithmétique binaire*. URL = http://ads.ccsd. cnrs.fr/docs/00/10/47/81/PDF/ p85_89_vol3483m.pdf; for an English translation, see

Strickland, L. (2007); URL = http://www. leibniz-translations.com/binary.htm, accessed 19/06/2013.

Leibniz's Calculating Machine, 2002. URL = http://www.gwleibniz.com/calculator/calculator.html, accessed 20/06/2013.

Lewes, G. (1875). *Problems of Life and Mind*. 2 Vols. London: Kegan Paul, French, Turbner and Co.

Lewis, M. (2006). *The Flood Myths of Early China*. Albany: State University of New York Press.

Li, W. and H. Poser (2006). Leibniz's Positive View of China. *Journal of Chinese Philosophy*, 33(1). 17–33.

**Liangyitaijitu* (2013). URL = http://baike. baidu.com/view/48746.htm, accessed 10/12/2013.

Littlejohn, R. (2012). "*Wuxing (wu-hsing)*". URL = http://www.iep.utm.edu/wuxing/, accessed 26/04/2013.

*Liu, C. (1980). 刘长林《内经的哲学和中医的方法》, 北京: 科学出版社. *The Philosophy of 'Neijing' and the Methodology of Chinese Medicine*. Beijing: Science Publications Press.

——— (2006).《中国象科学观: 易、道、与兵、医》上、下册, 北京：社会科学文献出版社. [*Chinese Science from the* Xiang *Perspective: Exploring Yi, Dao, Warfare and Medicine*. 2 Vols. Beijing: Social Sciences Academic Press .

——— (2008).《中国系统思维·文化基因探视》, 北京: 社会科学文献出版社. *Chinese Systemic Mode of Thought: An Exploratory Examination of Cultural Inheritance*. Beijing: Social Sciences Academic Press.

Liu, F., and J. Zhang (2013). A Note on Mohist Logic. URL = http://fenrong.net/archives/ MohistLogic.pdf, accessed 12/06/2013.

*Liu, L. (2003). 刘力红《思考中医》.（桂林, 广西师范大学出版社. *Exploring Chinese Medicine*. Guilin: Guangxi Normal University Press.

Lloyd, G. (1990). *Demystifying Mentalities*. Cambridge: Cambridge University Press.

——— (2004). *Ancient Worlds and Modern Reflections: Philosophical Perspectives on Greek and Chinese Science and Culture*. Oxford: Clarendon Press.

Lloyd, G. and N. Sivin (2002). *The Way and the Word: Science and Medicine in Early China and Greece*. New Haven and London: Yale University Press.

Loewe, M. (2011). *Dong Zhongshu: A "Confucian" Heritage and the* Chunqiu Fanlu. Leiden: Brill.

Loewe, M. and E. Shaughnessy (1999). *The Cambridge History of Ancient China*. Cambridge: University of Cambridge Press.

Loly, P. (2002). A Logical Way of Ordering the Hexagrams of the *Yijing* and the Trigrams of the *Bagua*. *The Oracle—The Journal of Yijing Studies*, 2(12), 2–13; Url = http://home.cc.umanitoba.ca/~loly/oracle.pdf, accessed 11/11/2012.

Loux, M. (2006). *Metaphysics: A Contemporary Introduction*. London: Routledge.

Lucas, T. (2005). Later Mohist Logic, *Lei*, Classes and Sorts. *Journal of Chinese Philosophy*, .32; URL = http://onlinelibrary.wiley.com/doi/10.1111/j.1540–6253.2005.00198.x/pdf, accessed 09/05/2013.

*Luo, D. (2014). 张锡纯, 中西医结合的奠基人 ("Zhang Xichun: Founding father of integrating Chinese and Western Medicines") URL = http://bbs.gdmm.com/thread-2779831–1–1.html, accessed 02/02/2016.

MacDonald, C. and MacDonald, G. (2010). Emergence and Downward Causation. In C. MacDonald and G. MacDonald (Eds., 2010).

MacDonald, C. and MacDonald, G. (2010). (Eds.). *Emergence in Mind*. Oxford: Oxford University Press.

McIntosh, R. (1985). *The Background of Ecology*: Concept and Theory. Cambridge: Cambridge University Press.

Major, J., S. Queen, A. Meyer and H. Roth (2010). (Trans. and Eds.). *Liu, An,* Huainanzi: *A Guide to the Theory and Practice of Government in Early Han China*. New York: Columbia University Press.

——— (2013). *The Essential Huainanzi*. URL = http://cup.columbia.edu/media/7299/major-essential-huainanzi.pdf, accessed 10/09/2013.

Maspero, H. (1938–1939). *Les instruments astronomiques des chinois. Mélanges chinois et bouddhiques*, 16, 183–370.

Mass (2013). URL = http://www.infoplease.com/encyclopedia/science/mass-physics.html, accessed 08/10/2013.

Mattos, G. and N. Jerry (2000). Early China. Berkeley: The Society for the Study of Early China and the Institute of East Asian Studies, University of California.

Maturana, H. and F. Varela (1980). *Autopoiesis and Cognition: The Organization of the Living*. Dordrecht/Boston: D. Reidel Publishing Company.

Meadows, D. (2009). *Thinking in Systems: A Primer*. London: Earthscan.

(The) Milky Way (2013). URL = http://starryskies.com/articles/ 2007/07/milky-way.html; URL = http://cultureofchinese.com/traditions/ folklore/ folklore-cowherd-and-the-weaver-girl/, accessed 20/11/2013.

Mill, J. (1843). *A System of Logic*. London: Longmans.

Minkowski, H. (1908). Space and Time. URL = https://todayinsci.com/QuotationsCategories/ S_Cat/Space-Time-Quotations.htm, accessed 23/08/2015.

Mitrophanove, A. and E. Groisman (2008). Positive feedback in cellular control systems". In *Bioessays*, 30(6), 542–555.

Mohaghegh, S. (2000). Virtual Intelligence Application in Petroleum Engineering: part 3, Fuzzy Logic. *Journal of Petroleum Technology*, November, 82–87.

Mokeur, (Prof). (2013). *History of the Atom from Democritus to Bohr and Schrödinger*. URL = http://profmokeur. ca/ chemistry/ history_of_the_atom.htm, accessed 25/10/2013.

Moore, C. (1967). Ed. *The Chinese Mind: Essentials of Chinese Philosophy and Culture*. Honolulu: East-West Center Press, University of Hawaii Press.

Morris, W. (1882). *Hopes and Fears For Art: Five Lectures: Delivered in Birmingham, London, and Nottingham, 1878–1881* .

*Mou Z. (1998). 牟宗三:《周易的自然哲学與道德的函義》, 台湾: 文泽出版社. *The Philosophy of Nature and the Ethical Meanings of the Book of Changes* .Taipei: Wenze Publishing Company.

Mumford, S. (2009). Causal Powers and Capacities. In Beebee (2009).

Mungello, D. (1977). *Leibniz and Confucianism: The Search for Accord*. Honolulu: University of Hawaii Press.

Munro, D. (1969). *The Concept of Man in Early China*. Stanford: Stanford University Press.

Nakayama, S. and N. Sivin (1973) Eds. *Chinese Science: Explorations of an Ancient Tradition*. Cambridge, MA: MIT Press..

Nagel, E. (1961). *The Structure of Science*. New York: Harcourt, Brace, and World.

Naess, A. and G. Sessions (1984). *Basic Principles of Deep Ecology*. URL = http://theanarchistlibrary.org/library/arne-naess-and-george-sessions-basic-principles-of-deep-ecology, accessed 26/02/2014.

Needham, J. (1969). The Great Titration. London: Allen and Unwin.

——— (1975).The Cosmology of Early China. In C. Blacker and M. Loewe (Eds.). *Ancient Cosmologies*. London: George Allen and Unwin Ltd..

——— (1981). *Science in Traditional China: A Comparative Perspective*. Cambridge, MA: MIT Press.

Needham, J., W. Pagel and F. Cornford (1936). *Background to Modern Science: Ten Lectures at Cambridge arranged by the History of Science Committee*. Cambridge: Cambridge University Press.

Needham, J. and L. Wang (1956). *Science and Civilisation in China*. Vol. 2. Cambridge: Cambridge University Press.

Needham, J. and G. Lu. (2000). *Medicine*. In N. Sivin (Ed. With An Introduction), Vol 6, Part VI of *Science and Civilisation in China*. Cambridge: Cambridge University Press.

Needham, J., K. Robinson and R. Huang (2004). *Science and Technology*. Vol. 7, Part 2. Of *Science and Civilisation in China*. Cambridge: Cambridge University Press.

Neolithic Burial Site (2013a). URL = http://www.chinanews.com/shipin/cnstv/2012/07–18/news79002.shtml, accessed 05/11/ 2013.

Neolithic Burial Site (2013b). URL = http://blog.sina.com.cn/s/blog_6a8164fd0100ukrf.html.

Neugebauer, O. (1962). *The Exact Sciences in Antiquity*. New York: Harper, 1962.

Ni, M. (1995). *The Yellow Emperor's Classic of Medicine: A New Translation of the Neijing Suwen with Commentary*. Boston, Mass., and London: Shambala.

Nisbett, R. and K. Peng. (2005). *The Geography of Thought: How Asians and Westerners Think Differently*. London: Nicholas Brealey Publishing.

O'Connor, J. and I. McDermott (1997). *The Arts of Systems Thinking*. London: Thorsons.

Odum (2014). URL = http://www.chattoogariver.org/ index. php? req= odum&quart=F2002, accessed 27/07/2014.

Oldenwald, S. (2013). What is a space time continuum? URL = http://einstein.stanford.edu/content/relativity/q411.html, accessed 07/03/2013.

——— (2013). What does the Word 'Spacetime' Mean? URL = http://einstein.stanford.edu/ content/relativity/a10385.html, accessed 07/03/2013.

Olshin, B. (2005). The '*I Ching*' or '*Book of Changes*': Chinese Space-time Model and a Philosophy of Divination. *Journal of Philosophy and Culture*. 2(2), 17–39; URL = http://www.ajol.info/index.php/jpc/article/view/36454, accessed 19/12/2012.

O'Neil, R. (2001). Is It Time to Bury the Ecosystem Concept (With Full Military Honours Of Course!)". *Ecology*, 82(12), 3275–3284; URL = http://www.esa.org/history/Awards/ /ONeill_RV_MA.pdf, accessed 21/01/2013.

.Overduin, J. (2007a). Spacetime Before Einstein. URL = http://einstein.stanford.edu/ SPACETIME/spacetime1.html, accessed 08/03/2013.

——— (2007b). Einstein's Spacetime. URL = http://einstein.stanford.edu/SPACE TIME/ spacetime2.html, accessed 08/03/2013.

Pais, A. (1991). *Niels Bohr's Times*. Oxford: Clarendon Press.

Palmer, J. (2012). Parmenides. In *The Stanford Encyclopedia of Philosophy*, E.N. Zalta (Ed.), URL = http://plato.stanford.edu/archives/sum2012/entries/parmenides/, accessed 23/08/ 2013.

*Pan, Y. 潘毅 (2013). *Xun hui zhongyi shiluo de yuan shen* 《寻回中医失落的元神》, 广东: 广东科技出版社, 2013 年. 2 Volumes. Guangdong: Guangdong Technology Publishers.

Pankenier, D. (2013). *Astrology and Cosmology in Early China: Conforming Earth to Heaven*. Cambridge: Cambridge University Press.

Peirce, C. (1974). Pragmatism and Critical Common-Sensism. In C. Hartshorne and P. Weiss (Eds.), *Collected Papers of Charles Sanders Peirce*. Vol. 5. Cambridge, Mass: Harvard University Press.

Peto, R. (2005). Nature, Nurture and Luck. URL = http://www.ctsu.ox.ac.uk/news/nature-nurture-luck-oxford-today-article.pdf/view, accessed 03/07/2013.

Photograph Capturing the Process of Converting Mass into Energy (2013). URL = http://www.aip.org/history/einstein/ae22.htm, accessed 08/10/2013.

Pike, O., F. Mackenroth, E. Hill and R. Rose. (2014). A photon-photon collider in a vacuum hohlraum. *Nature Photonics*, 8, 434–436; URL = http://www3.imperial.ac.uk/ newsandeventspggrp/imperialcollege/newssummary/news_16–5–2014–15–32–44, accessed 19/04/2014.

Pines, Y. (2002). *Foundations of Confucian Thought: Intellectual Life in the Chun Qiu Period, 722–453 BCE*. Hawaii: University of Hawaii Press.

Plumwood, V. (1993). *Feminism and the Mastery of Nature*. London: Routledge, 1993.

**Politics and Cosmology*. (2013). URL = http://baike.baidu.com/view/49959.htm. accessed 12/06/ 2013.

Popper, K. 1959). *The Logic of Scientific Discovery*. London: Routledge.

Porkert, M. (1974). *The Theoretical Foundations of Chinese Medicine: Systems of Correspondence*. Cambridge, MA.: MIT Press.

Priest, G. (1986). Contradiction, Belief, and Rationality. *Proceedings of the Aristotelian Society*, 86, 99–116.

——— (2003). *Beyond the Limits of Thought*. New York: Oxford University Press.

——— (2005). *Towards Non-Being: The Logic and Metaphysics of Intentionality*. Oxford: Oxford University Press.

——— (2008a). *An Introduction to Non-Classical Logic*. Cambridge: Cambridge University Press.

——— (2008b). Jaina Logic: A Contemporary Perspective. *History and Philosophy of Logic*, 29:3, 263–278. URL = http://dx.doi.org/10.1080/01445340701690233, accessed 17/02/2016.

Priest, G., R. Routley and J. Norman (1989). Eds. *Paraconsistent Logic: Essays on the Inconsistent*. Munich: *Philosophia Verlag.*

Priest, G. amd K. Tanaka (2009). Paraconsistent Logic. URL = http://plato.stanford.edu/ entries/logic-paraconsistent/, accessed 20/01/2014.

Priest, G. and F. Berto (2013). "*Dialetheism*", *The Stanford Encyclopedia of Philosophy*, E.N. Zalta (ed), URL = http://plato.stanford.edu/archives/sum2013/entries/dialetheism/, accessed 01/04/2016.

Priest, G., K. Tanaka and Z. Weber (2015). "Paraconsistent Logic", *The Stanford Encyclopedia of Philosophy*, E.N. Zalta (ed), URL = http://plato.stanford.edu/archives/spr2015/ entries/ logic-paraconsistent/, accessed 01/04/2016.

Prigogine, I. and I. Stengers (1985). *Order Out of Chao: Man's New Dialogue with Nature*. London: Flamingo.

——— (1997).*The End of Certainty: Time, Chaos and the New Laws of Nature*. New York: Free Press.

**Qi* (2013). URL = http://class.htu.cn/hzdam/05bkzl/hzyy/02yinianji x/yxkw08/yxkw08_ qi.htm, accessed 19/05/2013.

*Qian, C. and W. Hao 钱 超尘、郝万山, 整理. (2005). Eds.《伤寒论》。(北京: 人民卫生出版社). Shanghanlun. Beijing: The Peoples' Public Health Publishers.

Raphals, L. (2015). "Science and Chinese Philosophy". *The Stanford Encyclopedia of Philosophy*, E.N. Zalta (ed.). URL = http://plato.stanford.edu/entries/chinese-phil-science/, accessed 25/02/2016.

Reichenbach, H. (1938). *Experience and Prediction*. Chicago: The University of Chicago Press, Phoenix Books.

Rescher, N. (1997). *Process Metaphysics: An Introduction to Process Philosophy*. New York: SUNY Press.

——— (2000). *Process Philosophy: A Survey of Basic Issues*. Pittsburgh: University of Pittsburgh Press.

Restall, G. (2006). *Logic*. London: Routledge.

Richmond, B. (2005). *An Introduction to Systems Thinking*. URL = http://www.fi.muni.cz/ ~xpelanek/IV109/jaro07/IST.pdf, accessed 28/01/2013.

Robinet, I. (2008). Daojia. In F. Pregadio (Ed.), *Encyclopedia of Taoism*. London: Routledge.

Robins, D. (Spring 2014). Xunzi. In *The Stanford Encyclopedia of Philosophy*, Edward N. Zalta (Ed.), URL = http://plato.stanford.edu/entries/xunzi/, accessed 11/01/2013.

Robinson, H. (2014). Substance. In *The Stanford Encyclopedia of Philosophy*, E.N. Zalta (Ed.), URL = http://plato.stanford.edu/entries/substance/, accessed 20/10/2014.

Robinson, K. (2004). Ed. *Science and Technology*. Vol. 7, Part 2. Of *Science and Civilisation in China*. Cambridge: Cambridge University Press.

Robinson, T. (1987). *Heraclitus*. Toronto: University of Toronto Press.

*Rong, J. (2013a). *Wuxing*, URL = http://baike.baidu.com/view/4292.htm, accessed 04/10/2013.

——— (2013b). *Yinyang*, URL = http://blog.sina.com.cn/s/blog_69da04910101a5ls.html, accessed 04/10/2013.

Roth, H. (2014). Zhuangzi. In *The Stanford Encyclopedia of Philosophy*, E.N. Zalta (ed.), URL = <http://plato.stanford.edu/entries/zhuangzi/>, accessed 21/02/2017.

Russell, B. and A. Whitehead (1910–1913). *Principia Mathematica*, 3 Volumes. Cambridge: Cambridge University Press.

Rutt, R. (1999). Edward L Shaughnessy's Mawangdui 'Yijing': A Review Article. *The Oracle: Journal of Yijing Studies*, 2(8), 38–47; URL = http://www. biroco. com/yijing/mawangdui.htm, accessed 15/04/2013.

Ryan, J. (1996). Leibniz's Binary System and Shao Yong's 'Yijing'". *Philosophy East and West*. 46(1), 59–90.

Ryden, E. (2002). Trans. *Key Concepts in Chinese Philosophy*. (Beijing: Foreign Languages Press).

Rynasiewicz, R. (2014). Newton's Views on Space, Time and Motion. E.N. Zalta (Ed.), URL = <http://plato.stanford. edu/entries/newton-stm/>, accessed 28/11/2012.*

Sadi Carnot, 2013. URL = http://www.britannica.com/EBchecked/topic/96405/Sadi-Carnot, accessed 5/06/2013.

Sattler, R. (1986). *Biophilosophy Analytic and Holistic Perspectives*. Berlin and New York: Springer-Verlag.

——— (2011). *Healing Thinking Being*, URL = http://www.beyondwilber.ca/bookpre/healing/ healing_thinking_and_being.html, accessed 18/05/2014.

——— (2014). Either/or Logic and Beyond, URL = http://www.beyondwilber.ca/AQALmap/ bookdwl/files/WAQALMB_2.pdf., accessed 17/04/2014.

Sattler's Critique of Wilber (2014). URL = http://www.beyondwilber.ca/AQALmap/bookdwl/ files/ WAQALMB_2.pdf, accessed 20 April 2014.

Saunders, S. (2005). Complementarity and Scientific Rationality. *Foundations of Physics*, 35 (3), 417–447.

Scheid, V. (2002). *Chinese Medicine in Contemporary China: Plurality and Synthesis*. Durham: Duke University Press.

Schönfeld, M. (2006). Ed. Kant and Confucianism. *Journal of Chinese Philosophy*, 33(1), 1–157.

Schmitter, A. (2014). 17th and 18th Centuries on the Emotions. In *The Stanford Encyclopedia of Philosophy*, E.N. Zalta (Ed.), URL = http://plato.stanford.edu/entries/emotions-17th18th/ LD8Hume, accessed 25/01/2014.

Schwartz, B. (1985). *The World of Thought in Ancient China*. Cambridge, MA: Harvard University Press.

**(The) Scorpio Constellation* (2013). URL = http://www. youtube.com/watch?v=V0WbAaLkfrM ; URL = http://baike.baidu.com/view/157569.htm, accessed 05/11/2013.

Shapin, S. (1996). *The Scientific Revolution*. Chicago: University of Chicago Press.

Shaughnessy, E. (1998). Ever Changing Text: The Writing of the *Tradition of the Appended Statements* and the Making of the *Yijing*. URL = http://www.biroco

.com/yijing/ Shaughnessy_Xicizhuan.pdf (but entitled "The Writing of Xici Zhuan an(d) the Making of the Yijing"), accessed 14/02/2013.

———. (1999). Western Zhou History. In Loewe and Shaughnessy (1999).

Seibt, J. (2013). Process Philosophy. In *The Stanford Encyclopedia of Philosophy*, E.N. Zalta (ed.), URL = http://plato.stanford.edu/archives/fall2013/entries/process-philosophy/, accessed 27/8/2013.

Shu Xingbei (2013). URL = *http://baike.baidu.com/view/39883.htm, accessed 21/12/2013.

Silberstein, M. (2006). *In Defence of Ontological Emergence and Mental Causation*. In P. Clayton and P. Davies, 2006 (Eds.).

Sivin, N. (1987). *Traditional Medicine in Contemporary China*. Ann Arbor, MI: University of Michigan Center for Chinese Studies.

——— (1995a). *Medicine, Philosophy and Religion in Ancient China*. Aldershot: Avebury.

——— (1995b). Taoism and Science. URL = http://ccat.sas.upenn.edu/~nsivin/taos.pdf, accessed 13/01/2013.

——— (2005). Revised 1982, first published in *Chinese Science*, 5, 45–66). Why the Scientific Revolution Did Not Take Place in China—Or Didn't It? URL = http://ccat.sas.upenn.edu/~nsivin/scirev.pdf, accessed 15/12/2013.

**Six Strategies* (2013). URL = http://baike. baidu.com/view/39954.htm, accessed 12/12/2013.

Smith, K. (2003). Sima Tan and the Invention of Daoism, 'Legalism,' 'Et cetera.' *The Journal of Asian Studies*. 62(1), 129–156; URL = http://www.jstor.org/stable/3096138, accessed 08/01/2013.

Smith, P. (2003). *An Introduction to Formal Logic*. Cambrdige: Cambridge University Press.

Smith, R. (2008). *Fathoming the Cosmos and Ordering the World: The Yijing (I-Ching, or Classic of Changes) and Its Evolution in China*. Charlottesville and London: University of Virginia Press.

Spade, P. (2011). William of Ockham. In *The Stanford Encyclopedia of Philosophy*, Edward N. Zalta (Ed.), URL = < http://plato.stanford.edu/entries/ockham/>, accessed 03/05/2013.

Speed of Light May Not Be Constant (2013). URL = http://news.discovery.com/space/speed-of-light-einstein-physics-130428.htm, accessed 25/03/2014.

Spicker, S. (1978). Ed. *Organism, Medicine, and Metaphysics*. Dordrecht: D. Reidel Publishing Company.

Stengers, I. (2000).*The Invention of Modern Science*. Trans. D. W. Smith. Minneapolis: University of Minnesota Press.

——— (2002/2011). *Thinking with Whitehead: A Free and Wild Creation of Concepts*. Cambridge, Mass: Harvard University Press.

Stewart, B. (2008). The Science of Ecology. URL = http://geologyecology. suite101.com/ article.cfm/the_science_of_ecology, accessed 27/06/2013.

Stewart, B. and C. Wild (2014). Eds. *World Cancer Report 2014* (World Health Organization: International Agency for Research on Cancer).

Stöppler, M. (2013). *Genetic Disease Overview: Single Gene Inheritance, Multifactorial Inheritance*, URL = http://www.medicinenet.com/genetic_disease/article.htm, accessed 23/07/2013.

Suber, P. (1997). Non-contradiction and Excluded Middle, URL =. http://legacy.earlham.edu/~peters/courses/logsys/pnc-pem.htm, accessed 27/05/2013.

Theobald, U. (2014). *Dong Zhongshu*. URL = at http://www.chinaknowledge.de/History/ Han/ personsdongzhongshu.html, accessed 05/02/2014.

Thomas, E. (2014). Samuel Alexander. URL = http://www.iep.utm.edu/alex-sam/, accessed 16/05/2014.

Thorburn, W. (1915). Occam's Razor. *Mind*, 24, 287–88.

——— (1918). The Myth of Occam's Razor. *Mind*, 27, 345–53.

Tonomura, A., J. Endo, T. Matsuda, T. Kawasaki and H. Ezawa. (1989). Demonstration of single-electron buildup of an interference pattern. *American Journal of Physics*, 57, 117. See also URL = http://www.hitachi.com/rd/portal/research/em/doubleslit.html or URL =www.youtube.com/watch?v=ZJ-0PBRuthc, accessed 18/08/2014.

Three Laws of Thermodynamics (2013). URL = http://www.physicsplanet.com/articles/three-laws-of-thermodynamics; URL = http://www.zo.utexas.edu/courses/Thoc/ Thermodynamics.html, accessed 07/10/2013.

Tree Rings (2013). URL = http://ltrr.arizona.edu/about/treerings, accessed 01/12/2013.

Tsai, A. (2013). Where Does the Yin Yang Symbol Come From?. URL = http://www.chinesefortunecalendar.com/yinyang.htm, accessed 26/02/2013.

Unschuld, P. (1985). *Medicine in China: A History of Ideas*. Berkeley, CA: University of California Press.

Uritam, R. (1975). Physics and the view of nature in traditional China. In the *American Journal of Physics*, vol.43, No.2.

Van Helden, A. (1996). *Ptolomaic System*. URL = http://galileo.rice.edu/sci/theories/ptolemaic_ system.html, accessed 13/09/2012.

Van Inwagen, P. (2013). Metaphysics. In *The Stanford Encyclopedia of Philosophy*, E.N. Zalta (ed.), URL = <http://plato.stanford.edu/entries/metaphysics/>, accessed 05/07/2013.

Van Osta, P. (2011). A Human Cytome Project—discussion. URL = http://www.vanosta.be/humcyt.htm, accessed 13/08/2013.

Verderese, M. and H. Roth (2011). "Kekulé's Dream". URL = https://web.chemdoodle.com/kekules-dream/, accessed 21/10/2016.

Waldrop, M. (1992). *Complexity: The Emerging Science at the Edge of Order and Chaos*. New York and London: Simon and Schuster.

Walker. J. (2013). *Atoms*. URL = http://www.nobeliefs.com/atom.htm, accessed 25/10/2013.

Wang, A. (2000). *Cosmology and Political Culture in Early China*. Cambridge: Cambridge University Press.

Wang, M. (2013). Directions, Seasons, and Alterities: Notes on the Early History of Chinese Political Cosmology. In *Cosmos*, Vol. 29.

*Wang, Q. 王巧慧. (2009).《淮南子的自然哲学思想》(北京: 科学出版社, 2009.

Wang, Q.J. (2003). 'It-self-so-ing' and 'Other-ring' in Lao Zi's Concept of *Zi Ran*. URL = http://www.confuchina.com/05%20zongjiao/Lao%20Zi's%20Concept%20of%20Zi%20Ran.htm, accessed 25/03/2013.

Wang, R. (2012). *Yinyang: The Way of Heaven and Earth in Chinese Thought and Culture*. New York: Cambridge University Press.

———. (2005). Dong Zhongshu's Transformation of 'Yin-Yang' Theory and Contesting of Gender Identity. *Philosophy East and West*, 55 (2), 209–231.

Weinberg, S. (1992). *Dreams of a Final Theory*. New York: Vintage Books.

Welch, H. (1957). *Taoism: the Parting of the Way*. Boston: Beacon Press.

Whitehead, A. (1925). *Science and the Modern World*. Cambridge: Cambridge University Press.

——— (1929). *Process and Reality*. New York: Macmillan.

Wilczek, F. (2008). *The Lightness of Being: Big Questions, Real Answers*. London: Penguin Books.

Wiener, P. (1951). Ed. *Leibniz Selections*. New York: Charles Scribner's Sons.

Wilhelm, H. (1960). *Change*. Trans. Cary F. Baynes. New Jersey: Princeton University Press.

Wilhelm. R. (1975). *The I Ching or Book of Changes*. London: Routledge and Kegan Paul.

Wootton, D. (2015). *The Invention of Science: A New History of the Scientific Revolution*. (London: Allen Lane)

Wu, C. (2003). *The Essentials of the* Yi Jing. St. Paul, Minnesota: Paragon House.

*Wu, D. 吴东平. (2006).《汉字的故事: 一笔一故事, 一画一世界》. (北京: 新世界出版社, 2006). *Stories Which Hanzi Tells*. Beijing: New World Press.

*Wu, Y. (2006). 吴颐人.《汉字寻根》. (上海: 上海人民出版社, 2006). *Hanzi Seeking Its Roots*. Shanghai: Shanghai People's Press.

Xunzi. John Knoblock. links.jstor.org/ sici?sici=0161–9705(199012)12%3C135%3AXA TASO%3E2.0.CO%3B2–M .

Yates, R. (1997). *Five Lost Classics: Tao, Huang-Lao, and Yin-Yang in Han China*. New York: Ballantine Books.

**Yixue yu zhexue*. *Medicine and Philosophy*. Monthly journal. 辽宁省大连市: 中国自然辨证法研究会. URL = http://eng.oversea.cnki.net/kns55/oldnavi/n_CNKIPub.aspx? naviid=69&BaseID=YXZX&flg=local&NaviLink=Medicine+%26+Philosophy+(Humanistic+%26+Social+Medicine+Edition), accessed 09/04/2013.

Zadeh, L. (1965). Fuzzy Sets. *Information and Control*, 8, 338–353.

——— (1975). Fuzzy Logic and Approximate Reasoning. *Synthese*, 30, 407–428.

*Zeng, S-Q. 曾仕强. (2010). A series of lectures on *The Yijing*. Televised on CCTV (*Baijia jiangtan* 百家讲坛), accessed 14/09/2010.

Zhang, D. 张岱年. (1982).《中国哲学史大纲》.（北京：中国社会科学出版社, 1982). *Key Concepts in Chinese Philosophy*. Translated by Edmund Ryden. Beijing: Foreign Languages Press.

Zhang, W-R. (2009). Yin Yang Bipolar Relativity—A Unifying Theory of Nature, Agents and Life Science *International Journal of CBS*. 177–83.

Zhang, W-R, and S-S. Chen (2009). Equilibrium and Nonequilibrium Modeling of Yinyang Wuxing for Diagnositc Decision Support in Traditional Chinese Medicine. *International Journal of Information Technology and Decision Making* 8(3), 529–548.

Zhang, W-R. and L. Zhang (2004). Yinyang Bipolar Logic and Bipolar Fuzzy Logic." *Information Sciences*, 165(3–4), 265–287.

Zhang, X. 张锡纯 (1999). See Fruehauf (1999).

*Zhang, Z. 张再林 (2008). 《作为身体哲学的中国古代哲学》(Beijing: 中国社会科学出版社). *Traditional Chinese Philosophy as the Philosophy of the Body*. (Beijing: Chinese Social Sciences Publisher).

*Zhao, H. 赵化勇 (2006).《语林趣话》（四川: 四川出版集团）. *Yulin Quhua*. Sichuan: Sichuan Publishing Organisation.

ZhengXuan 郑玄 (2013). URL = http://history.cultural-china.com/en/49History13000.html, accessed 12/05/2013.

*Zhu, B. 朱伯昆崑 (2005).《易学哲学史》（北京: 昆仑出版社. *The History of the Philosophy of Yi*. 4 Vols. Beijing: Kunlun Publishers.

Ziporyn, B. (2009). Translation of *Zhuangzi: The Essential Writings, With Selections from Traditional Commentaries*. Indianapolis/Cambridge: Hackett Publishing Company, Inc.

——— (2012). *Ironies of Oneness and Difference: Coherence in Early Chinese Thought; Prolegomena to the Study of Li* 理. Albany: State University of New York Press.

——— (2013). On Sort of Knowing: The Daoist Unhewn. *Common Knowledge*, 19(1), 111–130; URL = http://muse.jhu.edu/journals/common_knowledge/v019/19.1.ziporyn.html, accessed 29/12/2013.

Glossary of Some Chinese Terms

Bagua/八卦/the trigrams
Bu/卜/divination based on producing cracks in bones and shells
Buji/不及/not enough
Cang/藏/to store
Cunzai/存在/existence
Dao/道/the Dao (left untranslated, but is often translated as the 'Way;' it is at once a metaphysical concept and a *Law of Nature*)
Daojia/道家 /Daoist *philosophy*
Daojiao/道教/Daoist religion
Di/地/Earth
Daoli/道理/Reason (in accordance with the Dao)
Dizhi/地支/Earthly Stems
Dui gua/兑卦/(left untranslated; complementary opposite of *gen gua*
Fanti/繁体 /traditional/unmodified script; *Jianti*/简体/modified script
Fang/方/direction, location, space
Fangshi/方士/practitioners of certain special arts such as alchemical, astrological, magical skills
Gen gua/艮卦(left untranslated; complementary opposite of *dui gua*)
Gongxing/共性/commonality behind diversities
Gua/卦/ (left untranslated; refers to a trigram, a *xiang* made up of three *yaos*, or a hexagram, a *xiang* made up of six *yaos*)
Han bao re/寒包热/"cold enveloping heat"
He$_1$/和/harmony, harmonious Wholeness

He$_2$/合/(organizational) unity
Houtiantu/后天图/Later Heaven Configuration
Hua/化/transform
Huainanzi/《淮南子》/the *Huainanzi*
Huangdi neijing/《黄帝内经》/*The Inner Canon of the Yellow Emperor*
Jiaguwen/甲骨文/Oracle Bone Script
Jinwen/金文/Bronze Script
Jishu/奇数/odd numbers
Kaishu/楷书/Standard Script
Kan gua/坎卦/(left untranslated); complementary opposite of *li gua*
Kun/坤/Pure *Yin* (three *yin yaos* constitute its trigram or six its hexagram); the complementary opposite of *Qian*
Laozi/《老子》/道德经》/the *Laozi* or the *Daodejing*
Li gua/离卦/(left untranslated); complementary opposite of *Kan gua*
Liangyitaijitu/两仪 太极图/the *Yinyang* icon of the "black" and "white" fishes
Lishu/隶书/Clerical Script
Liushisi gua/六十四卦/hexagrams
Mai/脉/(left untranslated as the word "pulse" does not yield its proper meaning in CCM)
Oushu/偶数/even numbers
Pi gua/否卦/(name of a hexagram, left untranslated but which stands for "bad portents")
Qi/气/(left untranslated, the fundamental ontological category in Chinese *philosophy* and cosmology)
Qi ju/气聚/*Qi*-in-concentrating mode
Qi san/气散/*Qi*-in-dissipating mode
Qingli/情理/reason (as informed by appropriate emotion(s))
Qixue/气血/*qi*-blood (an embodiment of *Yinyang*, as *qi* is *yang* and *xue* is *yin*)
Qian/乾/Pure *Yang* (three *yang yaos* constitute its trigram or six its hexagram), the complementary opposite of *Kun*
Ren/人/Humankind
Renhe/人和/harmony with fellow human beings
Ri/日/sun
Rujia/儒家/the Confucian School of *philosophy*
Sancai/天地人/the Three Talents or Powers—Heaven, Earth and Humankind
Shaoyang/少阳/(left untranslated but generally referred to as Lesser Yang)
Shaoyin/少阴/(left untranslated but generally referred to as Lesser Yin)
Sheng/生/engendering, giving birth
Shi/时/time
Shiji/《史记》/the *Historical Records* by the Han historian, Sima Qian

Shoulian/收敛/contract and conserve
Shi/蓍/yarrow stalks used in the divination practice called *zhan*/占
Shi yi/《十翼》/*The Ten Wings* or *The Yizhuan*
Sishi jielü/四时节律/*Law of Nature* about the four seasons in a year or in a day
Taigua/泰卦/(name of a hexagram, left untranslated, but stands for auspicious portents)
Taiguo/太过/too much
Taiji/太极/non-being, the Dao, the Nebulous Void which precedes the coming into existence of being itself
Taiyang/太阳/(left untranslated but known generally as Greater Yang)
Taiyin/太阴/(left untranslated but known generally as Greater Yin)
Tian/天/Heaven(s)
Tiangan/天干/(Ten) Heavenly Stems
Tianren-heyi/天人合一; *tianren-xiangying*/天人相应/Macro-micro-cosmic *Wholism* (but sinologically translated as "Correlative Thinking")
Tu/土/soil or earth
Wanwu/万物/(left untranslated, but has been translated as "the myriad things")
Wanwu zhi ling/万物之灵/refers to the uniqueness of human consciousness
Wangri/望日/fifteenth day of the lunar month (full moon); *shuori*/朔日/the first day of the lunar month (new moon).
Wu/无/the domain of great openness, the complementary opposite of *you*/有
Wuzang-liufu/五脏六腑/ensemble of the *yin* and *yang* visceral organ-systems
Wuwei/无为/action in accordance with *Tianren-heyi*, with the Dao
Wuxing/五行/(left untranslated; often translated as "five phases" but should be translated perhaps as "five Qi transformative phases")
Xiantiantu/先天图/Former Heaven Configuration, what accords with *Tianren-heyi*
Xiang /象/(left untranslated; but literally means a picture or a drawing)
Xiang ke/相克/Mutually Constraining
Xiang sheng/相生/ Mutually Engendering
Xiaozhuan/小篆/Lesser Seal Script
Xingershang/形而上/that which exists at the level above or beyond things with shape and size
Xie zhen/写真/"writing truth" via *xiang* (drawing)
Xing/形/"stuff" with shape and size, occupying space (location)
Xingerxia/形而下/that which exists at the level of shape and size
Xun gua/巽 卦/(left untranslated; complementary opposite of *zhen gua*
Yang/阳/standing for brightness, warmth, motion
Yang qi /阳气/(left untranslated; one of two types of *qi*, the polar contrast of *yin qi*)

Yang yao/阳爻/looking like this: — (unbroken)
Yao/爻/(left untranslated; refers to any component of a trigram or hexagram)
Yi/易/suddenly fine, suddenly cloudy (literal meaning), hence is translated as "change(s);" *Jian yi*/简易/Essence of *yi*; *bian yi*/变易/Change; *bu yi*/不易/ No change, that which is constant
Yi/意/meaning; *yi xiang* /意象/meaning embedded in and conveyed by *xiang*
Yijing/《易经》/the *Yijing*/the *Book of Changes*
Yin/阴/in the shadow, cold, concealed, tranquil, the complementary opposite of *yang*
Yin yao/阴爻/looking like this: - - (broken)
Yin qi/阴气/(left untranslated; one of two types of *qi*, the polar contrast of *yang qi*)
Yinyang/阴阳/(left untranslated)
Yizhuan/《易传》/*The Treatises Appended to the Yijing*
You/有/the domain of being, the complementary opposite of *wu*/无
Yuanqi/元气/Original *qi*
Yue/月/moon
Yuejing/月经/menstruation
Yuzhou/宇宙/the cosmos or universe
Zhan/占/divination based on using yarrow stalks
Zhang/长/growth, development
Zhen gua/震/(left untranslated; complementary opposite of *xun gua*)
Zhi/质/properties which "stuff" possesses such as solidity, impenetrability, with weight and mass
Zhong yi/中医/Chinese *Medicine*
Zhongyuan/中原/the Heartland of China occupied by what came to be called the Han people
Zhou er fu shi/周而复 始/Cyclic Reversion, a *Law of Nature*
Zhouye jielü/昼夜节律/*Law of Nature* about the daily rising and setting of the sun
Zhouyi/《周易》/the *Zhouyi* (the *Zhou Changes* which is the *Yijing* + the *Ten Wings*) commonly known as the *I Ching*
Zhuangzi/《庄子》/the *Zhuangzi*
Ziran/自然/(left untranslated but has been translated as "N(n)ature;" author prefers "self-engendering" or "autopoeisis"

Chinese Historical Periods and Dynasties

Palaeolithic Period 旧石器时代	ca. 1,7000,000–8000 BCE
Neolithic Period 新石器 时代 Yangshao Culture 仰韶文化 Hemudu Culture 河姆渡 文化 Dawenkou Culture 大汶口文化 Majiayao Culture 马家窑文化 Longshan Culture 龙山文化	ca. 8000–2000 BCE ca. 5000–3000 BCE ca. 5000–2500 BCE ca. 4300–2500 BCE ca. 3300–2050 BCE ca. 2300–1900 BCE
Xia Dynasty 夏代	ca. 21st–16th century BCE
Shang Dynasty 商代	ca. 16th–11th century BCE
Zhou Dynasty 周代 Western Zhou 西周 Eastern Zhou 东周 Spring and Autumn Period 春秋时代 Warring States Period 战国时代	ca. 11th century–221 BCE ca. 11th century–770 BCE 770–221 BCE 770–476 BCE 475–221 BCE
Qin Dynasty 秦代	221–207 BCE
Han Dynasty 汉代 Western Han 西汉 Eastern Han 东汉	206 BCE–220 CE 206 BCE–24 CE 25–220 CE
Three Kingdoms Period 三国时代	220–265 CE
Jin Dynasty 晋代	265–420 CE

Northern and Southern Dynasties 南北朝	420–589 CE
Sui Dynasty 隋代	581–618 CE
Tang Dynasty 唐代	618–907 CE
Five Dynasties 五代	907–960 CE
Song Dynasty 宋代 Northern Song 北宋 Southern Song 南宋	960–1279 CE 960–1127 CE 1127–1279 CE
Yuan Dynasty 元代	1279–1368 CE
Ming Dynasty 明代	1368–1644 CE
Qing Dynasty 清代	1644–1911 CE
The Republic of China 中华共和国 The People's Republic of China 中华人民共和国	1911–1949 CE 1949–

Index

About the Author

Keekok Lee is honorary research professor at Manchester University. Her extant publications cover numerous domains of philosophy including the philosophy of genetics and the philosophy of technology. She has of late focused on the philosophy of medicine.

www.ingramcontent.com/pod-product-compliance
Ingram Content Group UK Ltd.
Pitfield, Milton Keynes, MK11 3LW, UK
UKHW021905150926
475560UK00003B/197

9 781498 538879